MEDICAL
MANAGEMENT OF
HIV INFECTION

2000 Edition

MEDICAL MANAGEMENT OF HIV INFECTION

2000 Edition

John G. Bartlett, M.D.
Professor of Medicine,
Chief, Division of Infectious Diseases,
Department of Medicine,
Johns Hopkins University School of Medicine

Joel E. Gallant, M.D., M.P.H.
Associate Professor of Medicine,
Division of Infectious Diseases,
Director, Moore Clinic,
Director, Garey Lambert Research Center,
Johns Hopkins University School of Medicine

Baltimore, Maryland

retroviral infection, neonatal HIV infection, and patients in the window period following viral exposure. In most cases, confirmation of positive serology is accomplished simply by repeat serology. The sensitivity of tests for detection of HIV vary with the stage of disease and test technique, but are usually reported at >99% for DNA-PCR, 90-95% for quantitative HIV-RNA, 95-100% for viral culture of PBMC, and 8-32% for p24 antigen detection (J Clin Micro 1993;31:2557; NEJM 1989;321:1621; JAIDS 1990;3:1059; JID 1994;170:553; Ann Intern Med 1996;124:803). None of these tests should replace serology to circumvent the informed consent process.

Table 2-1. Tests for HIV-1

Assay	Sensitivity	Comments
Routine serology	99.9%	Readily available and inexpensive. Sensitivity >99.7% and specificity >99.9% (MMWR 1990;39:380; NEJM 1988;319:961; JAMA 1991;266:2861).
Rapid tests SUDS (Murex Diagnostics, Norcross,GA)	99.9%	Test results are available in ≤10 min. Specificity is 99.6%; positive tests should be confirmed. Highly sensitive; negative tests do not usually require confirmation. Other rapid tests are available but are not FDA approved (Int J STD AIDS 1997;8:192; Vox Sang 1997;72:11).
Peripheral blood mono-nuclear cell culture (PBMC - culture)	95-100%	Viral isolation by co-cultivation of patient's PBMC with PHA-stimulated donor PBMC with IL-2 over 28 days. Expensive and labor-intensive. May be qualitative or quantitative. Main use of qualitative technique is viral isolation for further analysis and for HIV detection in infants. Quantitative results correlates with stage: Mean titer is $2000/10^6$ cells in asymptomatic patients and $2,260/10^6$ cells in patients with AIDS (NEJM 1989;321:1621).
DNA PCR assay	>99%	Qualitative DNA PCR is used to detect cell-associated proviral DNA; primers are commercially available from Roche Laboratories. Sensitivity is >99% and specificity is 98%. This is not considered sufficiently accurate for diagnosis without confirmation (Ann Intern Med 1996;124:803). Main use is for viral detection in the case of neonatal HIV, the acute retroviral syndrome, and challenged or indeterminant serologic tests.
Salivary test (Orasure Test System)	99.9%	Salivary collection device to collect IgG for EIA and Western blot. Advantage is avoidance of phlebotomy. Sensitivity and specificity are comparable to standard serology (JAMA 1997;227:254).
Urine test (Calypte 1)	>99%	Used for EIA test only, so positive results must be verified by serology. Must be administered by a physician. Cost is low – about $4/test.
HIV RNA PCR	95-98%	False positive tests in 2-9%; usually at low titer. Sensitivity depends on VL threshold of assay and assumes no antiretroviral therapy

QUANTITATIVE PLASMA HIV RNA (VIRAL LOAD):

Techniques: (See Table 2-2, p. 14)

1. HIV RNA PCR (Amplicor HIV-1 Monitor versions 1.0 and 1.5, Roche Labs; 800-526-1247). Version 1.0 is FDA approved; version 1.5 is available commercially and is used for the non-B subtypes. Both the 1.0 and 1.5 versions are available in the "standard" assay and the "ultrasensitive" assay (JCM 1999;37:110).

2. Branched chain DNA or bDNA (Quantiplex HIV RNA 3.0 assay, Bayer, (800) 434-2447, formerly Chiron). Version 2.0 is being phased out.

3. Nucleic acid sequence-based amplification or Nuclisens HIV-1 QT (Organon Teknika), (800) 682-2666 x152.

Reproducibility: Commercially available assays vary based on the lower level of detection and dynamic ranges, as shown in Table 2-2 (J Clin Micro 1996;34:3016; J Med Virol 1996;50:293; J Clin Micro 1996;34:1058; J Clin Micro 1998;36:3392). Two standard deviations (95% confidence limits) with this assay are 0.3-0.5 log (2- to 3-fold) (J Infect Dis 1997;175:247; AIDS 1999;13:2269). This means that the 95% confidence limit for a value of 10,000 c/mL ranges from 3,100 to 32,000 c/mL. Recent studies indicate that the viral load in asymptomatic women is 2-fold lower than seen in men at the same CD4 counts and time to AIDS (Lancet 1998;352:1510). This difference is within the error of the test and will impact decisions based on standard guidelines for initiating therapy in only 1-2% of women. The gender difference in viral load disappears with disease progression (JID 1999;180:666). Quantitative results with the Amplicor (Roche), Quantiplex (Bayer version 3.0), and Nuclisens (Organon Teknika) assays are similar.

Cost: $80-292/assay

Indications: Quantitative HIV RNA is useful for diagnosing acute HIV infection, for predicting progression in chronically infected patients, and for therapeutic monitoring (Ann Intern Med 1995;122:573; NEJM 1996;334:426; J Infect Dis 1997;175:247).

- Acute HIV infection: Plasma HIV RNA levels are commonly employed to detect the acute retroviral syndrome prior to seroconversion. Most studies show high levels of virus (10^5-10^6 c/mL). Note that 2-9% of persons without HIV infection have false positive results, usually with low HIV RNA titers (Ann Intern Med 1999;130:37).

- Prognosis: The most comprehensive study of this assay for predicting natural history is the analysis of stored sera from the Multicenter AIDS Cohort Study (MACS) that showed a strong association between "set point" and rate of progression that was independent of the baseline CD4 count (Ann Intern Med 1995;122:573; Science 1996;272:1167; JID 1996;174:696; JID 1996;174:704; AIDS 1999;13:1305).

Table 2-2. Correlation Between Viral Load and Clinical Outcome

Viral load (c/mL)*	No. pts.	Relative Hazard**		Survival (median)	CD4 slope
		AIDS	Death		
<500	112	1.0	1.0	>10 yrs	-36
500-3,000	229	2.4	2.8	>10 yrs	-45
3,000-10,000	347	4.4	5.0	>10 yrs	-55
10,000-30,000	357	7.6	9.9	7.5 yrs	-65
>30,000	386	13.0	18.5	4.4 yrs	-77

MACS Data (Mellors J et al, Ann Intern Med 1997;126:946)

* The viral load analysis was done using the Chiron assay; these results should be multiplied by about 2 when extrapolating results for the Roche assay.

**Adjusted for baseline CD4 count, neopterin and thrush or fever.

- Therapeutic monitoring: There is a rapid initial decline in HIV RNA level (alpha slope), reflecting activity against free plasma HIV virions and HIV in acutely infected CD4 cells, followed by a second decline (beta slope) that is longer in duration (months) and more modest in degree. The latter reflects activity against HIV-infected macrophages, latently infected CD4 cells, and HIV released from other compartments, especially those trapped in follicular dendritic cells of lymph follicles. The maximum antiviral effect is seen at 4-6 months. Most authorities now believe that HIV RNA levels are the most important barometer of therapeutic response (NEJM 1996;335:1091; Ann Intern Med 1996;124:984).

- Unexpectedly low viral load: The Roche assay (RT-PCR) Version 1.0 uses primers designed primarily for detection of clade B strains of HIV, since this is the predominant clade in the U.S. and Europe where HAART is used. The result is that patients with non-clade B strains may show deceptively low plasma HIV RNA levels. The bDNA assay, the Roche 1.5 version test, or the Nuclisens HIV-1QT assay will give a more accurate quantitation of non-clade B strains, since these assays amplify subtypes A-G. None are accurate for the non-M subtypes (N or O) or HIV-2 strains.

Recommendations: Adapted from the International AIDS Society—USA (Nature Med 1996;2:625) and DHHS Guidelines (MMWR 1998;47[RR-3]:38).

- Quality assurance: Assays on individual patients should be obtained at times of clinical stability, at least 4 weeks after immunizations or intercurrent infections, and with use of the same lab and same technology.

- Frequency: Tests should be performed at baseline (x2) followed by routine testing at 3-4 month intervals. With new therapy and changes in therapy, assays should be obtained at 2-4 weeks (alpha slope), 12-16 wks, and at 16-

24 weeks. An optimal response to therapy should be associated with a 1.5-2 $\log_{10}$ decrease at 4 weeks, <500 c/mL at 12-16 weeks and <50 c/mL at 16-24 weeks.

- Interpretation: Changes of ≥50% (0.3 $\log_{10}$) are considered significant.

- Factors not measured by viral load tests: immune function, CD4 regenerative reserve, susceptibility to antivirals, infectivity, syncytial vs. non-syncytial inducing forms and viral load in compartments other than blood (e.g. lymph nodes, CNS, genital secretions).

- Factors that increase viral load:

  1. Progressive disease

  2. Failing antiretroviral therapy due to inadequate potency, inadequate drug levels, non-adherence, resistance, and/or drug interactions.

  3. Active infections: active TB increases viral load 5- to 160-fold (J Immunology 1996;157:1271); pneumococcal pneumonia increases viral load 3- to 5-fold.

  4. Immunization (Blood 1995;86:1082; NEJM 1996;335:817; NEJM 1996;334:1222).

- Specimens

II: Laboratory Tests

Table 2-3. Comparison Between Assay Methods for Viral Load

	Roche	Bayer (formerly Chiron)	Organon
Contact	(800) 526-1247	(800) 434-2447	(800) 682-2666 x 152
Technique	RT-PCR	bDNA	Nuclisens HIV-1 QT
Comparison of Results	Results with the RT-PCR assay are about 2x results with bDNA using version 2.0 assay	Results with bDNA are 50% of results with RT-PCR for the version 2.0 assay; the version 3.0 assay results are comparable to the Roche assay	Comparative results with RT-PCR
Advantages	Version 1.0 is FDA approved Fewer false positives compared to Chiron Version 1.5 amplifies subtypes A-G	Technician time demands are less Amplifies subtypes A-G	May be used with tissue or body fluids such as genital secretions Amplifies subtypes A-G Greatest dynamic range
Dynamic range	Standard: (1.0 & 1.5) 400 to 750,000 c/mL Ultrasensitive: (1.0 & 1.5) 50-75,000 c/mL	bDNA Version 3.0: 50-500,000 c/mL	Nuclisens HIV-1 QT: 40-10,000,000 c/mL depending on volume
Subtype amplified	Version 1.0: B only Version 1.5: A-G	A-G	A-G
Specimen Volume	Amplicor–0.2 mL Ultrasensitive–0.5 mL	1 mL	10 µL to 2 mL
Tubes	EDTA (lavender top)	EDTA (lavender top)	EDTA, heparin, whole blood, any body fluid, PMBC, semen, tissue, etc.
Requirement	Separate plasma <6 hr and freeze prior to shipping at -20°C or -70°C	Separate plasma <4 hr and freeze prior to shipping at -20°C or -70°C	Separate serum or plasma <4 hrs and freeze prior to shipping at -20°C or -70°C

SCREENING BATTERY: The usual screening battery advocated for patients with established HIV infection is summarized in Table 2-3, p. 16 (CID 1995;21 suppl 1:S13).

COMPLETE BLOOD COUNT: The CBC is especially important in patients with HIV infection since anemia, leukopenia, lymphopenia and thrombocytopenia are found in 30-40% of patients (JAIDS 1994;7:1134). The CBC should be repeated at 3-6 month intervals, in part because this is a necessary component of monitoring the CD4 cell count. More frequent testing is suggested in patients with symptoms suggesting marrow suppression, those receiving marrow suppressing drugs such as zidovudine, and those with marginal or low counts.

SERUM CHEMISTRY PANEL: The SMA-12, 14 or 20 is of limited value in a general health screen (Ann Intern Med 1987;106:403) but is commonly advocated in the initial evaluation of HIV infection due to high rates of hepatitis in patients at risk for HIV to obtain baseline values in patients who are also likely to have multisystem disease and as a baseline test in patients who receive multiple drugs that are potentially hepatotoxic. Studies of HIV-infected patients have shown that up to 75% have abnormal liver function tests, 20% have severe abnormalities of LFTs, and about half have elevated LDH levels (JAIDS 1994;7:1134).

SYPHILIS SEROLOGY: The usual screening test (VDRL or RPR) should be a performed at baseline and annually thereafter due to high rates of co-infection (MMWR 1988; 37:600). Up to 6% of patients with HIV infection have biologic false positive (BFP) screening tests. Risk factors for BFP results include injection drug use, pregnancy, and HIV infection (CID 1994;19:1040; JID 1992;165:1124; JAIDS 1994;7:1134; Am J Med 1995;99:55). False negative tests have been reported in patients with HIV infection (JID 1990;162:862; AIDS 1991;5:419; JID 1992;165:1020), but these are rare (Ann Intern Med 1990;113:872). The CDC suggest that both treponemal and non-treponemal tests should be interpreted "in the usual manner" (MMWR 1998;47[RR-1]:38). A lumbar puncture is recommended for patients with early syphilis (<1 year) when it is accompanied by neurologic signs or symptoms, when it is not treated with the standard regimen of 2.4 million units of benzathine penicillin, and in the setting of therapeutic failure. An LP is recommended for all patients with latent syphilis regardless of the clinical findings (MMWR 1998;47[RR-1]:39), although interpretation may be confounded by the presence of HIV-associated abnormalities of CSF including mononuclear cells and elevated protein. Relapse is common even with recommended therapy, so follow-up VDRL titers are advised at 3, 6, 9, 12 and 24 months for primary and secondary syphilis, and every 6 months thereafter until negative (MMWR 1998;47[RR-1]:39).

CHEST X-RAY: A routine chest x-ray is recommended by the CDC (MMWR 1986;35:448), both for detection of asymptomatic tuberculosis and as a baseline for patients who are at high risk for pulmonary disease. However, in a longitudinal study of 1,065 patients at various stages of HIV infection, routine x-rays performed at 0, 3, 6 and 12 months (Arch Intern Med 1996;156:191) detected an abnormality in only 123 (2%) of 5,263 x-rays. None of the asymptomatic patients (including 751 with anergy) had evidence of active tuberculosis; only one of 82 with a positive PPD had an abnormality on x-ray. The authors concluded that routine chest x-rays in HIV-infected patients with negative PPD skin tests are not warranted. DHHS Guidelines recommend an X-ray "when clinically indicated" (MMWR 1998;47[RR-1]:38).

PPD SKIN TESTING: The CDC recommends the Mantoux-method TST (Tuberculin Skin Test), using 5 TU of PPD, for HIV-infected patients who have not had a prior positive test. TST should be repeated annually if initial test(s) were negative and if the patient belongs to population with a high risk of tuberculosis (e.g., residents of prisons or jails, injection drug users, homeless). Some authorities recommend repeat TST following immune reconstitution (MMWR 1998;47 [RR-20]:37). Induration of 5 mm constitutes a positive test.

ANERGY TESTING: If anergy testing is performed, it should consist of two of the following skin test reagents: *Candida albicans*, tetanus toxoid, and/or mumps (MMWR 1991;49[RR-5]:1). Any induration constitutes a positive result. Most authorities no longer recommend anergy testing (MMWR 1995;44[RR-11]:1), and the U.S. Public Health Service-IDSA guidelines (Ann Int Med 1997;127:923) state that "anergy testing is not routinely recommended." This change in recommendations arose because of lack of standardization of the reagents, studies demonstrating inconsistent results in HIV-infected persons, and the failure of anergy to predict response to PPD (Ann Intern Med 1993;119:185; Am J Resp Crit Care Med 1996;153:1982; Arch Intern Med 1995;155:2111).

PAP SMEARS: The CDC and the Agency for Health Care Policy and Research recommend that a gynecological evaluation with pelvic exam and Pap smear be performed at baseline, repeated at six months and annually thereafter (MMWR 1998;47[RR-1]:98; JAMA 1994;271:1866; MMWR 1999;48[RR-10]:31) with management according to guidelines in Table 2-4, p. 19. More aggressive testing is recommended because of a several-fold increase in rates of SIL (33-45% HIV+ vs. 7-14% HIV2) and a 1.7 fold increase in rates of cervical cancer in young women with HIV (5th Retroviral Conference, 2/98, Abstracts 715 and 717; Obstet Gynecol Clin N Am 1996;23,861). Severity and frequency of cervical dysplasia increases with progressive immune compromise. There is a strong association between HIV infection and detectable and persistent human papilloma virus (HPV) infection; this association increases with progressive immunosuppression (CID 1995;21 suppl 1:S121; NEJM 1997; 337:1343).

Method: The cervix is scraped circumflexually using an Ayer spatula or a curved brush; a sample from the posterior fornix or the "vaginal pool" may also be included. The endocervical sample is taken with a saline-moistened cotton-tipped applicator or straight ectocervical brush that is rolled on a slide and immediately fixed in ethyl ether plus 95% ethyl alcohol or 95% ethyl alcohol alone. The yield is seven-fold higher with the brush specimen. Important steps in obtaining an adequate sample:

1. Collect Pap prior to bimanual exam.
2. Avoid contaminating sample with lubricant.
3. Obtain Pap before samples for STD testing.
4. If large amounts of vaginal discharge are present, carefully remove with large swab before obtaining Pap.

5. Obtain ectocervical sample before endocervical sample.
6. Small amounts of blood will not interfere with cytologic sampling but if patient is bleeding more heavily, Pap should be deferred.
7. Collected material should be applied uniformly to a slide, without clumping, and should be rapidly fixed to avoid air-drying; if spray fixatives are used, the spray should be held at least 10 inches away from the slide to prevent disruption of cells by propellant.

When performing speculum exam, if an ulcerative or exophytic lesion suspicious for invasive cancer is noted, the patient should be referred for possible biopsy.

Newer methods of cytologic evaluation using liquid-based collection and thin-layer processing may enhance sensitivity but have not yet been evaluated in HIV infected women.

Table 2-4. Recommendations for Intervention Based on Results of Pap Smear

Pap	Management
Severe inflammation	Evaluate for infection; repeat Pap preferably within 2-3 months
Atypia, ASCUS	Follow-up Pap without colposcopy q 4-6 mo x 2 years until 3 are negative; if second report of ASCUS colposcopy.
Low grade squamous intraepithelia; lesion (LSIL)	Colposcopy ± biopsy or follow with Pap smear q 4-6 months with colposcopy and biopsy if repeat smears are abnormal.
High grade squamous intraepithelial lesion (HSIL) (Carcinoma *in situ*)	Colposcopy with biopsy
Invasive carcinoma	Colposcopy with biopsy or conization; treat with surgery or radiation

II. Laboratory Tests

CD4 CELL COUNT: This is a standard test to stage the disease, formulate the differential diagnosis of patient complaints, (Table 1-2, p. 4) and to make therapeutic decisions regarding antiviral treatment and prophylaxis for opportunistic pathogens. It is also a relatively reliable indicator of prognosis that complements the viral load assay. These two assays independently predict clinical progression and survival (Ann Intern Med 1997;126:946). CD8 cell counts have not been found to predict outcome (NEJM 1990;322:166).

Technique: The standard method for determining CD4 count uses flow cytometers and hematology analyzers that are expensive and require fresh blood (<18 hrs. old). The cost of the test ranges from $50-$150. Alternative systems include: 1) FACSCount system (Becton Dickinson); 2) VCS Technology/ Coulter Cyto-Spheres (Coulter Corp.); 3) Zymmune CD4/CD8 Cell Monitoring Kit (Zynaxis Inc); and 4) TRAx CD4 Test Kit (T Cell Diagnostics) (JAIDS 1995;10:522).

Normal values for most laboratories are a mean of 800-1050/mm³, with a range representing two standard deviations of approximately 500 to 1400/mm³ (Ann Intern Med 1993;119:55).

Factors that influence CD4 cell counts include analytical variation, seasonal and diurnal variations, some intercurrent illnesses, and corticosteroids. Substantial analytical variations, which account for the wide range in normal values (usually about 500-1400/mm³), reflect the fact that the CD4 cell count is the product of three variables: the white blood cell count, % lymphocytes, and the % CD4 cells (lymphocytes that bear the CD4 receptor). There are also seasonal changes (Clin Exp Immunol 1991;86:349) and diurnal changes, with the lowest levels at 12:30 pm and peak values at 8:30 pm (JAIDS 1990;3:144); these variations do not clearly correspond to the circadian rhythm of corticosteroids. Modest decreases in the CD4 cell count have been noted with some acute infections and with major surgery. Corticosteroid administration may have a profound effect, with decreases from 900/mm³ to less than 300/mm³ with acute administration; chronic administration has a less pronounced effect. (Clin Immun Immunopath 1983;28:101). Acute changes are probably due to a redistribution of leukocytes between the peripheral circulation and the marrow, spleen, and lymph nodes (Clin Exp Immunol 1990;80:460). Co-infection with HTLV-1 may be responsible for a deceptively high CD4 cell count in the presence of immune suppression from HIV-1. Splenectomy may also cause deceptively high levels. The following have minimal effect on the CD4 cell count: gender, age in adults, risk category, psychological stress, physical stress, and pregnancy (Ann Intern Med 1993;119:55).

The CD4 cell percentage is sometimes used in preference to the absolute number, since this reduces the variation to one measurement (JAIDS 1989;2:114). In the ACTG laboratories, the within-subject coefficient of variation for % CD4 was 18% compared with 25% for the CD4 count (JID 1994;169:28). Corresponding CD4 cell counts are:

CD4 Cell Count	% CD4
>500/mm³	>29%
200-500/mm³	14-28%
<200/mm³	<14%

Precautions in the use and interpretations of CD4 cell counts include the need for both clinicians and patients to be aware of the fluctuations described above. Test results that represent "milestones" for therapeutic decisions should be repeated, especially if they show values that do not correlate well with prior trends. Prior studies show that 95% confidence ranges for a true count of 500/mm³ were 297-841/mm³ and 118-337/mm³ for a count of 200/mm³ (JAIDS 1993;6:537). Deceptively high CD4 cells are noted in patients with concurrent HTLV-1 infection, the agent of adult T cell leukemia and tropical spastic paraparesis. HTLV-1 is closely related to HTLV-2, and most serologic assays show cross reactivity, but only HTLV-1 causes deceptively high CD4 cell counts. Serologic studies in the U.S. show HTLV-1/2 infection rates of 7-12% in injection drug users and 2-10% in sex workers (NEJM 1990;326:375; JAMA 1990;263:60); 80-90% of these are accounted for by HTLV-2 in both populations. High rates of concurrent HIV and HTLV-1 have been reported in Brazil (JAMA 1994;271:353) and Haiti (JCM 1995;33:1735). Analysis of patients with co-infection suggest that CD4 counts were 80-180% higher than controls for comparable levels of immunosuppression (JAMA 1994;271:353). Splenectomy also causes deceptively high CD4 counts.

The CD4 cell count may be used as a **surrogate marker of HIV infection** in patients for whom serologic results are delayed or in patients who have refused the test. There are relatively few conditions associated with profound depletion of CD4 cell counts in patients with classic AIDS-indicator conditions included in their differential diagnosis. The median CD4 count at the time of an AIDS-defining diagnosis is 60/mm³, and only 10% have an AIDS-defining diagnosis with a CD4 count >200/mm³ (Am J Epidemiol 1995;141:645). Thus, a patient with a CD4 cell count of 800/mm³ with thrush, possible PCP, or cryptococcal meningitis is unlikely to have HIV infection. The total lymphocyte count may serve in a similar fashion, is readily available, and is advocated by WHO in settings where a CD4 cell count is not available. A total lymphocyte count of <1000/mL is strongly predictive of a CD4 count <200/mm³.

CD4 Repertoire: Progressive immunodeficiency in HIV infection is associated with both quantitative and qualitative changes in CD4 lymphocytes. There are two major categories of CD4 cells: naïve cells and memory cells. In early life all cells are naïve and express the isoform of CD45RA⁺. Memory cells (CD45RA⁺) represent the component of the T cell repertoire that has been activated by exposure to antigens. These are the CD4 cells with specificity for most opportunistic infections such as *P. carinii*, cytomegalovirus and *Toxoplasma gondii*. It is the depletion of these cells that accounts for the inability to respond to recall antigens, a defect

II. Laboratory Tests

noted relatively early in the course of HIV infection. Studies of HIV-infected patients show a preferential decline in naïve cells. With triple therapy using protease inhibitors there is a three phase component to the CD4 rebound. The initial increase is due primarily to redistribution of CD4 cells from lymphatic sites. The second phase is characterized by an influx of CD4 memory cells with reduced T cell activation and improved response to recall antigens. In the third phase there is an increase in naïve cells following at least 12 weeks of HAART (Nature Med 1997;5:533; Science 1997;277:112). By 6 months the CD4 repertoire is diverse; the competence of these cells is evidenced by favorable control of selected chronic infections such as cryptosporidiosis, microsporidiosis, and molluscum contagiosum, the ability to discontinue maintenance therapy for dissemminated MAC and CMV, and the ability to discontinue PCP and MAC prophylaxis in responders. Nevertheless, some patients with immune reconstitution have deficits in CTL responses to specific antigens that may result in PCP or relapses in CMV retinitis despite CD4 counts >300/mm³ (Hopkins HIV Report 2000;12:3; 7th CROI, Abstracts 272, 580, 581).

Idiopathic CD4 lymphocytopenia (ICL) is a syndrome characterized by a low CD4 cell count that is unexplained by HIV infection or other medical conditions. Criteria for the case definition are: 1) CD4 cell count less than 300/mm³ or a CD4 percent less than 20% on two or more measurements; 2) lack of laboratory evidence of HIV infection; and 3) absence of alternative explanation for the CD4 cell lymphopenia. Transient decreases in CD4 cells may occur with infections due to TB, *M. avium*, hepatitis B, EBV, toxoplasmosis, cryptococcosis, and CMV (Chest 1994;105:1335; Eur J Med 1993;2:509; Am J Med Sci 1996;312:240). The diagnosis of ICL requires persistence of the deficit. Through May 1993, there were 111 adults and 14 children reported to the CDC with ICL. Several conclusions can be drawn from the experience with these patients: 1) they lack risk factors for HIV infection; 2) there is no evidence of an infectious agent based on clustering or contact evaluations; 3) these patients often have the same opportunistic infections noted with HIV infection, though there are some differences, including higher rates of extrapulmonary cryptococcosis; 4) CD4 counts tend to remain stable; and (5) the prognosis is relatively good (Lancet 1992;340:273; NEJM 1993;328:373; NEJM 1993;328:380; NEJM 1993;328:386; NEJM 1993;328:393). Cases of this syndrome should be reported to local/state health departments instead of the direct reporting to the CDC that was originally advocated.

RESISTANCE TESTING: Resistance testing is an in vitro method to measure resistance of HIV to antiretroviral agents. Resistance testing can aid in antiretroviral drug selection, but has certain limitations: 1) Resistance assays measure only the dominant species at the time the test is performed; resistant variants that comprise less than 20% of the total viral population and species in "sequestered havens" (CNS, genital tract, etc.) are not detected; 2) there must be a sufficient viral load to do the test, usually ≥1,000 c/mL; and 3) genotypic assays are often difficult to interpret: Single mutations confer high level resistance to 3TC and NNRTIs, but multiple mutations are required for NRTIs other than 3TC and all PIs. As a result of these limitations:

- Resistance testing most reliably identifies drugs that should be avoided, but not necessarily the drugs that are most likely to be active.

- Testing should be done in the presence of the antiretroviral agents in question, since discontinuation of therapy often results in the proliferation of wild type virus that may deceptively suggest susceptibility. The time between discontinuation of HAART and the shift from resistant strains to wild type virus is usually 2-8 weeks, though there is considerable variation depending on the specific mutation.

- Interpretation of results in patients who have received prior antiretroviral agents is difficult. Resistance to previously used drugs may be present even if resistance assays indicate susceptibility.

- A viral load ≥1,000 c/mL is usually required.

Indications: The only clinical situation for which resistance testing has verified utility is in the selection of salvage regimens. The GART Study (CPCRA 046) (Baxter et al., 6th Retrovirus Conference, 1999, Chicago, LB 8) and the VIRADAPT study (Lancet 1999;353:2195) were prospective trials that demonstrated superior results when salvage regimens were selected based on genotype analysis compared to decisions based on history. Similar results were reported in a retrospective study from Stanford (Ann Intern Med 1999;131:813) and in VIRA 3001, a prospective trial that demonstrated the superiority of treatment decisions based on phenotype testing vs. standard of care (Cohen, et al., 7th CROI, San Francisco, CA 2000). Recommendations for use of resistance testing according to the DHHS Guidelines for 1/29/2000 are:

- Determination of baseline resistance patterns in patients presenting during or shortly after the acute retroviral syndrome

- Selection of antiretroviral agents after drug failure (assumes ≥8 weeks of therapy, a viral load ≥1,000 c/mL and testing during drug administration)

The test is **sometimes advocated** for the following indications:

- Drug selection in pregnant women (primarily to assess the presence of AZT resistance)

- Testing of the source patient when antiretroviral therapy is used for prophylaxis after HIV exposures

- Selection of initial therapy for treatment of naïve patients who are chronically infected (utility not demonstrated)

Test methods: There are two types of tests: genotypic and phenotypic assays. The most commonly used test is the genotypic assay, because results are available more quickly, the test is less expensive, and these assays are more readily available. A potential advantage of phenotypic assays is that results are more easily interpreted. Relative merits are shown below:

II. Laboratory Tests

Table 2-5: Comparison of Genotypic and Phenotypic Assays

Genotypic assays	
Advantages	**Disadvantages**
Widely available Less expensive ($360-$480/test) Short turn-around: 1-2 weeks May be preferred with failures of first regimen	Detects resistance only in dominant species (>20%) Interpretation requires knowledge of mutational changes, eg. expertise. Technician experience influences results. May show discrepancy with phenotype Requires VL >1000 c/mL
Phenotypic assays	
Advantages	**Disadvantages**
Interpretation more analogous to resistance testing of bacteria Assesses total effect including mutations, mutational interactions Reproducibility is good May be preferred in patients with extensive drug experience	More expensive (usually $800-$1000) Less readily available Longer delay in reporting: 2-3 weeks Thresholds to define susceptibility are arbitrary and non-standardized, and do not vary based on achievable drug concentrations. Detects resistance only in dominant species (>20%)

Genotypic assays: These assays are available from multiple commercial suppliers, and there are also a number of "home brews." Assays vary considerably based on cost, the number of mutations tested, and simplicity and accuracy of reporting. The methodology involves: 1) amplication of the reverse transcriptase (RT), protease (Pr) gene, or both by RT PCR; 2) DNA sequencing of amplicons generated for the dominant species (mutations are limited to those present in >20% of plasma virions); 3) reporting of mutations for each gene using a letter-number-letter standard, in which the first letter indicates the amino acid at the designated codon with wild type virus, the number is the codon, and the second letter indicates the amino acid substituted in the mutation (Table 2-6, p. 25). Thus, the RT mutation K103N indicates that asparagine (N) has substituted for lysine (K) on codon 103. The following table indicates the amino acids and corresponding letter codes used to describe mutations in genotype analyses. Updated information on resistance testing can be obtained at http://www.viral-resistance.com and http://hiv-web.lanl.gov

Table 2-6: Letter Designations for Amino Acids

A	Alanine	I	Isoleucine	R	Arginine
C	Cytosine	K	Lysine	S	Serine
D	Aspartic acid	L	Leucine	T	Threonine
E	Glutamic acid	M	Methionine	V	Valine
F	Phenylaline	N	Asparagine	W	Tryptophan
G	Glycine	P	Proline	Y	Tyrosine
H	Histidine	Q	Glutamine		

Amino acids and corresponding single letter codes used in describing genotypes.

Table 2-7: Resistance Mutations
adapted from Hirsch et al, JAMA (2000) 283:2417

Drug	Primary	Secondary
Nucleosides and Nucleotides		
AZT	70,215	41,67,210,219
3TC	44,118,184	–
ddC	65,69,74,184 (limited clinical data)	–
ddI	74	65,184
d4T	75 (selected *in vitro*, rarely seen in patients)	–
ABC	65,74,184	41,67,70,115,210,215,219
Multinucleoside Resistance – A	151	62,75,77,116
Multinucleoside Resistance – B	69 (insertion)	41,62,67,70,210,215,219
Non-nucleoside reverse transcriptase inhibitors		
NVP	103,106,108,181,188,190	100
DLV	103,181	236
EFV	103,188,190	100,108,225
Protease Inhibitors		
IDV	46,82 (usually selected in combination with other mutations	10,20,24,32,36,54,71,73,77 84,90
NFV	30,90	10,36,46,71,77,82,84,88
RTV	82	20,32,33,36,46,54,71,77,84,90
SQV	48,90	10,54,71,73,77,82,84
APV	50,84	10,32,46,47,54

Primary – usually develop first; associated with decreased drug binding
Secondary – also contributes to drug resistance; may affect drug binding *in vitro* less than primary
    mutations

II. Laboratory Tests

Phenotypic assays: Phenotype analysis involves insertion of the RT and protease genes from the patient's strain into a backbone laboratory clone by cloning or recombination. Replication is monitored at various drug concentrations and compared to a reference "wild type virus." This assay is comparable to conventional *in vitro* tests of antimicrobial sensitivity, in which the microbe is grown in serial dilutions of antiviral agents. The major difference is that the HIV strain *per se* is not used; instead, the RT and Pr genes of the test strain are inserted into a molecular HIV clone with standardized envelope and accessory genes. Results are reported as the IC_{50} or IC_{90} indicating the concentration necessary to inhibit 50% or 90% of the test strains, respectively. The ratio of the IC_{50} of the test strain and reference strain is reported as the fold increase in IC_{50} with 4x or 10x as commonly used thresholds. Interpretation of phenotypic assay results is complicated by the lack of knowledge about the true concentration or fold increase in IC_{50} that is associated with treatment failure for individual drugs. Thus, the thresholds used to define susceptibility are arbitrary, non-standardized, and not validated.

SEROLOGY FOR HEPATITIS B VIRUS (HBV): USPHS/IDSA Guidelines recommend screening for hepatitis B core antibody (anti-HBc) (MMWR 1999;48[RR-10]:41) with HBV vaccination of those who are susceptible. Antibody screening is advocated for high-risk populations to avoid the expense of unnecessary vaccination (MMWR 1991;40[RR-13]:1). HBV seroprevalence is 35-80% for gay men, 60-80% for injection drug users, 60-80% for hemophiliacs, 5-20% for heterosexuals with multiple partners, and 3-14% for the general population. The CDC recommends post-vaccination serology with anti-HB$_s$ in patients with HIV infection at 1-6 months after the third dose of vaccine to confirm an antigenic response. HIV-infected patients with abnormal liver function tests should be tested for hepatitis infection using a combination of HBV surface antigen (HBsAg) and hepatitis C antibody (anti-HCV).

TESTING FOR HEPATITIS C: USPHS/IDSA Guidelines recommend that all HIV infected persons should be tested for HCV infection using the EIA screening assay for anti-HCV antibodies; positive tests should be confirmed by either the recombinant immunoblot assay (RIBA) or by reverse transcriptase PCR (RT-PCR) for HCV RNA (MMWR 1999;48[RR-10]:33). The only test approved by the FDA for the diagnosis of HCV is anti-HCV, which detects ≥97% of infected persons, but does not distinguish acute, chronic or resolved infection and has a low predictive value in low prevalence populations (Hepatology 1997;26:435). Supplemental antibody testing with RIBA (recombinant immunoblot assay) or qualitative RT-PCR for HCV RNA is advocated to confirm the diagnosis; and may be done on the initial sample. Quantitative HCV RNA assays are not FDA approved but are widely available using RT-PCR or bDNA technology. These tests show a threshold of detection of 100-1,000 c/mL, and they are positive in 75-85% of persons with anti-HCV and >95% of persons with acute or chronic hepatitis C. Rigorous quality control is necessary for these assays in terms of specimen preparation for laboratory submission. This test and ALT levels are useful in determining candidates for treatment; they may be useful in judging response to treatment. Genotype assay identifies 6 genotypes and >90 subtypes. Genotype 1 accounts for 70% of HCV infected persons in the U.S., and is associated with a poor response to therapy compared to genotypes 2 and 3. The CDC recommended algorithm for detecting HCV is summarized in Figure 2-1, p. 27, and the tests to evaluate HCV are summarized in Table 2-8, p. 28. Patients coinfected with HCV and HIV should be:

- Advised not to drink excessive amounts of alcohol.

- Evaluated for HCV treatment with interferon plus ribavirin.

- Vaccinated for hepatitis A if susceptible.

Available data indicates that HCV-HIV co-infection causes more rapid progression of HCV, but there is no significant impact on the natural history of HIV (JID 1999;179:1254; Science 1999;285:26).

Home kit: The FDA has approved a home test kit for HCV. The consumer obtains blood by a lancet, which is placed on a filter strip and submitted by mail to a reading center. Results are available in 10 days. The cost is about $70/test.

Figure 2-1: Recommended Testing Algorithm (MMWR 1998;47[RR-20]:27)

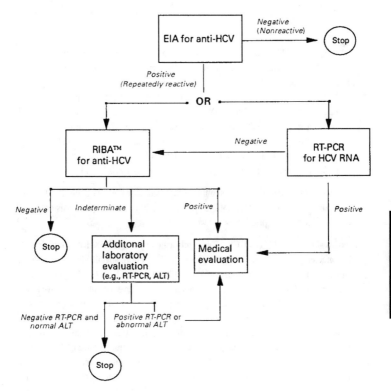

II. Laboratory Tests

Table 2-8: Tests for HCV

Test	Cost	Comment
Anti HCV EIA	$25-45	Includes EIA and RIBA; indicates past or present HCV infection. Sensitivity ≥97%; EIA lacks specificity in low prevalence populations – supplemental assay required for confirmation.
RIBA	$115-150	
HCV RNA (HCV RT-PCR)	$160-200	RT-PCR technology to detect HCV RNA; may have false positives and negatives.
Quantitative HCV PCR	$160-225	Determines concentration using RT-PCR or bDNA technology; less sensitive than qualitative RT-PCR. Threshold of detection is 500 c/mL; most patients with chronic HCV infection have 10^5-10^7 c/mL. These assays may predict response to therapy but are not useful yet for therapeutic monitoring. This assay has largely supplanted HCV RNA tests due to increased sensitivity and comparable cost.
Genotype	$200-250	6 genotypes – genotype 1 predominates in U.S. (70%) and shows poorest response to therapy.

TOXOPLASMOSIS SEROLOGY: *Toxoplasma* serology (IgG) is recommended to assist in the differential diagnosis of complications involving the central nervous system, to identify candidates for toxoplasmosis prophylaxis (Ann Intern Med 1992;117:163), and to counsel patients on preventive measures if seronegative. The preferred method is an agglutination assay for IgG; IgM assays are not useful, and the Sabin-Feldman dye test is less accurate than the agglutination assay. Toxoplasmosis seroprevalence among adults in the U.S. is 10-30%, and the seroconversion rate is up to 1%/year. Most infections in AIDS patients represent relapse of latent infection, which is noted in 20-47% with positive serology and no prophylaxis (CID 1992;15:211).

A negative *toxoplasma* serology should be repeated after the CD4 count is ≤100/mm³ if the patient cannot take TMP-SMX prophylaxis for PCP and toxoplasmosis encephalitis is considered with prior tests that were negative.

CYTOMEGALOVIRUS SEROLOGY: This is advocated by the USPHS/ IDSA Guidelines for HIV-infected persons who have low risk for CMV infection, specifically those who are not gay men or injection drug users (MMWR 1999;48[RR-10]:26). Possible applications for use of this information are to identify seronegative patients for counseling on CMV prevention (although the message is not different from the "safe sex message" for preventing HIV transmission), to assessing the likelihood of CMV disease in late-stage HIV infection, to identify candidates for CMV prophylaxis (not currently recommended), and to identify seronegative individuals who should receive CMV-antibody negative blood or leukocyte-reduced blood products for non-emergent transfusions. - Seroprevalence for adults in the United States is about 50%; in gay men and injection drug users it is >90% (JID 1985;152:243; Am J Med 1987;82:593).

GLUCOSE-6-PHOSPHATE DEHYDROGENASE LEVELS: G-6-PD deficiency is a genetic disease that predisposes to hemolytic anemia following exposure to oxidant drugs commonly used in patients with HIV infection. Over 150 G-6-PD variants are inherited on the X chromosome, but the most frequent are Gd^{A-}, which is found in 10% of black men and in 1-2% of black women, and Gd^{med}, found predominantly in men from the Mediterranean area (Italians, Greeks, Sephardic Jews, Arabs), India, and Southeast Asia. With most defects the hemolysis is mild and self-limited, because only the older red cells are involved and the bone marrow can compensate even with continued administration of the implicated drug. The important exception is Gd^{med}, which may cause life-threatening hemolysis. The limited hemolysis in patients with Gd^{A-} may be significant in patients with HIV infection who often have anemia from other causes. The severity of anemia also depends on the concentration of the drug in red cells and the oxidant potential of the inducing agent: The most likely offending agents are dapsone and primaquine. Sulfonamides cause hemolysis less commonly. G-6-PD deficiency may be partial, in which case the contraindication for oxidant drugs is relative. Options for screening include: 1) obtaining the test at baseline in all patients; 2) restricting testing to those most likely to have a defect; or 3) reserving testing for the occasional case of hemolytic anemia following exposure to typical inducing agents. Typical findings with this hemolysis include elevated bilirubin, elevated LDH, decreased haptoglobin, methemoglobinemia, reticulocytosis, and a peripheral smear showing the characteristic "bite cells." During hemolysis, G-6-PD levels are usually normal since the susceptible red cells are destroyed; testing must consequently be delayed until about 30 days after discontinuation of the offending agent. Some laboratories report results as units/gm Hgb, with less than three indicating severe deficiency, found in men and homozygous women; other labs report qualitative results.

Adverse drug reaction monitoring: Adverse drug reactions attributed to antiretroviral agents include diabetes mellitus, blood lipid changes associated with risks for coronary artery disease and stroke, and lactic acidosis/steatosis attributed to nucleoside analogs (DHHS Guidelines 2000, pg. 74-76).

Diabetes: Risk should be evaluated based on prior diabetes or family history of diabetes, and all patients should be warned of symptoms of hyperglycemia. The median reported time for detecting hyperglycemia attributed to protease inhibitors is at 63 days of treatment; some authorities recommend fasting blood glucose measurements at 3-4 month intervals.

Blood lipids: Changes include increases in triglycerides and/or cholesterol (total and LDL) with possible increased risk of premature coronary artery disease, cerebrovascular disease, pancreatitis, and cholelithiasis. Assessment should include evaluation of risk for cardiovascular disease, including family history, medical history, smoking history, weight, blood pressure, diabetes, baseline levels, and magnitude of lipid changes. Lipid changes usually take place within the first 3 months of therapy. Some authorities recommend monitoring fasting triglycerides and cholesterol levels at 3-4 month intervals with intervention when: 1) Triglyceride levels are >750-1000 mg/dL; 2) LDL cholesterol levels are >130 mg/dL with prior

II. Laboratory Tests

coronary disease or ≥2 risks (above); or 3) LDL cholesterol >160 mg/dL without prior coronary disease and ≤1 risk.

Lactic acidosis: Routine therapeutic monitoring is not recommended but lactic acidosis should be considered in patients who are receiving nucleoside analogs who have unexplained symptoms of lactic acidosis, including fatigue, dyspnea, abdominal pain, and vomiting. Tests to consider include anion gap, lactic acid levels, LDH, ALT, and CPK.

Table 2-9. Routine Laboratory Tests in Asymptomatic Patients

Test	Cost*	Frequency and Comment
HIV serology	$30-60	Repeat test for patients with positive test results and: 1) no confirmation available; 2) denial of commonly accepted risk factors; 3) test performed with techniques other than standard serology; and 4) other reason for concern such as undetectable viral load and normal CD4 count. Repeat test for indeterminate results at 3-6 months.
CBC	$6-8	Repeat at 3-6 months, more frequently for low values and with administration of marrow-toxic drugs.
VDRL or RPR	$5-16	Repeat annually.
CD4 cell count and %	$60-150	Repeat every 3-6 months, and repeat for results that represent "milestones" for therapeutic decisions (antiretroviral therapy and prophylaxis for opportunistic pathogens), and with results that are inconsistent with prior trends (see pages 31-34). Routine testing when counts are <50/mm³ is of minimal use except for monitoring response to antiretroviral therapy.
Chest x-ray	$40-140	Indicated for symptoms and signs suggesting pulmonary disease or newly detected positive PPD.
Serum chemistries	$10-15	Repeat annually or more frequently in patients with abnormal results and with administration of hepatoxic or nephrotoxic drugs.
Pap smears	$25-40	Repeat at 6 months and then annually if results are normal; some advocate Pap smear every 6 months if CD4 cell count is <500/mm³. Results reported as "inadequate" should be repeated. Refer to a gynecologist for results showing atypia or greater on the Bethesda scale (see pages 29-31).
PPD skin test	$1	Repeat annually in previously negative patients who have substantial risk for tuberculosis.
Hepatitis serology (see comments)	$10-15	Screen for vaccine candidates: anti-HBs or anti-HBc (see page 38). For HAV vaccine candidates : Total anti-HAV (IgG)
	$40-60	Abnormal liver function tests: HBsAg and anti-HCV.

II. Laboratory Tests

Table 2-9. Routine Laboratory Tests in Asymptomatic Patients (*Continued*)

Test	Cost*	Frequency and Comment
CMV IgG	$10-15	Sometimes advocated for low risk patients; seroprevalence in U.S. adults is 50-60% and for gay men and IV drug abuse patients it is ≥90%.
Toxoplasmosis serology (see comments)	$12-15	Screen all patients and repeat in seronegatives if: 1) CD4 count is ≤100/mm³ and patient does not take TMP-SMX for *P carinii* prophylaxis, and 2) symptoms suggesting toxoplasmosis encephalitis. Agglutination assays for IgG are preferred. IgM is not useful.
G-6-PD (optional — see comment)	$14-20	Test: 1) susceptible hosts: primarily men (X-linked) with the following ancestry: African-American, Italian, Sephardic Jew, Arabs, and those from India and SE Asia; 2) those receiving oxidant drugs, especially dapsone and primaquine; or 3) those with typical symptoms of G6 PD deficiency with testing following recovery (see pp. 40-41). Some authorities recommend screening all patients.
Fasting lipid profile	$20-40	Therapeutic monitoring recommended by some authorities for patients receiving antiretroviral regimens that include a PI or NNRTI; consider at baseline and at 3-4 months with subsequent measurements based on initial results and risks.

*Common charges based on survey of five laboratories.

III. Disease Prevention: Prophylactic Antimicrobial Agents and Vaccines

Recommendations of the U.S. Public Health Service and the Infectious Diseases Society of America Guidelines for the Prevention of Opportunistic Infections in Persons Infected with Human Immunodeficiency Virus (http://www.hivatis.org); MMWR 1999;48:[RR-10].

Table 3-1. Categories Reflecting Strength and Quality of Evidence

Category	Definition
	**Rating system for strength of recommendation and quality of evidence supporting the recommendation**

Category	Definition
Categories Reflecting the Strength of Each Recommendation	
A	Both strong evidence for efficacy and substantial clinical benefit support recommendation for use. Should always be offered.
B	Moderate evidence for efficacy — or strong evidence for efficacy, but only limited clinical benefit — supports recommendation for use. Should generally be offered.
C	Evidence for efficacy is insufficient to support a recommendation for or against use, or evidence for efficacy may not outweigh adverse consequences (e.g., toxicity, drug interactions, or cost of the chemoprophylaxis or alternative approaches). Optional.
D	Moderate evidence for lack of efficacy or for adverse outcome supports a recommendation against use. Should generally not be offered.
E	Good evidence for lack of efficacy or for adverse outcome supports a recommendation against use. Should never be offered.
Categories Reflecting Quality of Evidence Supporting the Recommendation	
I	Evidence from at least one properly randomized, controlled trial
II	Evidence from at least one well-designed clinical trial without randomization, from cohort or case-controlled analytic studies (preferably from more than one center), or from multiple time-series studies or dramatic results from uncontrolled experiments.
III	Evidence from opinions of respected authorities based on clinical experience, descriptive studies, or reports of expert committees.

III. Disease Prevention

STRONGLY RECOMMENDED AS STANDARD OF CARE

***Pneumocystis carinii* risk:** CD4 count <200/mm³, prior PCP or HIV-associated thrush or FUO x 2 wks. (A II)*

> **Preferred:** TMP-SMX 1 DS/day or 1 SS/day (A I)

> **Alternatives:**

>> TMP-SMX 1 DS 3 x/week (B I)

>> Dapsone 100 mg qd or 50 mg po bid (B I)

>> Dapsone 50 mg qd plus pyrimethamine 50 mg/wk plus leukovorin 25 mg/wk (B I)

>> Dapsone 200 mg/wk plus pyrimethamine 75 mg/wk plus leukovorin 25 mg/wk (B I)

>> Aerosolized pentamidine 300 mg q mo by Respirgard II nebulizer using 6 mL diluent delivered at 6L/min from a 50-psi compressed air source until reservoir is dry (usually 45 min) with or without albuterol (2 whiffs) to reduce cough and bronchospasm (B I)

>> Atovaquone 750 mg po bid with meals (NEJM 1998;339:1889) (B I)

Comments: Patients at risk given dapsone should be tested for G6PD deficiency. Data are inadequate to establish the efficacy and safety of parenteral pentamidine (4 mg/kg/month), or clindamycin-primaquine. Fansidar is rarely used due to possible severe hypersensitivity reactions. TMP-SMX has established efficacy for reducing the incidence of bacterial infections and toxoplasmosis. Patients who have a non-life threatening reaction to TMP-SMX should continue this drug if it can be tolerated. Those who have had such a reaction in the past should be rechallenged, possibly using desensitization (see page 269-270).

Immune reconstitution: Patients who have increases in CD4 count to >200/mm³ x 3-6 months may safely discontinue primary PCP prophylaxis (CII) (NEJM 1999;340:1301; Lancet 1999;353:1293; Lancet 1999;353:201). Data were inadequate to make this recommendation in patients receiving secondary PCP prophylaxis for prior PCP at the time they were written, but a subsequent report showed no PCP with 250 person-years of follow-up after discontinuing primary prophylaxis (7th CROI, Abst LB5).

***M. Tuberculosis* risk** (MMWR 1998;47[RR-20]): Positive PPD (≥5 mm induration) with prior treatment (A I), recent TB contact (A II), or history of inadequately treated TB that healed (A II).

> **Preferred:**

>> INH 300 mg/day + pyridoxine 50 mg/day ≥270 doses, 9 mos. or up to 12 mos. with interruptions (A II)

INH 900 mg + pyridoxine 100 mg twice weekly with directly observed therapy, ≥76 doses, 9 mos. or up to 12 mos. with interruptions (B I)

Patient not receiving PI or NNRTI:
Rifampin 600 mg/day + pyrazinamide 20 mg/kg/day with ≥60 doses x 2 mos. or up to 3 mos. with interruptions (A I).

Alternatives: Patients receiving a PI or NNRTI need rifabutin in place of rifampin/pyrazinamide 20 mg/kg and dose adjustment of the antiretroviral agent (B III).

- Amprenavir – standard; rifabutin – 150 mg/d

- Efavirenz – standard; rifabutin – 450 mg/d

- Indinavir – 1200 mg q8h; rifabutin – 150 mg/d

- Nelfinavir – 1000 mg tid; rifabutin – 150 mg/d

- Ritonavir – standard dose; rifabutin – 150 mg qod

Note: Rifabutin should not be combined with delavirdine and dose schedules are not available for Fortovase. Rifabutin should be combined with pyrazinamide 20 mg/kg/day with ≥60 doses x 2 mos. or up to 3 mos. with interruptions (B III).

Rifampin 600 mg qd x 4 mos. (B III)

Contact with INH resistant strain: Rifampin plus pyrazinamide x 2 mos. (above doses) (A I)

Alternative: Rifabutin/pyrazinamide (above doses x 2 mo.) (B III); Rifabutin 300 mg po qd x 4 mo. (C III).

Contact with strain resistant to INH and rifamycin: Use 2 agents with anticipated activity – ethambutol/pyrazinamide or levofloxacin/pyrazinamide

Pregnancy: INH regimens

***Toxoplasma gondii* risk:** CD4 count <100/mm³ plus positive IgG serology for *T. gondii*.

Preferred: TMP-SMX 1 DS/day (A II)

Alternatives: TMP-SMX 1 SS/day (B III)

Dapsone 50 mg po qd plus pyrimethamine 50 mg/wk plus leukovorin 25 mg/wk (B I)

Dapsone 200 mg po/wk plus pyrimethamine 75 mg po/wk plus leukovorin 25 mg po/wk

Atovaquone 1500 mg qd ± pyrimethamine 25 mg qd + leukovorin 10 mg qd (C III).

III. Disease Prevention

Immune Reconstitution: The number of patients with CD4 counts >100/mm^3 following HAART was considered inadequate to make discontinuation of prophylaxis a general recommendation in the USPHS/IDSA Guidelines for the 11/99 version. More recent studies now confirm the safety of discontinuing primary prophylaxis for toxoplasma when the CD4 count is >100/mm^3 for ≥3-6 months (7th CROI, Abst 230). Patients with prior toxoplasmosis should still receive lifelong secondary prophylaxis.

***M. avium* complex risk:** CD4 count <50 mm^3.

Preferred: Clarithromycin 500 mg or bid (A I) or azithromycin 1200 mg po weekly (A I).

Alternative: Rifabutin 300 mg po qd (B I) or azithromycin 1200 mg/wk plus rifabutin 300 mg qd (C I) (See rifabutin dose adjustment for use with PIs or NNRTIs – p. 46).

Immune Reconstitution: It appears safe to discontinue primary MAC prophylaxis when the CD4 count has increased to >100/mm^3 for 3-6 mos (CII) (NEJM 1998;338:853; 6th CROI Abst 692; 7th CROI Abst 242,246,247). Continuation of maintenance therapy is recommended for patients with prior MAC bacteremia, though discontinuation is currently under study.

***Varicella* risk:** Significant exposure to chickenpox or shingles who are either seronegative for VZV or have no history of primary or secondary VZV.

Preferred: VZIG 5 vials (6.25 mL) IM within 96 hours of exposure, preferably within 48 hours (A III).

Alternative: Prophylactic acyclovir was included in the 1995 USPHS/IDSA Guidelines, but was deleted from the 1999 version due to lack of supporting clinical evidence of efficacy.

GENERALLY RECOMMENDED

***S. pneumoniae* risk:** All patients (standard of care for patients with CD4 count >200/mm^3).

Preferred: Pneumovax 0.5 mL IM x 1 (CD4 >200/mm^3 – B II; CD4 <200/mm^3 – C III). Some authorities recommend repeating vaccination if CD4 count is >200/mm^3 or if it was low with the original vaccination. Some authorities recommend re-vaccination at 5 years.

Revaccinate: When CD4 count increases to >200/mm^3 if initial immunization was done with CD4 count <200/mm^3 (C III).

Alternative: The 7 valent protein-conjugated pneumococcal vaccine approved by the FDA in March, 2000 is recommended only for children, but studies in adults are ongoing since this may be a superior immunogen in immunosuppressed patients.

Hepatitis B risk: Negative anti-HBc screening test.

> **Preferred:** Recombivax HB 10 ug IM x 3 (B II) or Energix-B 20 µg IM x 3 (B II).

Influenza risk: All patients annually.

> **Preferred:** Influenza vaccine 0.5 mL IM each year preferably October - November (B III).

> **Alternative:** Amantadine 100 mg po bid (C III) or rimantadine 100 mg po bid (C III). (Note: zanamavir (Relenza) or osteltamivir (Tamiflu) should also be effective).

Hepatitis A risk: Susceptible patients with chronic hepatitis C infection.

> **Preferred:** Havrix 0.5 mL IM x 2 separated by 6 months (B III).

NOT RECOMMENDED FOR MOST PATIENTS; CONSIDER FOR SELECTED PATIENTS

Cryptococcosis risk: CD4 count <50/mm[3.]

> **Preferred:** Fluconazole 100-200 mg po qd (C I).

> **Alternative:** Itraconazole 200 mg po qd (C III).

Histoplasmosis risk: CD4 count <100/mm^3 plus residence in endemic area.

> **Preferred:** Itraconazole 200 mg po qd (C I).

CMV risk: CD4 count <50/mm^3 plus positive CMV serology.

> **Preferred:** Oral ganciclovir 1 gm po tid (C I).

> **Immune reconstitution:** For secondary prophylaxis, treatment may be stopped when the following criteria are met: CD4 >100-150/mm^3 for >3-6 mo., durable suppression of HIV RNA; nonsight-threatening lesion; vision adequate in contralateral eye and regular ophthalmic exam (CIII) (JID 1998;177:1182; JID 1998;177:1080; Ophthal 1998;105:1259).

Bacterial infection risk: Neutropenia.

> **Preferred:** G-CSF 5-10 µg/kg sc qd x 2-4 wks or GM-CSF 250 µg/m^2-IV over 2h qd x 2-4 wks (C II).

III. Disease Prevention

IV. Antiretroviral Therapy

I. RECOMMENDATIONS FOR ANTIRETROVIRAL THERAPY

Based on the recommendations of the Department of Health and Human Services/Kaiser Family Foundation as of April, 2000; [DHHS Panel on Clinical Practices for Treatment of HIV Infection Guidelines for Use of Antiretroviral Agents in HIV-infected Adults and Adolescents] http://www.hivatis.org. Print copies may be obtained from HIV/AIDS Treatment Information Service, P.O. Box 6303, Rockville, Maryland 20849-6303; Telephone: (800) 448-0440

GOALS OF THERAPY

Clinical goals: Prolongation of life and improved quality of life

Virologic goals: Reduction in viral load as much as possible (preferably <20 c/mL) for as long as possible to: 1) halt disease progression, and 2) prevent/reduce resistant variants

Immunologic goals: Achieve immune reconstitution that is quantitative (CD4 count in normal range) and qualitative (pathogen-specific immune response)

Therapeutic goals: Rational sequencing of drugs in a fashion that achieves virologic goals, but also: 1) maintains therapeutic options; 2) is relatively free of side effects; and 3) is realistic in terms of probability of adherence

Epidemiologic goals: Reduce HIV transmission

TERMS AND CONCEPTS

Class-sparing Regimens: Regimens that avoid exposure to drug classes, allowing the preservation of these agents for subsequent therapy. NNRTI/NRTI combinations are often referred to as "PI-sparing." NRTI based regimens, such as AZT/3TC/ABC or ddI/d4T/HU, spare both PIs and NNRTIs.

Cure: It is unfortunate that the cure theory was deemed plausible due to its impact on patient perceptions of the benefits of therapy. Virtually all studies show viral rebound within 12 weeks after discontinuing therapy despite no detectable virus for 2-3 years with HAART (NEJM 1999;340:1605; Nat Med 1999;5:512).

Drug holiday: Simultaneous discontinuation of antiretroviral drugs. This usually results in a viral rebound in 3-31 days (AIDS 1999;13:F79). The rebounding HIV strains are usually "wild-type;" the viral load usually rises rapidly to the pretreatment levels and immunologic deterioration with CD4 decline is rapid and substantial. S. Deeks reported that discontinuation of treatment in 18 patients with virologic failure resulted in a median viral load increase of $0.82 \log_{10}$ c/mL and a mean decrease in CD4 count of 94 cells/mm^3 at

12 weeks (7th CROI, Abstract LB10). Reversion to wild-type virus was noted at 12 weeks in most patients, suggesting that the resistant strains responsible for virologic failure were less fit, thus accelerated progression was observed after antiretroviral agents were discontinued and wild type virus reemerged.

GART: Genotypic antiretroviral resistance testing.

Genetic Barrier to Resistance: The mutations required by antiretroviral agents for evolution of phenotypic or clinically significant resistance. Examples of drugs with large genetic barriers include all protease inhibitors and all NRTIs except 3TC.

HAART (highly active antiretroviral therapy): An antiretroviral regimen that can reasonably be expected to reduce the viral load to <50 c/mL in treatment-naïve patients.

Immune-based Therapy: Treatment intended to achieve immune reconstitution that does not involve antiretroviral therapy. The most advanced forms of immune-based therapy in development through clinical trials are IL-2 and gp120 depleted inactivated HIV vaccine (Remune). Trials of IL-2 therapy show robust CD4 responses using doses of 5-7.5 MIU bid IM or SC x 5 days every 8 weeks; most studies have been carried out in patients with baseline CD4 counts >200/mm³ (Lancet 1999;353:1923). More recent studies show a modest response in patients with more advanced disease as well (JID 1999;180:56). Remune and other therapeutic vaccines are given to stimulate HIV-specific CTL response for improved immune regulation of HIV; preliminary results document immune response, but have not confirmed clinical benefit. Similarly disappointing preliminary results were obtained with a recombinant gp160 vaccine (Lancet 1999;353:1735).

Immune Reconstitution: The immune response to antiretroviral therapy is quantitative (CD4 response) and qualitative (antigen/microbe specific). The initial response is an increase in CD38+ MO+ (memory) cells, which is followed after 6 months by increases in CD38+ MA+ (naïve) cells including naïve cells of thymic origin. The biologic impact of immune reconstitution has been demonstrated by 1) an inflammatory response ascribed to immunologic reaction to selected microbial antigens; 2) the safety in discontinuation of prophylaxis for selected OIs; 3) control of several chronic, untreatable opportunistic infections as a result of HAART; and 4) an impressive decline in virtually all HIV-associated complications except lymphomas. With regard to the inflammatory reactions, the "immune reconstitution syndrome" has been observed with the following pathogens: *M. avium, M. tuberculosis, M. kanasii*, herpes simplex, herpes zoster, hepatitis and CMV. Chronic, relatively untreatable infections that can be controlled with immune reconstitution include Molluscum contagiosum, PML, CMV, cryptosporidiosis, and microsporidiosis. OI prophylaxis that may be suspended with adequate criteria for immune reconstitution according to the CDC/IDSA 1999 guidelines are primary PCP prophylaxis, primary MAC prophylaxis primary toxoplasmosis prophylaxis and secondary CMV prophylaxis (MMWR 1999;48:RR-10).

Intensification: The addition of antiretroviral agents to an existing regimen, usually due to failure to achieve a desired virologic response despite evidence of antiviral activity. This may be done in early treatment (VL >500 c/mL at 12-16 weeks), if optimal viral suppression has not been achieved (>20 c/mL at >20-24 weeks), or at the time of viral rebound.

Multi-drug Rescue Therapy: Salvage or rescue regimens containing ≥6 anti-retroviral regimens. Some of the drugs are "re-cycled." The rationale is that patients with multiple drug exposure and failures are unlikely to be infected with virus that is resistant to all drugs. Preliminary data from MDRT trials demonstrate some success with this approach; the main concerns are the need for extraordinary motivation, high rates of intolerance and cost.

Pharmacologic Barrier to Resistance: The achievement of tissue levels of pharmacologically active drugs substantially above the IC_{50} or IC_{90} for prolonged periods. Examples of drugs with large pharmacologic barriers include efavirenz, nevirapine and ABT-378/r.

Replicative (viral) fitness: The concept is that certain mutations, including mutations that confer resistance, may decrease the replicative capacity of HIV. This can be measured by comparative growth kinetics of strains with and without selected mutations or with a competitive assay (J Virol 1999;73:3744). An example is the RT 184 mutation which confers 3TC resistance but also reduces HIV fitness for replication. Data from *in vitro* studies of this phenomenon are inconsistent: protease mutations at codon 30 and 90 reduce *in vitro* replicative capacity, whereas multiply mutated strains resistant to indinavir showed no difference compared to wild-type virus (J Virol 1999;73:3744).

Resistance Testing: *Genotypic* resistance testing measures mutations on the reverse transcriptase and/or protease gene that impart partial or complete resistance to HIV. Results are interpreted on the basis of established patterns of mutations associated with phenotypic resistance, but assesses only the predominant strain(s), requires expertise for interpretation, and usually does not detect resistance to discontinued agents due to substitution by wild-type strains. *Phenotypic* resistance provides IC_{50}, IC_{90}, or IC_{95} data (concentration necessary to inhibit 50%, 90% or 95% of strains), and is most easily interpreted by care providers, but the test is expensive (~$900/test), results are not available for ≥3 weeks, only the dominant strains are tested and thresholds that define resistance are arbitrary and may not correlate with *in vivo* resistance. Despite the limitations, multiple studies show that resistance testing improves drug selection in "rescue regimens" including VIRADAPT (Lancet 1999;353:2191), CPCRA 046 (6th CROI, Abstract LB8), ACTG 372, the Stanford study (Ann Intern Med 1999;131:813), and VIRA 3001 (7th CROI, 2000 Abstract 237).

Salvage Therapy: Treatment regimens used in patients who have failed at least two antiretroviral regimens and have had extensive exposure to antiretroviral agents. Some prefer the term "rescue therapy," and some use these terms for any patient who has failed HAART.

Second Generation PIs and NNRTIs: Drugs currently in development that are active against HIV strains resistant to current members of that class.

Structured Treatment Interruption (STI): STI is the planned interruption of treatment by discontinuation of all antiretroviral drugs. There are two completely different reasons to consider STI: One is the "drug holiday" discussed above, in which the purpose is to relieve the patient of the inconvenience and toxicity of unsuccessful antiretroviral therapy while hoping to improve response to salvage therapy. A second rationale for STI is to reimmunize the patient to HIV in the hopes of regaining immunologic control through a regenerated HIV-specific immune response. This form of STI is usually studied in patients with optimal response to HAART. In patients with undetectable virus for sustained periods of 1-3 years, STI is associated with virologic rebound after approximately 2-8 weeks and a decrease in CD4 counts. These patients respond to reinstitution of treatment, and some studies have found that treatment can be stopped repeatedly with predictable response, to retreatment. *In vitro* data may demonstrate improved HIV-specific CTL responses and *in vivo* data suggests that some patients have longer mean replicative times correlating with improved *in vitro* HIV immune responses. This work, while promising, is still preliminary. So far, reports of long-term immunologic control as a result of STI have been purely anecdotal, as the case of the "Berlin patient" (NEJM 1999;340:1683).

Trial Analysis: Results of most clinical trials are presented in "intent-to-treat" analysis or "as-treated" analysis using virologic end points of <500 c/mL or <50 c/mL. In an "intent-to-treat analysis," the numerator is the number achieving the desired end point, and the denominator is all patients randomized to that treatment arm. Patients who discontinue the trial and those with missing data are counted as failures. In an "as-treated analysis," the numerator is the number who achieve the desired end point, and the denominator is the number continuing the trial to that time point. In this analysis, patients who change therapy due to treatment failure, discontinue the trial due to side effects, or have other reasons for missing data are excluded from the analysis. In trials of antiretroviral therapy, intent-to-treat analysis gives a better indication of "real world" issues, such as tolerability, convenience, and adherence, while as treated analysis may better reflect relative potency. In a review of 17 HIV therapeutic trials, A. Hill, et al [6th Conf. On Retroviruses, Chicago, 1999, Abstract #394] showed that the mean percent achieving "virologic success" was 81% by as treated analysis using <500 c/mL as the therapeutic goal, and 52% by intent-to-treat analysis using <50 c/mL as the therapeutic goal. This represents a 29% difference (a range of 15-46% for individual studies), emphasizing the impotance of understanding the form of analysis before attempting to compare results across trials.

Undetectable Virus or No Detectable Virus : This is the virologic goal of therapy, but the definition depends on the threshold of the assay used to determine plasma HIV RNA levels. Common thresholds are 400-500 c/mL or 20-50 c/mL.

Viral Load – CD4 Count Discordance: This term generally refers to the observation that many patients who fail to achieve adequate viral suppression, nevertheless have a robust CD4 cell response or sustained CD4 counts at high levels. For example, analysis of the Swiss Cohort showed that patients with persistent viral suppression had an average CD4 count increase of 138/mm³ compared to an increase of 130/mm³ in those with only a transient virologic response (Lancet 1998;351:723). In contrast, other studies have shown that discontinuation of antiretrovirals is associated with a precipitous fall in CD4 count. Similar conclusions result from analyses of opportunistic infections. 30 month follow-up data from 2674 patients treated with protease inhibitor combination regimens showed that the frequency of opportunistic infections was 6.6% for those with viral rebound, 20.1% for non-responders and about 55% for historic controls (Lancet 1999;353:863). These studies demonstrate that patients failing HAART often have immunologic responses to therapy and reduced clinical progression. In most cases there is also partial viral suppression, so that the "disconnect" component of the term may be inappropriate. However, benefit may be observed even when viral load returns to baseline, possibly due to reduced "fitness" of HIV. The durability of this benefit is unknown beyond the 1-2 years observed in the studies summarized above. Moreover, it is not known whether these observations apply to the antiretroviral regimens that do not contain protease inhibitors.

Virologic failure: Generally defined as detectable HIV RNA with an assay that has a threshold of detection of 20-50 c/mL after 20-24 weeks of initiating therapy or implementing a new regimen. HIV RNA levels >500 c/mL at ≥16-20 weeks also indicate virologic failure and levels >500 c/mL at 12-16 weeks generally predict virologic failure.

Wild-type Virus: The predominant virus in a region or population. At present, the majority of strains are pan-sensitive, but this could change with time.

A. ANTIRETROVIRAL THERAPY FOR HIV INFECTED PATIENTS (http://www.hivatis.org 4/2000)

The following represent the DHHS guidelines for antiretroviral therapy based on the document as of April, 2000 with minor modifications. This document makes recommendations for: 1) Indications to treat; 2) Recommended starting regimens; 3) Indications to change; 4) Regimens for salvage therapy. These four topics are presented in sequential order. In some cases, recommendations are also provided from the International AIDS Society-USA according to their consensus dated 12/99 (JAMA 2000;283:381).

1. Indications for Antiretroviral Therapy

Table 4-1a: Indications for the Initiation of Antiretroviral Therapy – DHHS Guidelines

Clinical Category	CD4+ T Cell Count and HIV RNA	Recommendation
Acute HIV or <6 months after seroconversion	All	Treat
Symptomatic (AIDS, thrush, unexplained fever)	All	Treat
Asymptomatic	CD4+ T Cells <500/mm³ or HIV RNA >10,000 (bDNA) or >20,000 (RT-PCR)	Treatment should be offered. Strength of recommendation is based on prognosis for disease-free survival (See Table 4-1b) and willingness of the patient to accept therapy.*
Asymptomatic	CD4+ T Cells >500/mm³ and HIV RNA <10,000 (bDNA) or <20,000 (RT-PCR)	Many experts would delay therapy and observe; however, some experts would treat.

* Some experts would observe patients with CD4+T cell counts between 350-500/mm³ and HIV RNA levels <10,000 (bDNA) or <20,000 (RT-PCR)

Table 4-1b: Indications for the Initiation of Antiretroviral Therapy – IAS-USA Recommendations

CD4 Count	Viral load (c/mL)		
	<5,000	5,000-30,000	>30,000
<350	Treat	Treat	Treat
350-500	Consider	Treat	Treat
>500	Defer	Consider	Treat

Table 4-2: Probability of an AIDS-Defining Opportunistic Infection Within 3 Years in the Absence of Antiretroviral Therapy Based on Baseline CD4 Count and Viral Load. Data from MACS (Mellors J, et al. Ann Intern Med 1997;126:946)

CD4 <350		% AIDS-Defining Complication		
VL (RT-PCR)*	n	3 years	6 years	9 years
1,500-7,000*	30	0	18.8	30.6
7,000-20,000	51	8.0	42.2	65.6
20,000-55,000	73	40.1	72.9	86.2
>55,000	174	72.9	92.7	95.6
CD4 350-500				
1,500-7,000	47	4.4	22.1	46.9
7,000-20,000	105	5.9	39.8	60.7
20,000-55,000	121	15.1	57.2	78.6
>55,000	121	47.9	77.7	94.4
CD4 >500				
<1,500	110	1.0	5.0	10.7
1,500-7,000	180	2.3	14.9	33.2
7,000-20,000	237	7.2	25.9	50.3
20,000-55,000	202	14.6	47.7	70.6
>55,000	141	32.6	66.8	76.3

* Plasma HIV RNA levels in c/mL using RT-PCR

Note: The recommendations of the DHHS Panel for therapy of asymptomatic patients define a group with the risk for an AIDS-defining complication in the absence of therapy of about 6% at 3 years, 25% at 6 years, and 50% at 9 years.

IV. Antiretroviral Therapy

2. Recommended Starting Regimens

Table 4-3a: Initial Regimen – DHHS Guidelines (One from column A and one from column B in the preferred category)

	Column A	Column B
Preferred	Efavirenz Indinavir Nelfinavir Ritonavir/Saquinavir	d4T/TC AZT/ddI AZT/3TC d4T/ddI
Alternative	Abacavir Amprenavir Delavirapine Nevirapine Ritonavir Saquinavir (Fortovase) Nelfinavir/Fortovase	ddI/3TC AZT/ddC
No recommendation (insufficient data)	Hydroxyurea Ritonavir/Indinavir Ritonavir/Nelfinavir	
Not recommended	Saquinavir (Invirase)	ddC/ddI ddC/d4T ddC/3TC AZT/d4T

Table 4-3b: Initial Regimen – IAS-USA (JAMA 2000;283:381)

Preferred:
- 2 nucleosides and a PI
- 2 nucleosides and a NNRTI

Under evaluation:
- 3 nucleosides
- Consider in patients with CD4 count <50/mm^3 or VL > 100,000 c/mL
  - 2 NRTIs + 2 PIs
  - 2 NRTIs + PI + NNRTI

a. **Factors that influence probability of prolonged viral suppression using regimens that are strongly recommended:**

Adherence: Obvious but critical, as demonstrated in a study that demonstrated a strong correlation between virologic response at 6 months and adherence as monitored by MEMS devices (ICAAC, 1998, San Diego, Abstract I-172).

Adherence to HAART*	VL <500 c/mL
>95% adherence	81%
90-95% adherence	64%
80-90% adherence	50%
70-80% adherence	24%
<70% adherence	6%

* No. doses prescribed/no. taken

Baseline CD4 count: A relatively high CD4 count (>200/mm³) is sometimes, but not invariably, associated with a superior viral response and a CD4 count <50/mm³ has a relatively poor probability of a good virologic response (JID 1999;180:659). Review of the Moore Clinic database in patients in the Hopkins HIV Care Program showed an inverse correlation between baseline CD4 count and probability of achieving a viral load <500 c/mL with HAART (7th CROI, Abstract 522):

Baseline CD4	No.	VL <400 c/mL	
		Ever	>6 mo
>350	176	81%	43%
200-350	125	74%	34%
<200	326	65%	28%

Similar results were noted with analysis of 4 protocols using indinavir/AZT/3TC. The probability of achieving VL <50 c/mL at 52 weeks with CD4 counts >500, 50-400, or <50 were 80%, 70%, and 45%, respectively (7th CROI, Abstract 521).

Baseline viral load: Most studies demonstrate a direct correlation between baseline viral load and probability of achieving viral suppression to <50 c/mL or <500 c/mL (AIDS 1999;13:187; CID 1999;29:75). In ACTG 175 a regimen of 2 NRTIs achieved a viral load <500 c/mL in approximately half of patients with baseline viral loads of ≤10,000 c/mL. Most studies show that even some recommended regimens (2 NRTIs + PI) are less effective in patients with a

IV. Antiretroviral Therapy

baseline viral load >100,000 c/mL; this was not the case in initial studies using efavirenz/2 NRTIs or ABT 378/r. The baseline viral load also predicts time required to reach undetectable virus (7th CROI, Abstract 520).

Prior exposure to antiretroviral agents: Multiple studies demonstrate a reverse correlation between response and the extent of prior antiretroviral therapy in terms of number of agents, number of classes and duration of treatment. The Swiss Cohort study (Lancet 1999;353:863), for example, showed that the probability of achieving a viral load <500 c/mL with HAART therapy was 91% in treatment-naïve patients compared to 75% in treatment-experienced patients. Among patients who achieved undetectable virus, the probability of retaining a viral load <500 c/mL at two years was 80% for treatment-naïve patients compared to 62% in treatment-experienced patients. The conclusion of many authorities is that the initial regimen is the most important regimen because it is associated with the greatest probability of achieving prolonged viral suppression.

Nadir of viral load: Multiple studies demonstrate that the nadir plasma HIV RNA level strongly predicts the durability of response and in fact may be the single most important predictor of a durable response.

Rapidity of viral load response: The trajectory of the viral load response predicts the nadir plasma HIV RNA level and consequently predicts the durability of HIV response. Expectations are that treatment-naïve patients treated with HAART will have a viral load <400 c/mL at 12 weeks and <50 c/mL at 16-24 weeks. In ACTG 320 the viral load response at 4 weeks strongly predicted long-term viral suppression. Thus, clinical and viral load evaluation at 4-8 weeks permits an estimate of the probability of viral suppression and affords an opportunity for enhanced counseling on adherence. The trajectory of the virologic response has less predictive value in patients receiving "salvage" or "rescue" regimens.

b. Regimens: Preferred regimens based on antiviral effect may be defined by clinical trial data showing a viral load <50 c/mL at ≥24 weeks for >40% of participants by intent-to-treat analysis. A number of regimens achieve this goal in treatment-naïve patients. Characteristic features of these regimens are the use of at least three drugs with a backbone of two nucleoside analogs combined with a PI or NNRTI (Table 4-4). (Note: These regimens should not be compared by outcome due to differences in enrollment criteria, patient characteristics, extent of adherence, etc.)

Table 4-4: Clinical Trials Showing HIV RNA Levels <50 c/mL After 24 Weeks in >40% of Patients by Intent-to-Treat Analysis*

Trial	Treatment	<50 c/mL at 24 weeks (ITT)
M97-720	2 NRTIs + ABT-378/r	89%
Danish PI	2 NRTIs + RTV + SQV	78%
Merck 035	2 NRTIs + IDV	66%
SPICE	2 NRTIs + NFV + SQV	65%
START-1	2 NRTIs + IDV	61%
DMP-006	2 NRTIs + EFV	59%
AVANTI-2	2 NRTIs + IDV	58%
START-1	2 NRTIs + IDV	55%
CNAB 3003	2 NRTIs + ABC	54%
AVANTI-3	2 NRTIs + NFV	53%
NV 15355	2 NRTIs + SQV	49%
DMP 005	2 NRTIs + EFV	49%
INCAS	2 NRTIs + NVP	45%
DMP 006	2 NRTIs + IDV	44%
SPICE	2 NRTIs + SQV	42%
SPICE	2 NRTIs + NFV	42%

* Trial results should not be compared due to differences in populations studied, entry criteria, and even definition of analysis by intent-to-treat

Table 4-5: Relative Merits of Early Therapy and Delayed Therapy

Advantages of early therapy	Advantages of delayed therapy
• Control viral replication	• Poor quality of life with treatment
• Prevent progressive immune deficiency	• Earlier drug resistance if not fully effective
• Delay progression to AIDS and death	• Limit future drug options
• Prevent resistance when fully effective	• Long term drug toxicity
• Better tolerability of drugs	• Duration of effectiveness is unknown
• Reduce viral transmission	• Risk transmission of resistant strains

IV. Antiretroviral Therapy

49

Table 4-6: Relative Merits of Antiretroviral Treatment Regimens

Regimen	Advantage	Disadvantage

2 NRTIs + a PI	Standard
	Extensively studied
	Durability >3 years
	  (Merck 035 trial)
	Genetic barrier to resistance
	NNRTI-sparing
		Cross-resistance among PIs
		Inconvenience: BID or TID regimens ± food requirements
		Toxicity: GI intolerance
		  Metabolic abnormalities
		  Agent-specific ADRs

2 NRTIs + NNRTI	Comparable to standard
	  (possibly better—EFV)
	Durability (≥1 year)
	PI-sparing
	Pharmacologic barrier to
	  resistance
	Good CNS penetration
	Convenience of qd dosing (EFV)
		Cross-resistance among NNRTIs
		Toxicity
		  CNS (EVF)
		  Rash
		  Lipid abnormalities (EFV)
		  Hepatic (NVP)

ABC + 3TC + AZT	PI- and NNRTI-sparing
	Comparable to standard
	  increased
	Potential for simplicity of single
	  pill bid
		Limited experience
		May have suboptimal response
		  with high baseline viral load
		Potential for extensive NRTI
		  resistance
		Hypersensitivity reactions (ABC)

ddI + 2nd NRTI + hydroxyurea	PI- and NNRTI-sparing
	Convenience of bid (and
	  possibly qd) dosing
		Limited published experience
		CD4 count increase blunted
		  (HU)
		Marrow toxicity (HU)
		Potentiation of ddI toxicity by HU

2 NRTIs + 2 PIs	Pharmacologic benefit with
	  reduced doses and longer
	  dosing intervals
	  (regimen dependent)
	Increased potency (?)
	Improved tolerability
		Cross-resistance among PIs
		Toxicity: GI intolerance
		  Metabolic abnormalities
		  Agent-specific ADRs
		Complex drug interactions with
		  multiple agents

2 NRTIs + PI + NNRTI	Increased potency (?)
	Reduced probability of
	  resistance (?)
		Risk resistance to PIs, NNRTIs
		Toxicity: ADRs of both classes
		Complex drug interactions with
		  multiple agents

3. When to Change Therapy

The goal of therapy is to reduce the level of HIV RNA to as low a level as possible for as long as possible, preferably using antiretroviral regimens that preserve future options, are relatively free of side effects, and are tailored to individual patient needs for adherence.

Analysis of virologic results from many studies indicates that the post treatment viral load nadir is the best predictor of the durability of a sustained viral response. Optimal results are achieved with undetectable virus using an assay with a threshold of 20 c/mL. Studies show that <5% of all AIDS-defining complications occur in patients with a viral load of <5,000 c/mL, suggesting that thresholds that define virologic failure and clinical failure may be different (AIDS 1999;13:1035). However, the assumption is that virologic failure will eventually lead to clinical failure. Unfortunately, clinical studies show that only 15-30% of patients in most urban clinics achieve a sustained level of <20 c/mL (Ann Int Med 1999;131:18; AIDS 1999;13:F35), and the HCSUS study suggests that only about 28% of persons in the U.S. who are receiving HIV care have a viral load <500 c/mL. Based on these observations, most authorities consider a reduction to <20-50 c/mL to be the ultimate goal of therapy, but this may be unrealistic in many patients. More importantly, the attempt to achieve unrealistic virologic responses may severely limit future therapeutic options due to the evolution of resistance.

The probability of achieving the goal of <50 c/mL with HAART in treatment naïve patients can be crudely predicted by the slope of the decay in plasma HIV RNA levels, which should show a decrease of 1.5-2.0 $\log_{10}$ c/mL at 4 weeks, <500 c/mL by 12 weeks and <50 c/mL at 16-24 weeks. The time required to reach undetectable levels correlates with the initial viral load with an average of 73 days to <50 c/mL in one study (7th CROI, Abstract 520). Once the goal of therapy has been achieved, therapy should be continued indefinitely with monitoring of HIV RNA levels at 3-4 month intervals and CD4 counts at 3-6 month intervals. The following guidelines apply:

Indications to change therapy: The major goal of antiretroviral therapy is viral suppression as indicated by HIV RNA levels. Changes based on inadequate virologic response should be confirmed using at least two viral load measurements at a time of clinical stability, bearing in mind that the 95% confidence interval for the test is about 3-fold. Therapeutic regimens may also require change due to adverse drug reactions or due to the complexity of the regimen that may threaten adherence.

CD4 counts: The CD4 response is generally a mirror image of the HIV RNA decay curve, with increases that average 100-200/mm³ in the first year after complete virologic suppression. Subsequent increases are more gradual but usually continuous. The lack of a CD4 response despite viral suppression is sometimes considered an indication to change therapy, but data to support this strategy are largely absent. The development of HIV-associated complications despite good viral suppression is usually not considered grounds for changing the antiretroviral regimen.

IV. Antiretroviral Therapy

Causes of virologic failure: Inadequate virologic response is ascribed to: 1) lack of adherence; 2) reduced potency of the regimen; 3) pharmacologic failure due to reduced drug delivery to the site of infection (absorption, protein binding, drug interactions); and 4) resistance. In general, most of the failure in the first 24 weeks of treatment using recommended HAART regimens in treatment-naïve patients is due to lack of adherence or inadequate potency, and most late failures that follow good virologic response are due to resistance.

Changes due to adverse drug reactions: An attempt should be made to use a regimen with equal potency if virologic success was achieved. If the offending agent is unclear or GI toxicity precludes adherence, it is appropriate to suspend all treatment and then restart a modified regimen. In patients who may be experiencing the abacavir hypersensitivity reaction, if possible, this drug should be discontinued and not restarted.

4. Regimens for Salvage Therapy: What to Change to

Changes in therapy can be divided into three categories: a) empiric selection of a new regimen based on history of drug exposure; b) changes based on resistance testing; or c) intensification. In all cases it is critical to evaluate adherence as a contributing factor to failure (Table 4-7).

Table 4-7a: Guidelines for Changing Antiretroviral Regimen (Modified from DHHS Guidelines, 4/2000)

- When change is due to a single viral load determination, confirm with repeat test.

- Changes based on adverse drug reactions or intolerance can be done with single agent substitution provided the patient has an appropriate virologic response to the regimen (?).

- Changes based on virologic failure should be based on resistance test results and history of prior exposures; empiric decisions should usually involve selection of a completely new regimen.

- Patients with virologic failure and limited options may do best with continuation of regimen that shows only partial viral suppression.

- Patients who fail HAART may require regimens containing 2 PIs or all drugs from three classes.

- Resistance tests are valid indicators only for drugs being taken at the time the test is performed, or within 2 weeks of discontinuation. Resistance should be suspected for drugs given previously during sustained periods with virologic failure.

- In making empiric decisions, assume cross resistance for NNRTIs and for the PIs after failure of ritonavir, indinavir or saquinavir; assume partial cross resistance or "after failure of retinavir or amprenavir"

Table 4-7b: Recommendations for Changing Therapeutic Regimen (Modified from IAS-USA Recommendations, JAMA 2000;283:381)

Clinical presentation	Recommendations
Toxicity	
Virologic success	Change offending drug
VL above target before 8-16 weeks	Change offending drug
VL above target after 8-16 weeks	Change entire regimen*
Virologic failure	
VL above target at 8-16 weeks	Continue regimen, check adherence and consider intensification
VL above target after 24-36 weeks	Change entire regimen*
Virologic "escape" after good suppression	Change entire regimen*

* A major difference between the DHHS guidelines and the IAS-USA guidelines is that the DHHS guidelines endorse resistance testing to facilitate regimen selection in patients with virologic failure. By contrast, the IAS-USA guidelines do not endorse resistance testing.

Empiric changes in NRTIs: the options may be limited by prior exposures or toxicity, but general recommendations are:

AZT + 3TC → ddI + d4T ± HU
AZT + ddI → d4T + 3TC
d4T + ddI → AZT + 3TC, AZT + ddC
d4T + 3TC → AZT + ddI ± HU
AZT + ddC → d4T + 3TC, d4T + ddI, ddI + 3TC

Note: Studies of abacavir in salvage regimens show little or no virologic response that can be independently ascribed to this agent in patients with heavy previous NRTI exposure, presumably due to cross resistance, but ABC may work after non-AZT containing regimens, or with low-level AZT resistance and it may be useful for intensification.

Empiric changes in PI containing regimens:

a. NNRTI in patients without prior exposure to this class

b. Dual PIs, usually RTV/SQV, RTV/IDV, RTV/APV or NFV/SQV with the following caveats: a) PI salvage from PI-containing regimens is most likely to be successful if the viral load is relatively low (<20,000 c/mL) and preferably <5000 c/mL) when the switch is made; b) indinavir and ritonavir demonstrate nearly complete cross resistance; and c) there are data suggesting that PIs are more likely to be effective following nelfinavir therapy than after failure of other PIs. NNRTI-containing regimens should be empirically changed to a PI-containing regimen. APV may be more active vs HIV strains resistant to other PIs and APV resistant strains may be more susceptible to other PIs.

c. Triple class regimens: The risk is exposure to all classes with the consequent impact on options if there is virologic failure with resistance. The lack of information about the pharmacology of some drug combinations and sparce clinical trial data is also limiting.

Suggested Empiric Regimens for Patients Who Failed Antiretroviral Therapy

Prior Regimen	New Regimen
2 NRTIs + PI	2 new NRTIs plus NNRTI or Dual PIs (RTV + SQV, RTV + IDV, NFV + SQV, RTV + APV) or Triple class regimen with 1-2 NRTIs plus NVP or EFV plus 1-2 PIs
2 NRTIs + NNRTI	2 new NRTIs + 1 or 2 PIs
ABC + AZT + 3TC	2 new NRTIs (ddI + d4T) + either PI or NNRTI
2 NRTIs	2 new NRTIs + PI or NNRTI
NRTI + NNRTI + PI	ddI + HU + 2 PIs or megaHAART

Selection based on resistance testing: Initial results from trials in which salvage regimens were selected by genotypic resistance test results show two major benefits compared to decisions based on ART history: 1) virologic outcome appears to be superior with analysis at 16-24 weeks, and 2) the number of drugs changed is reduced due to knowledge that resistance is problematic only for selected components of the initial regimen (CPCRA 046, 6th CROI, Abstract LB8; 7th CROI, Abstract 237; Lancet 1999;353:2195; AIDS 1999;13:1861). It is anticipated that resistance testing will be widely used for selecting salvage regimens with the following caveats: a) Resistance is determined as due to the agents that are being taken at the time testing is done; replacement by wild-type virus usually takes place at 2-8 weeks after antiretroviral agents responsible for resistance have been discontinued (AIDS 1999;13:F123; AIDS 1999;13:2541); b) Results are limited to the dominant strains (those making up ≥20% of the total population for the individual); c) A viral load of ≥1000 c/mL is generally required; d) Genotypic testing does not necessarily reveal all relevant mutations; e) Interpretation of genotypic test results is complex due to the multiplicity of mutations necessary to impart clinically relevant resistance to PIs and NRTIs other than 3TC and due to complex interactions between mutations; f) Phenotypic resistance is limited by arbitrary and non-standardized thresholds to define resistance that does not have clinical correlates; g) Interpretation of all resistance testing requires substantial expertise; and h) Resistance testing is more accurate when selecting regimens after first regimen failures compared to subsequent failures (see Tables 2-5 on pg. 24 and 2-6 on pg 25).

Intensification: This refers to the addition of one or two agents to an existing regimen that has resulted in incomplete suppression of viral load. Typical indications include failure to reach targeted threshold or confirmed rebound in a patient with previously undetectable virus. There are few studies that systematically assess the benefits and risks of intensification; however, common practices include: a) addition of hydroxyurea to a ddI-containing regimen; b) addition of a second PI to a PI-containing regimen; or c) addition of a third NRTI such as abacavir or 3TC.

Interrupted therapy: Patients who require discontinuation of components of treatment due to toxicity, non-availability or other reasons, should usually suspend the entire treatment regimen. If drugs are held in the presence of near complete viral suppression, most patients will experience a prompt viral rebound, with high levels of HIV RNA within 1-3 weeks.

Therapeutic drug monitoring: This is not an issue with NRTIs since only intracellular concentrations are relevant. Levels are also not relevant for NNRTIs, since high concentrations relative to IC_{90} are achieved. Levels may be useful with some PIs in single PI containing regimens since these drugs often have highly variable levels that may be subtherapeutic in some patients; levels should not be considered for many dual PI regimens containing ritonavir due to the high and sustained levels achieved. An exception is level measurements with three way interactions of uncertain pharmacologic effect on selected components, eg., IDV levels with RTV/IDV/EFV. IAS-USA does not recommend any therapeutic monitoring (JAMA 2000;283;381).

IV. Antiretroviral Therapy

B. RECOMMENDATIONS FOR ANTIRETROVIRAL THERAPY IN PREGNANCY

1. Prevention of Perinatal Transmission

ACTG 076

ACTG 076 showed that AZT reduced the rate of perinatal transmission from 22.6% to 7.6% (NEJM 1996;335:1621). Multiple uncontrolled studies have confirmed the benefit of AZT in reducing perinatal transmission (JID 1995;172:353; CID 1995;20:1321) and subsequent surveillance studies in the U.S. showed substantial declines in the rates of perinatally acquired HIV that accompanied use of AZT in pregnant women (MMWR 1997;46:1986). Initial recommendations for women were based on ACTG 076 and were designed to prevent perinatal transmission only using the following three-part protocol (MMWR 1994;43,[RR-11]:1-20):

- **Before delivery:** AZT (300 mg bid, 200 mg tid or 100 mg 5x/day) initiated at 14-34 weeks of gestation and continued to onset of labor.

- **During labor:** IV AZT (loading infusion of 2 mg/kg IV for one hour followed by continuous infusion 1 mg/kg per hour until delivery)

- **Infant:** AZT for the newborn (AZT syrup at 2 mg/kg every six hours) for the first six weeks of life beginning 8-12 hours after birth.

Current Recommendations: The current DHHS recommendations (Revised guidelines April, 2000; http://www.hivatis.org) are based on the philosophy that "pregnancy *per se* should not preclude use of optimal therapeutic regimens. However, the choice of drugs is subject to unique considerations, including potential changes in dosing requirement due to the physiologic changes associated with pregnancy and the potential effects of the antiretroviral drugs on the fetus and newborn." In essence, pregnant women should be treated according to standard guidelines for antiretroviral therapy in adults, with the objective of reducing the viral load to as low as possible for as long as possible. This is optimal for the health of the pregnant woman, and appears to be optimal for reducing perinatal transmission as well. Exceptions to the use of standard regimens noted in Tables 4-3 and 4-7 are the following:

AZT Issues: When feasible, AZT should be included in the regimen since this is the only drug with established merit for reducing HIV perinatal transmission. If AZT is contraindicated because of intolerance or by the need to use d4T, which cannot be combined with AZT due to pharmacologic antagonism, part 2 and part 3 of the 076 protocol should be followed, e.g., the pregnant woman should receive AZT intravenously during labor and the newborn infant should receive oral AZT for 6 weeks.

Safety of Antiretroviral Agent: Antiretroviral drugs that should be avoided during pregnancy, and in women who may become pregnant are hydroxyurea and efavirenz, because of teratogenic concerns. Some consider indinavir to be relatively contraindicated in late pregnancy because of theoretical concerns related to possible hyperbilirubinemia and renal stones in the neonate. All PIs may increase the pregnancy-related risk for hyperglycemia; periodic monitoring of glucose levels is indicated.

The only antiretroviral drugs that have undergone pharmacokinetic studies in pregnant women are AZT, 3TC and nevirapine; all three show pharmacokinetics that are similar to those observed with non-pregnant women.

Teratogenicity and mutagenicity of antiretroviral agents has been examined in animals with variable results (Table 4-8). Safety data in patients is limited, although follow-up of 734 infants exposed to prophylactic antepartum AZT and followed for a median of 4.2 years showed no adverse outcomes that could be ascribed to AZT in terms of rate of progression to AIDS or death, or differences in neurodevelopment, or rate of malignancies. All of the current FDA approved antiretroviral agents other than hydroxyurea are FDA pregnancy category B or C, including efavirenz. The Antiretroviral Pregnancy Registry has provided data from 916 pregnant women given antiretroviral agents, including 136 given PIs and 343 treated in the first trimester. The rate of birth defects was 2.0/100 live births for women treated in the first trimester. This is consistent with CDC surveillance data showing rates of 2.2/100 for women without HIV; there were no consistent patterns for birth defects (7th CROI, Abstract 68). There is one report from France of 8 infants with mitochondrial damage ascribed to NRTIs (Lancet 1999;354:1084), but no such cases were found in a review of 20,000 infants exposed to prenatal AZT in the U.S. (http://www.hivatis.org).

First Trimester Issues: Some authorities recommend that therapy be delayed or interrupted during the first trimester when the fetus is most vulnerable to malformations. This should be a clinical decision based on theoretical concerns and safety data that are preliminary. Recommendations should be made based on clinical findings (CD4 count, viral load, symptoms, etc.) and the patient's decision after being informed about the theoretical concerns and available data.

Breastfeeding: A meta-analysis of 5 studies performed in developing countries indicated that the risk of HIV transmission with breastfeeding is about 15% in the absence of antiretroviral therapy (Lancet 1992;340:385; JAMA 2000;283:1167). The risk appears to be greatest in the first 4-6 months (JAMA 1999;282:744). A randomized study of breastfeeding vs. formula feeding by HIV-infected mothers in Kenya showed two-year infant mortality rates that were surprisingly similar: 20% vs. 24% (JAMA 2000;283:1167). Nevertheless, breast milk substitutes were strongly recommended for the first 6 months (JAMA 2000;283:1175).

Viral load: In ACTG 076 AZT was associated with a mean decrease in plasma HIV RNA levels of only 0.24 logs. This antiviral effect explained less than 17% of the treatment effect on vertical transmission. In a subsequent AZT trial in

Thailand AZT recipients had a 0.56 log decrease in plasma HIV RNA levels, explaining about 80% of the reduction in perinatal transmission (Lancet 1999;353:773). In ACTG 185 there was no perinatal transmission among 43 patients who maintained HIV RNA levels <500 c/mL (JID 1999;179:567). An analysis of 552 mother-infant pairs in The Women and Infants Transmission Study (WITS) found no transmission when maternal viral loads at delivery were <1000 c/mL (NEJM 1999;341:394). There was a direct correlation between viral load and transmission rate ranging from 32/194 (17%) with 1,000-10,000 c/mL to 24/64 (41%) with viral load >100,000 c/mL). Similar results were noted in ACTG 185 (NEJM 1999;341:385). Most authorities conclude that the primary objective in treating pregnant women should be a reduction in viral load to prevent HIV progression in the mother and also to reduce perinatal transmission. Nevertheless, there are exceptions in which transmission has occurred despite undetectable virus in the mother. Some feel this is due to discordance between HIV levels in plasma and genital secretions (AIDS 1999;13:1377; JID 1999;179:871).

Table 4-8: Safety of Antiretroviral Agents in Pregnancy

Antiretroviral Drug	FDA Pregnancy Category*	Placental Passage Newborn: Maternal Drug Ratio	Long-Term Animal Carcinogenicity Studies	Rodent Teratogen
zidovudine** (AZT)	C	Yes (human) [0.85]	Positive (rodent, vaginal tumors)	Positive (near lethal dose)
zalcitabine (ddC)	C	Yes (rhesus) [0.3-0.50]	Positive (rodent, thymic lymphomas)	Positive (hydrocephalus at high dose)
didanosine (ddI)	B	Yes (human) [0.5]	Negative (no tumors, lifetime rodent study)	Negative
stavudine (d4T)	C	Yes (rhesus) [0.76]	Not completed	Negative (but sternal bone calcium decreases)
lamivudine (3TC)	C	Yes (human) [~1.0]	Negative (no tumors, lifetime rodent study)	Negative
abacavir (ABC)	C	Yes (rats)	Not Completed	Positive (anasarca and skeletal malformations at 1000 mg/kg during organogenesis)
saquinavir (SQV)	B	Unknown	Not Completed	Negative
Indinavir (IDV)	C	Yes (rats) ("Significant" in rats, low in rabbits)	Not Completed	Negative (but extra ribs in rats)
ritonavir (RTV)	B	Yes (rats) [mid-term fetus, 1.15; late term fetus, 0.15-0.64]	Not Completed	Negative (but crytorchidism in rats)†
nelfinavir (NFV)	B	Unknown	Not Completed	Negative
amprenavir	C	Unknown	Not Completed	Positive (thymicelongation; incomplete ossification of bones; low body weight)
nevirapine (NVP)	C	Yes (human) [~1.0]	Not Completed	Negative
delavirdine (DLV)	C	Yes (rats) [late-term fetus, blood, 0.15 Late-term fetus, liver 0.04]	Not Completed	Ventricular septal defect
efavirenz (EFV)	C	Yes (cynomolgus monkeys, rats, rabbits) [~1.0]	Not Completed	Anencephaly; anophthalmia; microphthalmia (cynomolgus monkeys)

IV. Antiretroviral Therapy

* FDA Pregnancy Categories are:

　B – Animal reproduction studies fail to demonstrate a risk to the fetus and adequate, well-controlled studies of pregnant women have not been conducted;

　C – Safety in human pregnancy has not been determined, animal studies are either positive for fetal risk or have not been conducted, and the drug should not be used unless the potential benefit outweighs the potential risk to the fetus.

** Despite certain animal data showing potential teratogenicity of ZDV when near-lethal doses are given to pregnant rodents, considerable human data are available to date indicating that the risk to the fetus, if any, is extremely small when ZDV is given to the pregnant mother after 14 weeks gestation. Follow-up for up to 6 years of age for 734 infants born to HIV-infected women who had in utero exposure to ZDV has not demonstrated any tumor development. However, no data are available on longer follow-up for late effects.

† These effects seen at only maternally toxic doses.

2. Recommendations

All women should be counseled on the risks and benefits of antiretroviral therapy for the mother and for the newborn infant.

HIV Infected Women Without Prior Antiretroviral Therapy

- The three-part AZT regimen to prevent perinatal transmission should be followed.

- If the woman satisfies criteria for therapy (CD4 <500/mm^3 or HIV RNA level >10,000-20,000 c/mL) recommendations of DHHS should be followed, usually with an AZT-containing regimen.

- Women in the first trimester may wish to delay initiating therapy until after the first trimester due to concern for possible teratogenic effects of these drugs during the most vulnerable part of pregnancy. This is an unknown risk and must be weighed against the possible consequences of delayed suppression of viral load.

- AZT and d4T should not be taken concurrently. Women who receive d4T in place of AZT should receive only the intrapartum and newborn components of AZT prophylaxis.

HIV Infected Women Receiving Antiretroviral Therapy

1. If the regimen does not include AZT, this drug should be added or substituted, but should not be added to a regimen that includes d4T (see above).

2. If therapy is to be suspended during the first trimester, all drugs should be discontinued simultaneously and reintroduced simultaneously.

3. Intrapartum and newborn AZT is recommended regardless of the antiretroviral regimen.

HIV Infected Women in Labor Without Prior Therapy

1. Single dose nevirapine (200 mg po) at onset of labor and a single dose of nevirapine (2 mg/kg po) to the infant at 48-72 hours;

2. Oral AZT/3TC during labor and then one week of therapy with AZT/3TC for the infant;

3. AZT IV during delivery and po to the infant (076 protocol); or

4. Nevirapine/AZT IV followed by the 6 wk AZT regimen for the newborn.

Infant Born to Women who Received no Treatment During Pregnancy or Intrapartum

1. Treat the infant with the 6 week course of AZT + an additional antiretroviral agent.

2. Postpartum evaluation of the woman for standard therapy.

IV. Antiretroviral Therapy

3. Antiretroviral Pregnancy Registry

Care providers with HIV-infected pregnant women should report cases of prenatal exposure to the Antiretroviral Pregnancy Registry. This registry collects observational data, patients are anonymous and the Registry obtains birth outcome data. The Registry is contacted at:

> Antiretroviral Pregnancy Registry
> 115 N. Third St., Suite 306
> Wilmington, NC 28401
> TEL: (800) 258-4263 or (910) 251-9087
> FAX: (800) 800-1052

4. Caesarean section:

Elective caesarean section reduces perinatal transmission in all studies that address this issue. Mandelbrot retrospectively reviewed data for C-section in women receiving prophylactic AZT (JAMA 1998;28:55). Occurrence of perinatal transmission was as follows: elective C-section – 0.8%, emergent C-section – 11.4%, vaginal delivery – 6.6%. Kind reported transmission of 17% with AZT alone compared to 0% in women given AZT + C-section (AIDS 1998;12:235). In a meta-analysis of 15 studies with 8,533 mother-infant pairs, occurrence of perinatal transmission was as follows: no AZT or C-section – 19%, C-section and no AZT – 10%, AZT (076 protocol) and no C-section – 7%, and AZT (076 protocol) + C-section – 2% (NEJM 1999;340:977). The authors concluded that C-section reduced the rate of HIV transmission by about 50%. The European Mode of Delivery Collaboration has completed a multicenter prospective study in which pregnant HIV-infected women were randomly assigned to elective C-section or vaginal delivery (Lancet 1999;353:1035). There was a significant reduction in perinatal transmission with elective C-section: Among 170 infants in this group, three (1.8%) had HIV infection versus 21 of 200 (10.5%) in the vaginal delivery group. The authors reported few postpartum complications or serious adverse events in either group.

The problem with all of these studies is that none examined the impact of viral load or HAART therapy on rates of perinatal transmission. Studies cited above show that the risk of transmission with a viral load <1000 c/mL is very low but not zero. Several reports indicate that C-sections are associated with an increase in complications in women with HIV infection, a risk that is inversely related to the CD4 count (JAMA 1999;281:1946; Lancet 1999;354:1612).

ACOG Committee Opinion

"Scheduled Cesarean Delivery and the Prevention of Vertical Transmission of HIV Infection" [ACOG Committee Opinion #219, August 1999]: The American College of Obstetrics and Gynecologists (ACOG) has issued an official statement regarding the issue of elective C-section to reduce vertical transmission of HIV infection.

- HIV-infected women should be offered elective caesarean section.

- Data are inadequate to demonstrate benefit in caesarean section in women with viral loads <1,000 c/mL.

- No reduction of transmission is noted if caesarean delivery is performed after onset of labor or rupture of membranes.

- Patients should be informed that AZT therapy reduces the risk of HIV transmission from 25% to 5-8%, and the addition of elective caesarean section further reduces the risk to 2%.

- The patient should have autonomy in making this decision.

- HIV-infected women should receive antiviral therapy according to guidelines of DHHS and guided by findings from the ACTG 076 protocol. Women should receive intravenous AZT beginning three hours before C-section.

- Prophylactic antibiotics should be considered during C-section due to increased morbidity in HIV-infected women.

- C-section is recommended at 38 weeks of gestation (which is earlier than the 39 weeks recommended for other populations).

- Amniocentesis to determine fetal lung maturity should be avoided when possible.

- Current recommendations for monitoring viral load and CD4 cell count should be followed during pregnancy.

5. Developing countries

The three phase 076 protocol is not considered implementable and is too expensive for developing countries, which account for >95% of perinatal transmissions. This has led to searches for alternative regimens to reduce perinatal transmission:

IV. Antiretroviral Therapy

Table 4-9: Prevention of Perinatal Transmission

Trial	Citation	Regimen	Transmission	Efficacy
076	NEJM 1994;331:1173	Pregnancy: AZT 500 mg/d starting wk 14-34 Labor: AZT IV Infant: AZT x 6 wks Breast feeding: not allowed	AZT – 8% Placebo – 26%	68%
Thai	Lancet 1999;353:773	Pregnancy: AZT 300 mg bid starting wk 36 Labor: AZT 300 mg q3h Infant: none Breast feeding: not allowed	AZT – 9% Placebo – 19%	51%
Ivory Coast	Lancet 1999;353:781	As above, except breast feeding allowed	AZT – 16% Placebo – 25%	37%
PERTA	1999; 6th Conf. on Retroviruses and Opportunistic Infections, Abstract S-7	Group 1 – Pregnancy: AZT/3TC 36 wks – 1 wk postpartum + infant: AZT/3TC 1 wk Group 2 – AZT/3TC during labor: 1 wk postpartum + infant: AZT/3TC 1 wk Group 3 – AZT/3TC in labor Group 4 – placebo/placebo	Gr 1 – 9% Gr 2 – 11% Gr 3 – 18% Gr 4 – 17%	42% 37% –
DITRAME	Lancet 1999;353:786	Pregnancy: AZT 300 mg bid starting wk 36-38 Labor: 600 mg Infant: none Postpartum: AZT 300 mg bid x 1 wk Breast feeding: allowed	AZT – 18% Placebo – 28%	38%
HIVNET 012	Lancet 1999;354:795	Group 1 – Nevirapine Labor: NVP 200 mg po Infant: NVP 2 mg/kg within 72 hrs Group 2 – AZT Labor: AZT 600 mg then 300 mg q 3 h until delivery Infant: AZT 4 mg/kg/d x 7 days	NVP – 13.1% AZT – 21.5%	

It is estimated that 1,600 infants with HIV infection are born daily; over 90% are born in developing countries. The studies summarized above show that AZT is beneficial even with brief courses given orally at a cost of about $50 (Thai course). Efficacy is reduced with breast feeding, and this is not improved with postpartum AZT, although the timing of this treatment may have been suboptimal (Lancet 1999;353:786). When treatment is restricted to the intrapartum and post-partum period, a single 200 mg intrapartum oral dose of nevirapine and a single dose of nevirapine given within 72 hours to the infant is significantly superior to AZT given in an analogous fashion (Lancet 1999;354:795). The nevirapine regimen is $4, making it the least expensive effective regimen. The challenges are to test pregnant women, make antenatal care accessible, give prophylaxis in a fashion that is logistically feasible using a regimen that is affordable, and deal effectively with the complexities of breast feeding (Lancet 1999;353:766).

C. POST-EXPOSURE PROPHYLAXIS FOR HEALTH CARE WORKERS (MMWR 1998;47:1-14)

1. Risk for Transmission

A total of 23 studies of needle sticks among health care workers demonstrate HIV transmission in 20 of 6,135 (0.33%) exposed to an HIV-infected source (Ann Intern Med 1990;113:740). With mucosal surface exposure, there was one transmission in 1,143 exposures (0.09%), and there were no transmissions in 2,712 skin exposures. As of December 1997, there were a total of 54 health care workers in the U.S. who had occupationally-acquired HIV infection as indicated by seroconversion in the context of an exposure to an HIV-infected source. There are an additional 132 health care workers who had possible occupationally-acquired HIV; these latter health care workers did not have documented seroconversion in the context of an exposure. Of the 54 confirmed cases: 1) the major occupations were nurses (22), laboratory technicians (19), and physicians (6); 2) all transmissions involved blood or bloody body fluid except for three involving laboratory workers exposed to HIV viral cultures; 3) exposures were percutaneous in 46, mucocutaneous in five and both in two; and 4) to date there are no confirmed seroconversions in surgeons and no seroconversions with exposures to a suture needle.

A retrospective case control study of needle stick injuries from an HIV-infected source by the CDC included 33 cases who seroconverted and 739 controls (MMWR 1996;45:468; NEJM 1997;337:1485). Results showed that risks for seroconversion included: 1) deep injury; 2) visible blood on the device; 3) needle placement in a vein or artery; and 4) a source with late stage HIV infection (presumably reflecting high viral load). There was also evidence that AZT prophylaxis was associated with a 79% reduction in transmission rates. On the basis of this experience, revised preliminary guidelines recommending more aggressive antiretroviral therapy were published in June 1996 (MMWR 1996;45:468) and updated in 1997 (Am J Med 1997;102:117).

2. **Management** (Public Health Service Statement on the Management of Occupational Exposures to HIV and Recommendations for Postexposure Prophylaxis [MMWR, 47:RR-7].)

- **Post-exposure prophylaxis hotline:** (888) 448-4911 (24 hours/day)

- **Immediate treatment:** Skin should be washed with soap and water; mucous membranes should be flushed with water.

- **Assessment:** Source should be evaluated for HIV, HBV, and HCV, the major bloodborne pathogens. Exposure considered potential sources of HIV are blood, bloody body fluids, semen, vaginal secretions, cerebrospinal, pleural, peritoneal, pericardial, synovial and amniotic fluid, tissue or viral cultures.

- **PHS recommendations for Post-Exposure Prophylaxis (PEP)**

    Step 1: Determine the exposure code (see figure 4-1, p. 67)

    Step 2: Determine the HIV status code (see figure 4-2, p. 68)

    Step 3: PEP recommendations based on exposure category (EC) and HIV RNA level in the source. (Table 4-10, p. 69)

Figure 4-1

STEP 1: Determine the Exposure Code (EC)

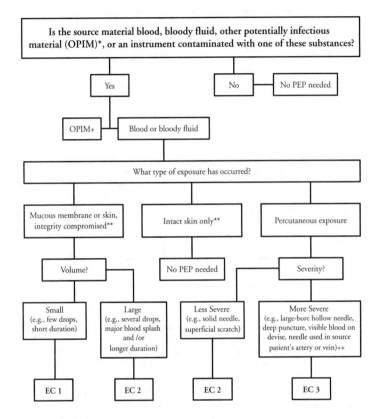

* OPIM = Semen; vaginal secretions; cerebrospinal, synovial, pleural, peritoneal, pericardial and amniotic fluids; tissue.

+ Exposures to OPIM must be evaluated on a case-by-case basis. In general, these body substances are considered a low risk for transmission in health care settings. Any unprotected contact to concentrated HIV in a research laboratory or production facility is considered an occupational exposure that requires clinical evaluation to determine the need for PEP.

** Skin integrity is considered compromised if there is evidence of chapped skin, dermatitis, abrasion or open wound.

Contact with intact skin is not normally considered a risk for HIV transmission. However, if the exposure was to blood, and the circumstance suggests a high volume exposure (e.g., an extensive area of skin was exposed or there was prolonged contact with blood), the risk of HIV transmission should be considered.

++ The combination of these severity factors (e.g., large-bore hollow needle and deep puncture) contribute to an elevated risk for transmission if the source is HIV positive.

Figure 4-2

STEP 2: Determine the HIV Status Code (HIV SC)

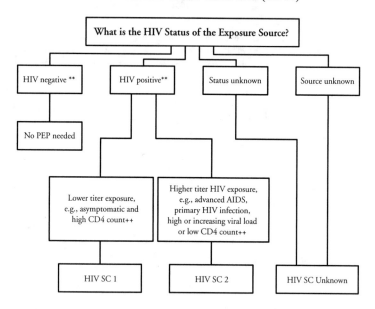

** A source is considered to be negative for HIV infection if there is laboratory documentation of a negative HIV antibody, HIV PCR or HIV p24 antigen test result from a specimen collected at or near the time of exposure and there is no clinical evidence of an acute or recent retroviral-like illness. A source is considered to be infected with HIV (HIV Positive) if there has been a positive laboratory result for HIV antibody, HIV PCR or HIV p24 or physician-diagnosed AIDS.

++ Examples are used as surrogates to estimate the HIV titer in an exposure source for purposes of considering PEP regimens and do not reflect all clinical situations that may be observed. Although a high HIV titer (status code 2) in an exposure source has been associated with an increased risk of transmission, the possibility of transmission from a source with a low HIV titer also must be considered.

Table 4-10: Step 3: PEP Recommendations Based on Exposure Category and HIV RNA Level in the Source

Exposure Category (EC)	HIV RNA (source)	PEP Recommendation*
1	1 (low)	PEP may not be warranted. Exposure risk of drug toxicity may outweigh risk of HIV transmission.
1	2 (high)	Consider AZT/3TC. Exposure poses negligible risk
2	1 (low)	Recommend AZT/3TC. Most exposures are in this category, but no increased risk of transmission has been observed.
2	2	Recommend AZT/3TC + indinavir or nelfinavir. Increased risk of transmission has been
3	1 or 2	observed.

* Recommended treatment is 4 weeks with AZT (200 mg tid or 300 mg bid) + 3TC (150 mg bid) + Indinavir (800 mg po tid 1 hr before meal and 2 hrs after meal, or with low fat snack plus >1.5 L fluids/day) or AZT + 3TC (above doses) + nelfinavir (750 mg po tid with meal or snack)

Table 4-11: Management of PEP

Drug	Testing	Side Effects	Comment
AZT	CBC at baseline, 2 and 4 weeks	Nausea, vomiting, headache, fatigue, insomnia, anemia, and neutropenia (rare). All side effects are reversible.	Intolerance is common; marrow suppression is rare. For GI intolerance: Take with meals or multiple small doses (100 mg po q 4h while awake). For severe intolerance, substitute d4T (40 mg po bid)
3TC	None	GI intolerance	Usually well tolerated
Indinavir	LFTs, urinalysis, renal function, glucose at baseline, 2 and 4 weeks	Renal calculi or nephrotoxicity, GI intolerance, hepatitis, glucose intolerance/diabetes	Must ingest >1.5 L/day fluids Must take q 8h on empty stomach or with small low fat snack
Nelfinavir	LTFs, glucose at baseline, 2 and 4 weeks	Diarrhea, glucose intolerance/diabetes	Most frequent side effect is diarrhea that usually responds to imodium. Must take bid or tid with meal

IV. Antiretroviral Therapy

Step 4: Monitoring (added by the author)

Testing source: If there is no prior positive or negative serology, a rapid test is preferred, since results should be available in ≤10 minutes. Standard serologic tests may take 3-7 days, but a negative EIA screening assay is usually available in 24-48 hours and is adequate for the decision to discontinue PEP. Some states permit testing the source of an HCW exposure without informed consent; about half require informed consent. If the source has had an illness compatible with acute HIV syndrome, testing should include plasma HIV RNA levels.

Testing healthcare worker: HIV serology should be performed at the time of injury, and repeated at 6 wks., 3 months and 6 months; testing at one year is optional. There have been 3 healthcare workers who seroconverted at >6 months post exposure. This represents about 4% of confirmed seroconversions in healthcare workers (Am J Med 1997;102:117). Most health care workers who seroconverted had symptomatic acute HIV syndrome, usually 2-6 weeks post exposure.

Caution: The healthcare worker should be advised to practice safe sex or abstain until serology is negative at six months post-exposure.

Time: PEP should be initiated as quickly as possible, preferably within 1-2 hours of exposure. The median time from exposure to treatment in 432 HCW with HIV exposure from 10/96 to 8/98 was 1.8 hours (ICAAC 9/98, Abstract I-161).

Side effects: For healthcare workers who receive PEP, about 74% experience side effects primarily nausea (58%), fatigue (37%), headache (16%), vomiting (16%), or diarrhea (14%). About 53% discontinue treatment before completion of the 4 week course due to multiple factors including side effects of drugs (ICAAC 9/98, Abstract I-161).

Management of Common Side Effects

Drug	ADR	Solution
AZT	GI intolerance	Take with food Take 3-5x/day Antiemetic Switch to d4T
	Asthenia	Symptomatic treatment
	Headache	Symptomatic treatment
	Insomnia	Switch to d4T
	Marrow suppression	Monitor CBC (Marrow suppression rare in PEP)
IDV	GI intolerance	Take with low fat snack Switch to NFV
	Nephrolithiasis	Increase fluid intake or Switch to NFV
NFV	Diarrhea	Fiber supplements, then imodium

Pregnancy: There is evidence of carcinogenicity ascribed to AZT using 12-15x the standard dose in rodents. The relevance of this experience to patients is unknown. An NIH panel judged that these findings are of uncertain significance, and AZT should be given to HIV infected pregnant women due to the known benefit for reducing perinatal transmission. The risk:benefit ratio in pregnant healthcare workers with occupational exposure may be quite different. Counseling healthcare workers with childbearing capacity should include a discussion of this risk as well as a discussion about the limited data regarding safety of any antiretroviral agents during the first trimester and the limited studies of protease inhibitors in pregnant women. CDC guidelines state that pregnancy should not preclude PEP (MMWR 1998;47:1).

Breast feeding: Consider temporary discontinuation of breastfeeding antiretroviral therapy

Confidentiality: This is considered critical

Agent selection: AZT is advocated because it has been used extensively and has established merit for preventing transmission. Safety in this setting appears well established, and efficacy appears to be about 80%. AZT use in pregnancy suggests efficacy even when the implicated source strain shows genotypic resistance to AZT, although efficacy is reduced. Other agents in the standard PEP regimen are suggested based on enhanced antiretroviral potency and toxicity profile. NNRTIs are generally avoided due to the potential for toxicity with a one month exposure: nevirapine causes high rates of rash and occasional cases of Stevens-Johnson Syndrome; efavirenz causes CNS toxicity and possible teratogenic effects in pregnancy. Protease inhibitors are generally considered to be of equal potency, the preference for indinavir and nelfinavir was based on availability and experience at the time the CDC recommendations were written. Anticipated or proven resistance in the source strain may pose a dilemma in terms of drug selection. Many authorities advocate that regimens be selected on the basis of drug history and response in the source; i.e. a high viral load in the face of AZT/3TC/indinavir therapy suggests resistance to these drugs, necessitating an alternative regimen comparable to one that would be chosen as a salvage treatment in the host. There is also increasing enthusiasm for nevirapine due to the favorable results in preventing perinatal transmission, its rapid activity, and its long half-life. Some speculate that a single dose would be as effective as the currently recommended three drug regimen. This has not been tested, and a regimen that includes AZT for one month is generally preferred.

Resistance testing: Some advocate testing resistance of the source strain to facilitate drug selection in the exposed HCW. The obvious problem is the time required for test results and the importance of rapid institution of prophylaxis. Most authorities recommend that decisions be based on the drug history and viral load of the source. In a review of 52 patients who were the source of occupational exposures, 39% had major mutations conferring resistance (7th CROI, Abstract 469).

IV. Antiretroviral Therapy

Post exposure registry:
The Registry is closed effective June 30, 1999 (MMWR 1999;48:194).

3. **PEP: experience in the U.S.:** (Summarized by L. A. Wang et al., ICAAC, 9/98, I-161)

Period reviewed: 10/96-8/98

Number injuries reviewed: 432

Type of exposure: percutaneous 85%
                   mucocutaneous 10%

Fluid: Blood – 71%
       Bloody fluid – 13%
       HIV culture – 2.3%

Time to initiate PEP antiviral: 1.8 hrs (median)

Treatment: 3 drugs – 59%, 2 drugs – 36%, 4 drugs – 4%

Side effects: Any – 74, nausea – 58%, fatigue – 37%, headache – 13%, vomiting – 16%, diarrhea – 14%

Number who completed 4 week course: 47%

4. **Healthcare worker to patient transmission:** This became a topical issue in 1990 with the case of Dr. Acer, a Florida dentist, who was identified as the source of HIV infection for six dental patients (Ann Intern Med 1992;116:798; Ann Intern Med 1994;121:886). The source of the virus was established by genetic sequencing (J Virol 1998;72:4537), but the mechanism of transmission was never established. This disclosure led to a series of "look backs," in which serologic tests were performed on over 22,000 patients who received care from 59 health providers with known HIV infection. No transmissions were identified (Ann Intern Med 1995;122:653). Since this time there has been one additional case, an orthopedic surgeon in France who may have transmitted HIV infection to a patient during a total hip replacement in 1992 (Ann Intern Med 1999;130:1).

Management: The incident with the Florida dentist raised great concern about this issue and led to a recommendation for review of practices by HIV-infected providers who "performed invasive procedures in a blind body cavity." It was felt that performing surgery in anatomical sites that could not be visualized would be most likely to result in injuries, with the potential for patient exposure to provider blood. The standard based on these recommendations was to review such practices on a case-by-case basis. The probable outcome was that HIV infected physicians would be forced to abandon surgical careers or be required to explain risks to potential surgical patients.

A recent review by Julie Gerberding of the CDC did not mention these recommendations regarding management of HIV-infected healthcare workers (Ann Intern Med 1999;130:64), but did emphasize the following:

Patients who have exposures analogous to what would be defined as a potentially high-risk occupational exposure in a health-care worker should be managed by standard guidelines with respect to counseling, serologic testing, and antiretroviral therapy. This means that a patient exposed to blood from an HIV infected surgeon, such as an accidental needle injury resulting in contamination of the surgical field with the surgeon's blood, needs counseling regarding the exposure and the option of antiretroviral treatment. One issue that is often overlooked is that anonymity is an ethical and legal requirement for the HCWs dealing with HIV-infected patients, but there are no such restrictions on the patient who is notified about a HCW with HIV. Disclosure of a surgeon's serologic status may end his/her career.

D. POST EXPOSURE PROPHYLAXIS FOR SEXUAL CONTACT OR NEEDLE SHARING

1. CDC Recommendations (MMWR 1998;47[RR-17])

a. Conclusion: The Public Health Service is unable to recommend for or against prophylaxis after non-occupational exposure due to the lack of data.

b. If prophylaxis is attempted, the health care provider must:

- inform the patient about the lack of data

- make judicious use of antiretroviral agents (no specific regimen is recommended)

- address patients' needs for risk reduction

- restrict use of post-exposure prophylaxis to high risk exposures: unprotected receptive and or vaginal intercourse with a known HIV-infected source.

c. Miscellaneous issues

- Cost: $800 (estimate for 28 day course of antiretroviral agents)

- Current practice guidelines: British Columbia Centre for Excellence in HIV/AIDS published "A Guideline for Accidental Exposure to HIV" which recommends antiretroviral agents for rape victims. The Center provides a "starter kit" with a 5 days supply of AZT and 3TC to emergency rooms.

- Registry: The CDC has established a new Nonoccupational HIV Postexposure Prophylaxis Registry that includes 6 forms and 17 pages. All information can be provided by telephone (877) 448-1737, on the website (HYPERLINK http://www.hivpepregistry.org www.hivpepregistry.org), or by hardcopy (Nonoccupational HIV PEP Registry, John Snow Inc., 44 Farnsworth St., Boston, MA 02210-1211; fax (877) 448-7737.) The provider incentive is a $10 gift certificate to a national chain.

Table 4-12: Risk of HIV Transmission with Single Exposure From an HIV-infected Source

Exposure	Probability/10,000 exposures*
Needle sharing	67
Percutaneous (occupational exposure)	30
Receptive anal intercourse	10-30
Receptive vaginal intercourse	8-20
Insertive vaginal sex	3-9
Insertive anal sex	3

* (Am J Med 1999;106:324; Ann Intern Med 1996;125:497; Jaids 1992;5:1116; NEJM 1997;336:1072)

2. **Recommendations of M. Katz and J. Gerberding, San Francisco Dept. Public Health and UCSF (Ann Intern Med 1998;128:306 and Am J Med 1999;106:323)**

   a. **Recommendations for post exposure prophylaxis:**

   - Risk is high: unprotected receptive anal intercourse, unprotected receptive vaginal intercourse; unprotected insertive vaginal intercourse; unprotected insertive anal intercourse or unprotected receptive fellatio with ejaculation *and*

   - Patient's partner is known to have HIV infection or to be in a high risk category (gay male, injection drug use, sex worker, etc.) *and*

   - Exposure is an isolated event and patient has made a commitment to safer sex in the future *and*

   - The exposure occurred ≤72 hours of presentation for care

   b. **Treatment regimens x 4 weeks**

   Standard: AZT (200 mg tid or 300 mg bid) plus 3TC (150 mg bid)

   Alternative: d4T (40 mg bid) plus ddI (200 mg bid)

   Protease inhibitor: Consider adding nelfinavir (750 mg tid or 1250 mg bid with meals) or indinavir (800 mg tid on empty stomach) if source has viral load >50,000 c/mL, advanced HIV disease, or has been treated with one or both NRTIs

   c. **Testing of exposed patient:** (Pregnancy test if appropriate) HIV, HCV, HBV, gonorrhea, syphilis, *Chlamydia trachomatis*; baseline tests for post-exposure prophylaxis—CBC, liver function tests, renal function tests.

d. Cost: Estimated at $500 for the two NRTI regimen and $1,100-$1,200 for the PI containing regimen. Medical care and laboratory testing add about $500 for a total of $1,000-$1,700.

e. Preliminary experience reported at ICAAC 9/98 by J. N. Martin (Abstract I-160):

Number treated: 202

Type of exposure: Sexual exposure – 91%, needlesharing – 0.5%

Treatment: AZT/3TC – 82%, d4T/ddI – 11%, PI containing regimen – 3%

Number who discontinued regimen prior to 4 weeks – 8%

II. ANTIRETROVIRAL AGENTS

Table 4-13: Antiretroviral Drugs Approved by FDA for HIV

Generic Name (abbreviation)	Brand Name	Firm	FDA Approval Date
zidovudine, AZT	Retrovir	Glaxo Wellcome	March 87
didanosine, ddI	Videx	Bristol Myers-Squibb	October 91
zalcitabine, ddC	Hivid	Hoffman-La Roche	June 92
stavudine, d4T	Zerit	Bristol Myers-Squibb	June 94
lamivudine, 3TC	Epivir	Glaxo Wellcome	November 95
saquinavir, SQV, hgc	Invirase	Hoffman-La Roche	December 95
ritonavir, RTV	Norvir	Abbott Laboratories	March 96
indinavir, IDV	Crixivan	Merck & Co., Inc.	March 96
nevirapine, NVP	Viramune	Boehringer Ingelheim	June 96
nelfinavir, NFV	Viracept	Agouron Pharmaceuticals	March 97
delavirdine, DLV	Rescriptor	Pharmacia & Upjohn	April 97
zidovudine and lamivudine	Combivir	Glaxo Wellcome	September 97
saquinavir, SQV, sgc	Fortovase	Hoffman-La Roche	November 97
efavirenz, EFV	Sustiva	DuPont Pharmaceuticals	September 98
abacavir, ABC	Ziagen	Glaxo Wellcome	February 99
amprenavir, APV	Agenerase	Glaxo Wellcome	April 99

IV. Antiretroviral Therapy

Table 4-14: Nucleoside Analogs

Generic Name	Zidovudine (AZT, ZDV)	Didanosine (ddI)	Zalcitabine (ddC)	Stavudine (d4T)	Lamivudine (3TC)	Abacavir (ABC)
Trade Name	Retrovir	Videx	Hivid	Zerit	Epivir	Ziagen
How Supplied	100 and 300 mg tabs IV vials –10 mg/mL 300 mg + 3TC 150 mg as Combivir 10 mg/mL oral soln	25, 50, 100 and 150 mg tabs; 100, 167 and 250 mg powder packets 200 mg tabs for once daily dosing. Pediatric powder with 4 gm/8 oz.	0.375 & 0.75 mg tabs	15, 20, 30, and 40 mg caps 1 mg/mL oral soln	150 mg tabs 150 mg with AZT 300 mg as Combivir 10 mg/mL oral soln	300 mg tabs
Dosing Recommendations	300 mg bid or 200 mg tid (or with 3TC as Combivir 1 tab bid)	Tablets or oral solution† >60kg: 400 mg qd or 200 mg bid (tabs) or 250 mg bid (powder) <60kg: 250 mg qd or 125 mg bid (tabs) or 167 mg bid (powder)	0.75 mg tid	>60kg: 40 mg bid <60kg: 30 mg bid	150 mg bid or with AZT as Combivir (1 tab bid) <50kg: 2 mg/kg bid	300 mg bid
Oral bio-availability	60%	30%-40%	85%	86%	86%	83%
Food effect	None	Levels ↓ 55% Take 1/2 hr before or 1 hr after meal	None	None	None	None Alcohol ↑ ABC levels 41%
Serum half-life	1.1 hour	1.6 hours	1.2 hour	1.0 hour	3-6 hours	1.5 hours
Intracellular half-life	3 hours	25-40 hours	3 hours	3.5 hour	12 hours	3.3 hours
CNS penetration (% serum levels)	60%	20%	20%	30-40%	10%	Good

Table 4-14: Nucleoside Analogs (Continued)

Generic Name	Zidovudine (AZT, ZDV)	Didanosine (ddI)	Zalcitabine (ddC)	Stavudine (d4T)	Lamivudine (3TC)	Abacavir (ABC)
Trade Name	Retrovir	Videx	Hivid	Zerit	Epivir	Ziagen
Elimination	• Metabolized to AZT Glucuronide (GAZT) • Renal excretion of GAZT	Renal excretion – 50%	Renal excretion – 70%	Renal excretion – 50%	Renal excretion unchanged	• Metabolized • Renal excretion of metabolites – 82%
Major toxicity Class toxicity***	• Bone marrow suppression: Anemia and/or neutropenia • Subjective complaints: GI intolerance, headache, insomnia asthenia	• Pancreatitis • Peripheral neuropathy • GI intolerance nausea, diarrhea	• Peripheral neuropathy • Stomatitis	Peripheral neuropathy	(Minimal toxicity)	Hypersensitivity (2-5%), with fever, nausea, vomiting, anorexia, cough, dyspnea, malaise, morbilliform rash. May be life-threatening with rechallenge
Drug Interactions	Ribavirin may reduce AZT activity	Methadone ↓ ddI levels 41%, consider ddI dose increase	Methadone ↓ d4T levels 27%. No dose adjustment.	None	None	None
Mutations conferring resistance (codon)	41*, 67, 69*, 70*, 151*, 210, 215*, 219, 333	65, 69*, 74*, 75, 151*, 184	69*, 74, 151*, 184	41, 50, 69*, 70, 75, 151*	69*, 184***, 333	65*, 69*, 74, 115*, 151*, 184*

† For adults, ddI pediatric oral solution can be mixed by the pharmacist with liquid antacids. See package insert for instructions

* Mutations considered most clinically significant. The RT 151 codon mutation and the 69 insertion mutation confer class resistance to nucleoside analogues; adefovir retains activity with the 151 mutation.

** RT codon 184 mutation confers high level resistance to 3TC, but increases activity of AZT and adefovir.

*** Lactic acidosis with hepatic steatosis is a rare, but potentially life-threatening toxicity with all NRTIs (see Table 4-20 on pg 106).

IV. Antiretroviral Therapy

B. NON-NUCLEOSIDE REVERSE TRANSCRIPTASE INHIBITORS (NNRTI)

Table 4-15: Non-Nucleoside Reverse Transcriptase Inhibitors (NNRTIs)

Generic Name	Nevirapine	Delavirdine	Efavirenz
Trade Name	Viramune	Rescriptor	Sustiva
Form	200 mg tabs	100 mg and 200 mg tabs	50, 100, 200 mg caps
Dosing Recommendations	200 mg po qd x 14 days, then 200 mg po bid	400 mg po tid	600 mg po qd at hs
Oral bioavailability	>90%	85%	42%
Food Effect	No effect	No effect	Increased 50% with high fat meal; avoid after high fat meal
Serum half-life	25-30 hours	5.8 hours	40-55 hours
Elimination	Metabolized by cytochrome P450 (3A inducer); 80% excreted in urine (glucuronidated metabolites, <5% unchanged), 10% in feces	Metabolized by cytochrome P450 (3A inducer); 51% excreted in urine (<5% unchanged), 44% in feces	Metabolized by cytochrome P450 enzymes (3A mixed inhibitor/inducer); 14-34% excreted in urine, 16–61% in feces
Drug interactions (See Tables 4-17, 4-18 and 4-19)	• Induces cytochrome P450 enzymes • PI interactions: See Table 4-16 • Methadone AUC decreased 60%-titrate methadone dose • Not recommended: Ketoconazole and rifampin • Caution: Anticonvulsants	• Inhibits cytochrome P450 enzymes • Contraindicated drugs: terfenadine, astemizole, simvastatin, lovastatin, ergot derivatives, triazolam, midazolam, cisapride, rifabutin, rifampin, H2 blockers, proton pump inhibitors • Delavirdine increases levels of clarithromycin, dapsone, quinidine, warfarin, anticonvulsants, sildenafil • Antacids and didanosine: separate administration by >1 hr • PI interactions: See Table 4-16	• Inhibits and induces cytochrome P450 3A4 enzymes • Contraindicated drugs: astemizole, midazolam, triazolam, cisapride, ergot alkaloids, terfenadine • Possibly important drug interactions: rifampin, rifabutin, clarithromycin, phenobarbital, ethinyl estradiol, anticonvulsants, warfarin • PI interactions: See Table 4-16 • Methadone AUC decreased 60% – titrate methadone dose

Generic Name	Nevirapine	Delavirdine	Efavirenz
Trade Name	Viramune	Rescriptor	Sustiva
Major toxicity	Rash (15-30%) may require hospitalization; rare cases of Stevens-Johnson syndrome; hepatitis	Rash; headaches Increased transaminase levels	Dizziness, "disconnectedness," somnolence, insomnia, bad dreams, confusion, amnesia, agitation, hallucinations, poor concentration – 40%, usually resolves after 2 weeks; take hs. Rash - severe in 5%; rare reports of Stevens-Johnson syndrome; Teratogenic in cynomalgus monkeys (See Table 4-8). Avoid in pregnancy and women should use adequate contraception methods. False positive drug screening test for cannabinoids (marijuana)
Class Toxicity**			

* Rash; severe rash in about 5%; cases of Stevens-Johnson syndrome reported (See Table 4-20 on pg 90)

IV. Antiretroviral Therapy

C. PROTEASE INHIBITORS

Table 4-16: Protease Inhibitors

Generic Name	Indinavir	Ritonavir	Saquinavir		Nelfinavir	Amprenavir
Trade Name	Crixivan	Norvir	Invirase	Fortovase	Viracept	Agenerase
Supplier	Merck	Abbott	Hoffman-LaRoche	Hoffman-LaRoche	Agouron	Glaxo Wellcome
Form	200, 333, 400 mg caps	100 mg caps 600 mg/7.5 mL po – solution	200 mg caps (Hard gel caps)	200 mg caps (Soft gel caps)	250 mg tablets 50 mg/g oral powder	50, 150 mg caps 15 mg/mL
Usual Dose	800 mg q 8h Separate ddI dose by 1 hr	600 mg bid* Separate ddI dose by 2 hr	800 mg tid (not recommended) 400 mg bid with RTV	1200 mg tid	1250 mg bid 750 mg tid or	1200 mg bid
Food effect	Levels decreased 77%; take 1 hr before or 2 hours after meals; may take with low fat snack or skim milk	Levels increased 15%; take with food if possible to improve tolerability	No food effect when taken with RTV	Levels increase 6x; take with large meal unless taken with RTV	Levels increase 2–3x; take with meal or snack	High fat meal decreases AUC 20%; can be taken with or without food, but high fat meal should be avoided.
Bioavailability	65% (on empty stomach)	Not determined	4%	Not determined	20-80%	89%, based on clinical studies.
Storage	Room temperature	Soft gel cap and liquid formulation – room temperature	Room temperature	Room temperature or refrigerate	Room temperature	Room temperature
Serum half-life	1.5-2 hours	3-5 hours	1-2 hours	1-2 hours	3.5-5 hours	7-10 hours
CNS penetration	Moderate	Poor	Poor	Poor	Moderate	Moderate

Generic Name	Indinavir	Ritonavir	Saquinavir		Nelfinavir	Amprenavir
Trade Name	Crixivan	Norvir	Invirase	Fortovase	Viracept	Agenerase
Elimination	Biliary metabolism P450 cytochrome 3A4 inhibitor	Biliary metabolism P450 cytochrome 3A4>2D6; most potent 3A4 inhibitor	Biliary metabolism P450 cytochrome 3A4 inhibitor	Biliary metabolism P450 cytochrome 3A4 inhibitor	Biliary metabolism P450 cytochrome 3A4 inhibitor	Biliary metabolism P450 cytochrome 3A4 inhibitor (similar to indinavir and nelfinavir)
Side Effects	GI intolerance (10-15%); nephrolithiasis or nephrotoxicity (10-15%); headache; asthenia; dizziness; rash; metallic taste; ITP.; alopecia; lab: increase indirect bilirubinemia (inconsequential) Class side effects**	GI intolerance (20-40%); paresthesias-circumoral and extremities (10%); taste perversion (10%); lab; triglycerides increase in 60% and transaminase increase in 10-15%, CPK and uric acid increase Class side effects**	GI intolerance (10-20%); headache; transaminase increase Class side effects**	GI intolerance (20-30%); headache; transaminase increase hypoglycemia; Class side effects**	Diarrhea (10-30%) Class side effects**	GI intolerance (10-30%); rash (20-25% – usually at 1-10 wks) Stevens-Johnson syndrome (1%); paresthesias (10-30% – perioral or peripheral) Increase in liver function tests. Class side effects**
Drug interactions (See Tables 4-17, 4-18 and 4-19)	• Inhibition of P450 enzymes (less than ritonavir) • Contraindicated drugs: rifampin, terfenadine, astemizole, cisapride, triazolam, midazolam, ergot alkaloids, simvastatin, lovastatin, St. John's wort	• Potent inhibition of CYP$_3$A$_4$ enzymes • Ritonavir reduces levels of warfarin, anticonvulsants, divaproex, lamotrigine, atovaquone, methadone 37% (titrate dose), ethinyl estradiol 40% (use alternative contraception), theophylline 47% (monitor levels).	• Inhibits CYP$_3$A$_4$ enzymes • Saquinavir levels increased by: RTV 5x (standard dose), ketoconazole 3x (standard dose) grapefruit juice, NFV 3-5x, DLV 5x, clarithromycin 45% • Saquinavir levels reduced by: rifampin 84%, rifabutin 40%, phenobarbital, phenytoin, dexamethasone and carbamazepine, NVP 25%, EFV 62%		• Inhibition of CYP$_3$A$_4$ • Nelfinavir levels reduced by rifampin 81% and rifabutin 32%, possibly by anticonvulsants • Contraindicated drugs: rifampin, triazolam, midazolam, ergot alkaloids, astemizole, terfenadine, cisapride, simvastatin, lovastatin	• Inhibition of CYP$_3$A$_4$ • Contraindicated drugs: astemizole, beoridil, cisapride, ergot alkaloids, midazolam, triazolam, rifampin, simvastatin, lovastatin

IV. Antiretroviral Therapy

Table 4-16: Protease Inhibitors (Continued)

Generic Name	Indinavir	Ritonavir	Saquinavir		Nelfinavir	Amprenavir
Trade Name	Crixivan	Norvir	Invirase	Fortovase	Viracept	Agenerase
Drug interactions (continued)	• Indinavir levels increased by ketoconazole, DLV, NFV, RTV • Indinavir levels reduced by rifampin 89%, rifabutin 32%, (IDV 1000 mg tid; RFB 150 mg/d) NVP 28%, EFV 31%, possibly anticonvulsants (monitor levels) and grapefruit juice • Didanosine reduces indinavir absorption unless taken ≥1 hr apart • Indinavir increases levels of clarithromycin 53% (no dose change), estradiol 24% (no dose change)	• Didanosine reduces ritonavir absorption take ≥2 hours apart • Ritonavir increases ketoconazole levels 3x (reduce dose), rifabutin 4x (RFB dose 150 mg qod), clarithromycin 71% (standard dose) desipramine 145%, ethinyl estradiol 40% (use alternative contraceptive) sildenafil 2-11x (≤25 mg/48 hr) • Ritonavir levels increased by DLV 70%, EFV 18%	• Contraindicated drugs: terfenadine, astemizole, cisapride, ergot alkaloids, rifampin, rifabutin, simvastatin, lovastatin, midazolam, triazolam • Saquinavir increases levels of clarithromycin 45% (standard dose), nelfinavir 20%, sildenafil (3.1x)		• Nelfinavir decreases levels of ethinyl estradiol 47% (use alternative methods), DLV 50% • Nelfinavir increases levels of rifabutin 2x (150 mg qd), SQV 3-5x and IDV 50%, sildenafil 2-11x (≤25 mg/48 hrs)	• Amprenavir levels increased by abacavir 30-50%, ketoconazole 31%, clarithromycin 18%, IDV 33%, ketaconazole 31% • Amprenavir levels decreased by rifampin 82%, rifabutin 15%, saquinavir 32% • Amprenavir increases levels of rifabutin 193%, ketoconazole 44%, sildenafil 2-11x (≥25 mg/48 hrs) • Potentially important drug interactions: anticonvulsants, statins, methadone, oral contraceptives, tricyclic antidepressants, oral anticoagulants, amiodarone, quinidine

Generic Name	Indinavir	Ritonavir	Saquinavir		Nelfinavir	Amprenavir
Trade Name	Crixivan	Norvir	Invirase	Fortovase	Viracept	Agenerase
Codon mutations associated with resistance; bold indicates most significant	10, 20, 24, 32, 36, **46**, 48, 54, 63, 71, 73, **82**, 84, 90	10, 20, 32, 33, 36, 46, 54, 63, 71, **82**, 84	10, 36, 20, 24, 30, 36, 46, **48**, 54, 63, 71, 73, 82, 84, **90**		**30**, 36, 46, 63, 71, 77, **88**, 90	10, 36, 46, 47, **50**, 54, 63, 71, 82, 84, **90**

* Dose escalation for ritonavir: day 1-2: 300 mg bid; day 3-5: 400 mg bid; day 6-13: 500 mg bid; day 14: 600 mg bid. Combination treatment regimen with saquinavir (400 mg as Invirase or Fortovase po bid) plus ritonavir (400 mg po bid)

** Class adverse reactions: See Table 4-20

IV. Antiretroviral Therapy

Table 4-17: Drugs that Should not be Used with Protease Inhibitors or NNRTIs*

Drug Category**	Indinavir	Ritonavir	Saquinavir	Nelfinavir	Delavirdine	Elfavirenz	Amprenavir
Analgesics	(none)	meperidine, piroxicam, propoxyphene	(none)	(none)	(none)	(none)	(none)
Cardiac	(none)	amioderone, encainide, flecainide, propafenone, quinidine, bepridil	(none)	(none)	(none)	(none)	bepridil
Lipid lowering agents	simvastatin, lovastatin	simvastatin, lovastatin	simvastatin, lovastatin	simvastatin, lovastatin	simvastatin, lovastatin	(none)	simvastatin, lovastatin
Anti-Mycobacterial	rifampin	rifampin (?)	rifampin, rifabutin	rifampin	rifampin, rifabutin	(none)	rifampin
Ca++ channel blocker	(none)	bepridil	(none)	(none)	(none)	(none)	bepridil
Antihistamine	astemizole, terfenadine	astemizole, terfenadine	astemizole, terfenadine	astemizole, terfenadine	astemizole, terfenadine	astemizole, terfenadine	astemizole terfenadine
GI	cisapride	cisapride	cisapride	cisapride	cisapride, H$_2$ blockers	cisapride	cisapride
Antidepressant	(none)	bupropion	(none)	(none)	(none)	(none)	(none)
Neuroleptic	(none)	clozapine, pimozide	(none)	(none)	(none)	(none)	(none)
Psychotropic	midazolam, triazolam	midazolam, triazolam	midazolam, triazolam	midazolam, triazolam	midazolam, triazolam	midazolam, triazolam	midazolam, triazolam
Ergot Alkaloid (vasoconstrictor)	dihydroergotamine, ergotamine (various forms)	dihydroergotamine, ergotamine (various forms)	dihydroergotamine, ergotamine (various forms)	dihydroergotamine, ergotamine (various forms)	dihydroergotamine, ergotamine (various forms)	dihydroergotamine, ergotamine (various forms)	dihydroergotamine, ergotamine (various forms)

** Alternatives: Analgesics – ASA, oxycodone, acetaminophen; Rifabutin (MAC) – clarithromycin, ethambutol, azithromycin; Antihistamine – loratadine, fexofenadine, cetirizine Antidepressant – fluoxetine, desipramine; Psychotropic – temazepam, forazepam; Lipid-lowering – atorvastatin, pravastatin, fluvastatin, cervastatin

Table 4-18: Drug Interactions Requiring Dose Modifications or Cautious Use

Drugs Affected	Indinavir (IDV)	Ritonavir (RTV)	Saquinavir* (SQV)
ANTIFUNGALS Ketoconazole	Levels: IDV ↑ 68% Dose: IDV 600 mg tid	Levels: keto. ↑ 3x Dose: use with caution	Levels: SQV ↑ 3x Dose: Standard
ANTI-MYCOBACTERIALS Rifampin	Levels: IDV ↓ 89% Contraindicated	Levels: RTV ↓ 35% May increase hepato-toxicity	Levels: SQV ↓ 84% Contraindicated
Rifabutin	Levels: IDV ↓ 32% Rifabutin ↑ 2x Dose: ↓ rifabutin to 150 mg qd IDV 1000 mg tid	Levels: Rifabutin ↑ 4x Dose: ↓ rifabutin to 150 mg qod or dose 3x/wk	Levels: SQV ↓ 40% Not recommended
Clarithromycin	Levels: Clari. ↑ 53% No dose adjustment	Levels: Clari. ↑ 77% Dose adjust for renal insufficiency	Levels: Clari. ↑ 45% SQV ↑ 177% No dose adjustment
ORAL CONTRACEPTIVES	Levels: Norethindrone ↑ 26% ethinylestradiol ↑ 24% No dose adjustment	Levels: ethinyl estradiol 40% Use alternative method	No data
ANTICONVULSANTS Phenobarbitol Phenytoin Carbamazepine	Unknown but may decrease IDV levels substantially	Unknown Use with caution	Unknown but may decrease SQV levels substantially
METHADONE	No data	Methadone ↓ 37%, May require dose increase	No data
MISCELLANEOUS	Grapefruit juice ↓ IDV levels by 26% Sildenafil: potential for increased concentrations and side effects. Do not exceed 25 mg/48 hr.	Desipramine ↑ 145%, Reduce dose Theophylline ↓ 47%, monitor theo. levels Many possible interactions (see product insert) Sildenafil: potential for increased concentrations and side effects. Do not exceed 25 mg/48 hr.	Grapefruit juice increases SQV levels Dexamethasone decreases SQV levels Sildenafil: potential for increased concentrations and side effects. Do not exceed 25 mg/48 hr.

* Some drug interaction studies were conducted with INVIRASE. May not necessarily apply to use with FORTOVASE.

IV. Antiretroviral Therapy

Table 4-18: Drug Interactions Requiring Dose Modifications or Cautious Use (Continued)

Drugs Affected	Nelfinavir (NFV)	Amprenavir (APV)	Nevirapine (NVP)
ANTIFUNGALS Ketoconazole	No dose adjustment necessary	Levels: keto. ↑ 44% APV ↑ 31%; combination under investigation	Levels: Keto. ↓ 63% Dose: Not recommended
ANTI-MYCOBACTERIALS Rifampin	Levels: NFV ↓ 82% Contraindicated	Levels: APV ↓ 82% Contraindicated	Levels: NVP ↓ 37% Not recommended
Rifabutin	Levels: NFV ↓ 32% Rifabutin ↑ 2x Dose: ↓ rifabutin to 150 mg qd NFV to 1000 mg tid	Levels: APV ↓ 15% Rifab ↑ 193% Dose: ↓ rifabutin to 150 mg qod, APV Dose: standard	Levels: NVP ↓ 16% No data for rifabutin
Clarithromycin	No data	Levels: APV ↑ 18% Clari. no change Dose: usual	Levels: NVP ↑ 16% Clari. ↓ 30% Dose: usual
ORAL CONTRACEPTIVES	Levels: Norethindrone ↓ 18%, ethinylestradiol ↓ 47% Use alternative method	Not studied Use alternative method	No data
ANTICONVULSANTS Phenobarbitol Phenytoin Carbamazepine	Unknown but may decrease NFV levels substantially	Unknown but may decrease APV levels substantially Monitor anticonvulsant level	Unknown Monitor anticonvulsant level
METHADONE	No data	No data	NFV unchanged Methadone ↓ 60% Titrate methadone dose
MISCELLANEOUS	Sildenafil: potential for increased concentrations and side effects. Do not exceed 25 mg/48 hr.	Abacavir: APV ↑ 30% Sildenafil: potential for increased concentrations and side effects. Do not exceed 25 mg/48 hr.	

Table 4-18: Drug Interactions Requiring Dose Modifications or Cautious Use (Continued)

Drugs Affected	Delavirdine (DLV)	Efavirenz (EFV)
ANTIFUNGALS Ketoconazole	Not studied	Not studied
ANTI-MYCOBACTERIALS Rifampin	Levels: DLV ↓ 96% Contraindicated	Levels: EFV ↓ 25% Dose adjustment unclear—
Rifabutin	Levels: DLV ↓ 80% Rifabutin ↑ 100% Not recommended	EFV unchanged Rifabutin ↓ 35% Dose ↑ rifabutin to 450 mg/d
Clarithromycin	Levels: clari. ↑ 100% DLV ↑ 44% Dose adjust for renal failure	Levels: clari. ↓ 39% Alternative recommended
ORAL CONTRACEPTIVES	No data	Levels: Ethinyl estradiol ↑ 37%
ANTICONVULSANTS Phenobarbitol Phenytoin Carbamazepine	Unknown but may decrease DLV levels substantially Monitor anticonvulsant levels	Unknown Use with caution Monitor anticonvulsant levels
METHADONE	No data	Methadone levels decreased – tritrate methadone dose
MISCELLANEOUS	May increase levels of dapsone, warfarin and quinidine Sildenafil: potential for increased levels and side effects. Do not exceed 25 mg/48 h	Monitor warfarin when used concomittantly

IV. Antiretroviral Therapy

Table 4-19: Drug Interactions: Protease Inhibitors and Non-nucleoside Reverse Transcriptase Inhibitors Effect of Drug on Levels (AUCs)/Dose

Drug Affected	Ritonavir	Saquinavir	Nelfinavir	Amprenavir	Nevirapine	Delavirdine	Efavirenz
Indinavir (IDV)	Levels: IDV ↑ 2-5x Dose: IDV 400 mg bid + RTV 400 mg bid, or IDV 800 mg bid + RTV 100-200 mg bid	Levels: IDV no effect SQV ↑ 4-7x** Dose: Insufficient data	Levels: IDV ↑ 50% NFV ↑ 80% Dose: Limited data for IDV 1200 mg bid + NFV 1250 mg bid	Levels: IDV ↓ 38% APV ↑ 53% Dose: IDV 800 mg tid, APV 800 mg tid	Levels: IDV ↓ 28% NVP no effect Dose: IDV 1000 mg q 8h	Levels: IDV ↑ 40% DLV: no effect Dose: IDV 600 mg q 8h; DLV: standard	Levels: IDV ↓ 31% Dose: IDV 1000 mg q 8h EFV 600 mg hs
Ritonavir (RTV)	—	Levels: RTV no effect SQV ↑ 20x*·** Dose: Invirase or Fortovase 400 mg bid + RTV 400 mg bid	Levels: RTV no effect NFV ↑ 1.5x Dose: Limited data for RTV 400 mg bid + NFV 500-750 mg bid	Levels: APV ↑ 2.5x Dose: APV 600 mg bid + RTV 100 mg bid or APV 1200 mg qd + RTV 200 mg qd (limited data)	Levels: RTV ↓ 11% NVP no effect Dose: Standard	Levels: RTV ↑ 70% DLV No effect Dose: No data	Levels: RTV ↑ 18% EFV ↑ 21% Dose: RTV 600 mg bid (500 mg bid for intolerance)
Saquinavir (SQV)		—	Levels: SQV 3-5x NFV ↑ 20%** Dose: Standard NFV Fortovase 800 mg tid or 1200 bid	Levels: APV ↓ 32% SQV** ↓ 19% Dose: SQV 800 mg tid, APV 800 mg tid	Levels: SQV ↓ 25% NVP no effect Dose: No data	Levels: SQV ↑ 5x** DLV no effect Dose: Fortovase 800 mg tid, DLV standard (monitor transaminase levels)	Levels: SQV ↓ 62% EFV ↑ 12% Co-administration not recommended
Nelfinavir (NFV)			—	Levels: NFV ↑ 15% APV ↑ 1.5x Dose: NFV 750 mg tid, APV 800 mg tid	Levels: NFV ↑ 10% NVP no effect Dose: Standard	Levels: NFV ↑ 2x DLV ↓ 50% Dose: No data (monitor for neutropenic complications)	Levels: NFV ↑ 20% Dose: Standard

Drug Affected	Ritonavir	Saquinavir	Nelfinavir	Amprenavir	Nevirapine	Delavirdine	Efavirenz
Amprenavir (APV)				—	No Data	No Data	APV ↓ 36% Dose: APV 1200 mg tid as single PI or APV 1200 mg bid + RTV 200 mg bid + EFV 600 mg qd

*Conducted with Invirase   **Conducted with Fortovase

IV. Antiretroviral Therapy

Table 4-20: Class Adverse Drug Reactions to Antiretroviral Agents
(DHHS Guidelines Supplement 11/98 with additions by author)

Several class-related adverse events have been recognized with antiretroviral drugs during the post-marketing period. For nucleoside analog reverse transcriptase inhibitors (NRTIs), lactic acidosis with hepatomegaly and hepatic steatosis has been reported. For protease inhibitors reports of hyperglycemia/diabetes mellitus, increased bleeding episodes in patients with hemophilia, and fat redistribution with and without serum lipid abnormalities have been received. Because these events were identified based on spontaneous reports and other uncontrolled data, the actual incidence of these events and the causal association with these drugs have not been definitively established. Controlled and/or population-based epidemiologic studies evaluating these potential class adverse events are warranted.

NUCLEOSIDE ANALOGS

Lactic Acidosis/Hepatic Steatosis

The occurrence of lactic acidosis and severe hepatomegaly with steatosis during use of nucleoside analog reverse transcriptase inhibitors (NRTIs) appears to occur at a low frequency, but with a high case fatality risk. (Lancet 1994;343:1494). One retrospective database analysis showed an incidence of 1.3 per 1000 patient-years among patients who received NRTIs. The incidence may be as high as 5-10% with more aggressive diagnostic evaluations using serum lactate levels (39th ICAAC, San Francisco, 9/99, Abstract 1285; 7th CROI Abst S21, 42, 55, 56, 57). Patients typically present with fatigue, nausea, vomiting, abdominal pain, weight loss, dyspnea, and/or a low serum bicarbonate. Evaluation shows lactic acidosis with elevated CPK, ALT, and/or LDH, and abdominal CT scans or liver biopsy often shows steatotosis. The initial clinical manifestations of lactic acidosis are variable and may include nonspecific gastrointestinal symptoms without dramatic elevation of hepatic enzymes, and in some cases dyspnea. Fatalities have been reported despite intensive supportive treatment; in other cases the adverse event has resolved after discontinuation of NRTIs. Treatment should be suspended if clinical or laboratory manifestations suggestive of lactic acidosis or otherwise unexplained pronounced hepatotoxicity occur. All NRTIs have been implicated, although some studies suggest higher rates with d4T or ddI/hydroxyurea. It is quite possible that other clinical expressions of mitochondrial toxicity include myopathy, cardiomyopathy, neuropathy, pancreatitis, asthenia, and/or lipoatrophy (7th CROI, Abstract 521). The most important therapeutic intervention is NRTI withdrawal; the safety of substituting alternative drugs in this class is not known. One report suggests response to 50 mg riboflavin (Lancet 1998;252:292).

NON-NUCLEOSIDE REVERSE TRANSCRIPTASE INHIBITORS

Rash

Rash is a relatively common toxicity encountered during use of NNRTIs. A significant minority (occurring in up to approximately 5% of patients receiving NNRTIs) of these rashes are severe, and potentially fatal cases of Stevens-Johnson syndrome have been reported.

PROTEASE INHIBITORS

Fat redistribution, hyperlipidemia, and insulin resistance have been associated with protease inhibitor use with variable frequency. These changes may occur together or as isolated observations. The etiologic role of PIs is not considered established by some and the long term consequences are generally unclear. Recommendations for monitoring and intervention are also unclear at the present time.

Hyperglycemia

Hyperglycemia, new onset diabetes mellitus, diabetic ketoacidosis, and exacerbation of existing diabetes mellitus in patients receiving protease inhibitors have been reported (Lancet 1997;350:317; Ann Intern Med 1997;127:947; Ann Intern Med 1997;127:948). Among these reports, symptom onset occurred a median of 63 days (range 2-390 days) following initiation of protease inhibitor therapy. Hyperglycemia resolved in some patients who discontinued protease inhibitor therapy; however, the reversibility of these events is currently unknown due to limited data. Some patients continued protease inhibitor therapy and initiated treatment with oral hypoglycemic agents or insulin. Clinicians are advised to monitor HIV-infected patients with pre-existing diabetes closely when protease inhibitors are prescribed, and to be aware of the risk for drug-related new-onset diabetes in patients without a history of diabetes (*BIII*). Patients should be advised about the warning signs of hyperglycemia (i.e. polydipsia, polyphagia, and polyuria) when these medications are prescribed. Some authorities recommend routine fasting blood glucose measurements at 3–4 month intervals during treatment (*CIII*). Routine use of glucose tolerance tests to detect this complication is not recommended (*DIII*). There are no data to aid in the decision to continue or discontinue drug therapy in cases of new-onset or worsening diabetes; however, most experts would recommend continuation of highly active antiretroviral therapy in the absence of severe, life-threatening diabetes (*BIII*).

Fat Redistribution

Changes in body fat distribution, sometimes referred to as "lipodystrophy syndrome," "fat redistribution syndrome," or "pseudo-Cushing's syndrome" have been observed in patients taking protease inhibitors. Clinical findings include central obesity and peripheral fat wasting. The changes may include visceral fat accumulation, dorsocervical fat accumulation ("buffalo hump"), extremity wasting with venous prominence, facial thinning, breast enlargement, and lipomatosis (Lancet 1998;351:871; Lancet 1998;351:867; Lancet 1997;350:1596; Lancet 1998;352:1881; JAIDS 1999;21:107). Some patients may have a cushingoid appearance despite the absence of measurable abnormalities in adrenal function. It is unclear whether the various clinical manifestations represent distinct entities with different etiologies, or whether they occur as a result of a single pathologic process. Similar findings have also been reported in HIV-infected patients not receiving protease inhibitors (Lancet 1998;351:867); however, the number of reports has increased concomitant with the widespread use of protease inhibitor-containing antiretroviral regimens. There are sparse data on management recommendations, although dose reduction of PIs is not recommended.

IV. Antiretroviral Therapy

Discontinuation of PI therapy has been successful in the resolution of symptoms in some cases.

Hyperlipidemia

Changes in triglycerides and/or cholesterol have occurred with or without the clinical findings of fat redistribution. In clinical studies, all PIs have been implicated, but ritonavir has been shown to produce substantial increases in triglycerides and cholesterol most frequently. Although the long-term consequences of fat redistribution are unknown, substantial increases in triglycerides or cholesterol are of concern because of the possible association with cardiovascular events and pancreatitis. In this regard, case reports have appeared describing premature coronary artery disease, cerebrovascular disease, and cholelithiasis in patients receiving PI therapy. Some authorities recommend monitoring of serum levels of cholesterol and triglycerides at 3–4 month intervals during PI therapy (*CIII*). Assessment should include evaluation for independent risks for cardiovascular disease (i.e. family history, medical history, smoking, diet, weight, etc.) and the magnitude of lipid changes. Intervention is often recommended for triglyceride levels >750–1,000 mg/dL and or LDL cholesterol levels >130 mg/dL (in individuals without known coronary disease and with 2 or more coronary risk factors) or >160 mg/dL (in individuals without known coronary disease and with fewer than 2 coronary risk factors). The effectiveness of dietary modification and lipid lowering drugs such as gemfibrozil and niacin is not clear. Some patients have had resolution of serum lipid abnormalities with discontinuation of PIs; however, this decision requires a risk-benefit analysis.

Table 4-21: National Cholesterol Education Program Indications for Dietary Therapy or Hyperlipidemia

	Threshold for diet therapy		Threshold for drug therapy	
	Cholesterol	LDL	Cholesterol	LDL
0-1 Risks*	>240**	<160	>275	<190
>2 Risks*	>200	<130	>240	<160
Cardiovascular disease	>160	<100	>200	<130

* Risks: Age (men >45 yrs, women post-menopausal); hypertension, smoking, diabetes mellitus, hx of cardiovascular disease in first degree relatives (<55 yrs for men and <65 yrs for women), or serum HD cholesterol <35 mg/dL.

** mg/dL

Increased Bleeding Episodes in Patients with Hemophilia

Increased spontaneous bleeding episodes in patients with hemophilia A and B have been observed with the use of protease inhibitors. Most of the reported episodes involved joints and soft tissues; however, more serious bleeding episodes including intracranial and gastrointestinal bleeding have been reported. the bleeding episodes occurred a median of 22 days after initiation of protease inhibitor therapy. Some patients received additional coagulation factor while continuing protease inhibitor therapy.

Avascular necrosis

Avascular necrosis is another possible late complication of HAART. Reported rates are 0.3 to 1.3% (39th ICAAC, San Francisco, 9/99, Abstracts 1131 and 1312). The most common site is the femoral head; many patients have other risk factors including alcohol abuse, hyperlipidemia, corticosteroid use and hypercoaguability.

IV. Antiretroviral Therapy

Table 4-22: HIV-Related Drugs with Overlapping Toxicities

Bone Marrow Suppression	Peripheral Neuropathy	Pancreatitis	Nephrotoxicity	Hepatotoxicity	Rash	Diarrhea	Ocular Effects
cidofovir	didanosine	cotrimoxazole	adefovir	delavirdine	abacavir	didanosine	ethambutol
cytotoxic chemotherapy	isoniazid	didanosine	aminoglycosides	efavirenz	cotrimoxazole	clindamycin	rifabutin
dapsone	stavudine	lamivudine (children)	amphotericin B	fluconazole	dapsone	nelfinavir	cidofovir
fluctosine	zalcitabine	pentamidine	cidofovir	isoniazid	NNRTIs	ritonavir	
ganciclovir		ritonavir	foscarnet	ketoconazole	protease inhibitors		
hydroxyurea			indinavir	nevirapine			
interferon-α			pentamidine	NRTIs			
pentamidine			ritonavir	protease inhibitors			
pyrimethamine				rifabutin			
ribavirin				rifampin			
sulfadiazine							
TMP-SMX (high dose)							
trimetrexate							
zidovudine							

Table 4-23: Dosing of Antiretroviral Agents in Renal and Hepatic Failure

Drug Name	Usual Adult Dose	Dosing for GFR >50 mL/min	Dosing for GFR 10–50 mL/min	Dosing for GFR <10 mL/min	Dosing in Hemodialysis	Dosing in Peritoneal dialysis	Hepatic Failure
Zidovudine (Retrovir; AZT)	300 mg bid	300 mg bid	300 mg bid	300 mg qd	300 mg qd*	300 mg qd	200 mg bid
Didanosine (Videx; ddI)	Wt >60 kg dose: 400 mg qd or 200 mg bid. Wt <60 kg dose: 250 mg qd or 125 mg bid	Usual dose	50% of usual dose	25% of usual dose	25% of usual dose* qd*	25% of usual dose	Consider empiric dose reduction
Stavudine (Zerit; d4T)	Wt >60 kg dose: 40 mg bid Wt <60 kg dose: 30 mg bid	Usual dose	Wt >60 kg dose: 20 mg q12-24h. Wt <60 kg dose: 15 mg q12-24	Wt >60 kg dose: 20 mg q24h. Wt <60 kg dose: 15 mg q24	25% of usual dose*	25% of usual dose*	Usual dose (no data)
Zalcitabine (Hivid; ddC)	0.75 mg tid	0.75 mg tid	0.75 mg bid	0.75 mg qd	0.75 mg qd* **	0.75 mg qd* **	Usual dose
Lamivudine (Epivir; 3TC)	150 mg bid	150 mg bid	150 mg qd	50 mg qd	25-50 mg qd* **	50 mg qd* **	Usual dose (no data)
Abacavir (Ziagen)	300 mg bid	Usual dose	Usual dose likely**	Usual dose likely**	Usual dose likely**	Usual dose likely**	Usual dose (no data)
Efavirenz (Sustiva)	600 mg qd	Usual dose**	Usual dose likely**	Usual dose likely**	600 mg qd**	No data	Consider empiric dose reduction
Nevirapine (Viramune)	200 mg qd x 14 days then 200 mg bid	Usual doses**	Usual doses likely**	Usual doses likely**	Usual dose likely**	Unlikely to be removed in dialysis due to high protein binding**	Consider empiric dose reduction

Table 4-23: Dosing of Antiretroviral Agents in Renal and Hepatic Failure (Continued)

Drug Name	Usual Adult Dose	Dosing for GFR >50 mL/min	Dosing for GFR 10–50 mL/min	Dosing for GFR <10 mL/min	Dosing in Hemodialysis	Dosing in Peritoneal dialysis	Hepatic Failure
Delavirdine (Rescriptor)	400 mg tid	Usual dose**	Usual dose likely**	Usual dose likely**	Usual dose likely**	Unlikely to be removed in dialysis due to high protein binding**	Consider empiric dose reduction
Nelfinavir (Viracept)	750 mg tid or 1250 mg bid	Usual dose likely**	Usual dose likely**	Usual dose likely**	Usual dose likely**	No data: Usual dose likely**	Consider empiric dose reduction
Indinavir (Crixivan)	800 mg tid	Usual dose likely**	Usual dose likely**	Usual dose likely**	Usual dose likely**	No data: Usual dose likely**	600 mg q 8h
Ritonavir (Norvir)	600 mg bid	Usual dose likely**	Usual dose likely**	Usual dose likely**	Usual dose likely**	No data: Usual dose likely**	Consider empiric dose reduction
Saquinavir (Invirase, Fortovase)	Invirase 400 mg bid Fortovase 1200 mg tid, 1600 mg qd or 400 mg bid	Usual dose likely**	Usual dose likely**	Usual dose likely**	Usual dose likely**	No data: Usual dose likely**	Consider empiric dose reduction
Amprenavir (Agenerase)	1200 mg bid	Usual dose likely**	Usual dose likely**	Usual dose likely**	Usual dose likely**	Usual dose likely**	Impairment moderate – 450 mg bid; severe – 300 mg bid

* Administer daily dose after dialysis.

** There are limited or no data on dosing in renal failure; the major mechanism of elimination of these drugs is hepatic metabolism and this accounts for the recommendation of standard doses

Table 4-24: Characteristics of Antiretrovirals During Dialysis

	Volume of Distribution (L/kg)	Protein Binding (%)	Size (Molecular Weight) (Dalton)	Prediction based on drug characteristics
Zidovudine (Retrovir, AZT)	1.6 L/kg	34-38%	267 Dalton	Unlikely to be dialysed out
Didanosine (Videx, ddI)	0.8-1 L/kg	<5%	236 Dalton	Possibly dialysed
Stavudine (Zerit, d4T)	0.5-1 L/kg	<5%	224 Dalton	Likely to be dialysed out
Zalcitabine (Hivid, ddC)	0.54-0.64 L/kg	<4%	211 Dalton	Likely to be dialysed out
Lamivudine (Epivir, 3TC)	0.9-1.7 L/kg	<36%	229 Dalton	Unlikely to be dialysed out
Abacavir (Ziagen)	0.86 L/kg	50%	671 Dalton	Unlikely to be dialysed out
Efavirenz (Sustiva)	2-4 L/kg (in animal studies	99.5-99.75%	315 Dalton	Unlikely to be dialysed out
Nevirapine (Viramune)	1.4 L/kg	50-60%	266 Dalton	Unlikely to be dialysed out
Delavirdine (Rescriptor)	No data	98-99%	552 Dalton	Unlikely to be dialysed out
Nelfinavir (Viracept)	2-7 L/kg	99%	663 Dalton	Unlikely to be dialysed out
Indinavir (Crixivan)	No data	60% (variable)	712 Dalton	Low probability of small amount being dialysed
Ritonavir (Norvir)	0.41 L/kg	98-99%	721 Dalton	Low probability of small amount being dialysed
Saquinavir (Invirsase, Fortovase)	10 L/kg	98%	767 Dalton	Unlikely to be dialysed out

Vd>Protein Binding>Size

Likely to be removed
 Vd <0.7 L/kg
 Protein Binding <80%
 Size <1,500 Dalton

Unlikely to be removed
 Vd >0.7 L/kg
 Protein Binding >80%
 Size >1,500 Dalton

IV. Antiretroviral Therapy

V. MANAGEMENT OF OPPORTUNISTIC INFECTIONS IN PATIENTS WITH HIV INFECTION

	Preferred regimen(s)	Alternative regimen(s)	Comment
FUNGAL INFECTION			
Pneumocystis carinii Acute infection	• Trimethoprim 15 mg/kg/day + sulfamethoxazole 75 mg/kg/day po or IV x 21 days in 3-4 divided doses (typical oral dosage is 2 DS tid)	• Trimethoprim 15 mg/kg/day po + dapsone 100 mg po/day x 21 days • Pentamidine 4 mg/kg/day IV x 21 days (usually reserved for severe cases) • Clindamycin 600 mg IV q8h or 300-450 mg po q6h + primaquine* 30 mg base po/day x 21 days • Atovaquone 750 mg suspension po with meal bid x 21 days • Trimetrexate 45 mg/m² IV/day plus folinic acid 20 mg/m² po or IV q6h	• Some recommend trimethoprim-sulfamethoxazole/dapsone in dose of 20 mg/kg/day (trimethoprim). • In a comparative trial (ACTG 108) TMP-SMX, trimethoprim-dapsone and clindamycin-primaquine were equally effective in patients with mild-moderate PCP (Ann Intern Med 1996;124:792). • Resistance of *P. carinii* to sulfonamides by mutations on the dihydropteroate synthase gene have been noted and appear to correlate with both sulfanamide exposure and clinical failure (Lancet 1999;354:1347; JID 1999;180:1169). • Intolerance to TMP-SMX is noted in 25-50%, primarily skin rash ± fever (Lancet 1991;338:431). • Patients with moderately severe or severe disease (PO₂<70 mm Hg or A-a gradient >35 mm Hg) should receive corticosteroids (prednisone 40 mg po bid x 5 days, then 40 mg qd x 5 days, then 20 mg/day to completion of treatment). Side effects include CNS toxicity, thrush, cryptococcosis, *H. simplex* infection, tuberculosis, and other OIs (JAIDS 1995;8:345).

	Preferred regimen(s)	Alternative regimen(s)	Comment
Pneumocystis carinii (_continued_) Prophylaxis (JAIDS 1993;6:46) Initiation and discontinuation	• Trimethoprim/sulfa-methoxazole po (1 DS/day, 1 SS/day)	• Dapsone 100 mg po qd • Aerosolized pentamidine 300 mg q month via Respirgard II nebulizer ± ß₂ agonist (albuterol, 2 whiffs) • Dapsone 50 mg/day po plus pyrimethamine 50 mg/wk po plus leukovorin 25 mg/wk po or dapsone 200 mg plus pyrimethamine 75 mg plus leucovorin 25 mg po q week • Atovaquone 1500 mg qd • Trimethoprim-sulfamethoxazole, 1 DS 3x/wk. • **Other regimens** without established efficacy: Dapsone 50 mg/day po, pentamidine 4 mg/kg IM or IV q 4 wks, Fansidar 1-2 x/wk.	• **Indications:** History of _Pneumocystis_ pneumonia, CD4 count <200-250/mm³ (or <14%), thrush, or unexplained fever >2 weeks. • **Discontinuation:** Primary prophylaxis may be discontinued in patients with HAART when the CD4 count is >200/mm³ x >3-6 mo (NEJM 1998;339:1889; Lancet 1999;353:201; Lancet 1999;353:1293). Patients with prior PCP may also discontinue prophylaxis when immune reconstitution takes place (7th CROI, Abstract LB5). • TMP-SMX is superior in efficacy for PCP prophylaxis compared to aerosolized pentamidine and also prevents toxoplasmosis and bacterial infections (NEJM 1995;332:693; NEJM 1992;327:1842; JID 2000;181:158). • Adverse drug reactions requiring drug discontinuation are noted in 20-40% receiving TMP-SMX, 20-40% receiving dapsone, and 2-5% given aerosolized pentamidine. • Patients who have mild or moderate reactions to TMP-SMX may be rechallenged or desensitized. • Regimen of 1DS 3x/wk is inferior to 1 DS/day (CID 1999;29:775). • Regimens that provide prophylaxis for PCP and toxoplasmosis are the TMP-SMX, dapsone/pyrimethamine and atovaquone (Ann Intern Med 1997;122:755).

			• A CPCRA/ACTG trial showed that atovaquone was equivalent to dapsone for PCP prophylaxis (NEJM 1998;339:1889)
Aspergillosis Invasive pulmonary infection	• Amphotericin B 0.7-1.4 mg/kg/day • Lipid formulation of amphotericin: Amphotec, Abelset or AmBisome	• Itraconazole 200 mg po tid x 3 days, then 400 mg/d • Surgery for localized disease	• Prognosis is poor without immune reconstitution (CID 1992;14:141). • Endobronchial lesions respond well to itraconazole (Chest 1993;105:1314). • Promising new agents: voriconazole, SCH 56592, and pradimicins. • Predisposing factors: Corticosteroids: decrease or stop if possible; neutropenia: G-CSF and avoid 5-FC; marijuana.
Candida Oropharyngeal (Thrush) Initial infection	• Clotrimazole oral troches 10 mg 5x/day • Nystatin 500,000 units gargled 5x/day	• Fluconazole 100 mg po qd • Amphotericin B oral suspension 1-5 mL qid swish & swallow • Amphotericin B 0.3-0.5 mg/kg/day IV • Itraconazole 200 mg/day (tabs) or 100 mg/day oral suspension	• Treat until symptoms resolve (usually 10-14 days). • Fluconazole 100 mg/d and itraconazole 200 mg/d are comparable to ketoconazole 400 mg/d in efficacy and show reduced side effects (Rev Inf Dis 1990;12:S364). • Amphotericin B (oral or IV) and itraconazole are usually reserved for patients who fail with other oral regimens; most common with chronic azole administration and azole-resistant Candida species. • Itraconazole in liquid formula at half dose appears to be as effective as fluconazole for treatment and prophylaxis (Am J Med 1998;104:33).

V. Opportunistic Infections

	Preferred regimen(s)	Alternative regimen(s)	Comment
Candida (continued)			• *In vitro* resistance is most common with prior azole exposure, late stage HIV infection and non-albicans species. • Some report high rates of response (48/50) to fluconazole despite *in vitro* resistance (JID 1996;174:821). Doses up to 800 mg/day may be tried. Alternatives are oral amphotericin and itraconazole 200 mg bid.
Maintenance (optional or as needed: see Comments)	• Clotrimazole (above dose); Nystatin (above dose) • Fluconazole 100 mg po/day or 200 mg 3x/wk	• Itraconazole 200 mg (tabs)/day or 100 mg oral suspension qd • Ketoconazole 200 mg/day po	• Advantage of fluconazole for maintenance treatment is prevention of deep fungal infection: cryptococcosis, and Candida esophagitis with CD4 count <100/mm³ (NEJM 1995;332:700) and reduction of frequent relapses. • Concerns with continuous treatment with fluconazole are azole-resistance by Candida species, drug interactions and cost. Risks for azole-resistant Candida infections are prolonged azole exposure and low CD4 count (JID 1996;173:219). • Fluconazole is superior to clotrimazole in preventing relapses of thrush. • Most patients will relapse within 3 mos post therapy if treatment is discontinued in absence of immune reconstitution. Options are treatment of each episode or maintenance.

			Comments
Prophylaxis	• Not recommended		• Efficacy of fluconazole (200 mg/d) is established for AIDS patients with CD4 counts <100/mm³; this is not generally advocated because the study showed no survival benefit, treatment of cryptococcosis is generally effective, the cost is high, and there is concern for azole-resistant Candida infections (NEJM 1995;332:700). Weekly fluconazole (400 mg) is less effective and offers no advantage (CID 1998;27:1369).
Vaginitis	• Intravaginal miconazole suppository 200 mg x 3 days or cream (2%) x 7 days • Clotrimazole cream (1%) x 7-14 days or tabs: 100 mg qd x 7 days or 100 mg x 2/d x 3 days or 500 mg x 1 • Fluconazole 150 mg po x 1	• Ketoconazole 200 mg/d po or bid x 5-7 days or 200 mg po bid x 3 days	• May require continuous treatment to prevent relapse: Ketoconazole 100 mg/d po, fluconazole 50-100 mg/d po or fluconazole 200 mg/wk po. • Clotrimazole and miconazole (both cream and 100 mg tabs) are available over the counter. • Weekly fluconazole (200 mg) appears to be effective without risk of azole resistance in women with CD4 count >300/mm³ • Treatment is identical with and without HIV infection (MMWR 1998;47: [RR-1]:78).
Esophagitis: Initial infection	• Fluconazole 200 mg/d po; up to 400 mg/day x 2-3 wks	• Ketoconazole 200 mg/day po • Itraconazole 200 mg/day po (tabs) or 100 mg/day oral solution	• Fluconazole is clinically superior to ketoconazole as initial treatment. • Relapse rate is 84% within 1 yr. in absence of prophylaxis post therapy.
Maintenance	• Fluconazole 100-200 mg/d po	• Ketoconazole 200 mg/day po • Itraconazole 200 mg/day po (tabs) or 100 mg/day oral solution	• Consider maintenance therapy in all patients with recurrent esophagitis, although this increases the probability of resistance (JID 1996;173:219).

V. Opportunistic Infections

	Preferred regimen(s)	Alternative regimen(s)	Comment
Cryptococcal meningitis Initial treatment (NIAID Mycosis Study Group recommendations 4/2000)	• Amphotericin B 0.7-1.0 mg/kg/day IV ± flucytosine 100 mg/kg/d x 10-14 days po then fluconazole 400 mg/day x 8-10 wks	• Fluconazole 400-800 mg/d po ± flucytosine 100 mg/kg/d po x 6-10 wks.	• Amphotericin B is preferred for initial treatment, but total dose prior to fluconazole maintenance is arbitrary. Fluconazole is acceptable as initial treatment only for patients with normal mental status. Other favorable prognostic findings are cryptococcal antigen <1:32 and CSF WBC >20/mm³. • Cryptococcal antigen is nearly always detected in CSF and is somewhat useful in monitoring response; sensitivity of serum antigen is 95%, but it is useless in monitoring response. • Flucytosine use may reduce relapse rates; it does not reduce mortality or speed recovery (NEJM 1997;337:15). • Fluconazole/flucytosine for initial treatment shows promise, but experience is limited (CID 1994;19:741). • Itraconazole: In ACTG 159 itraconazole (400 mg/d) was as effective as fluconazole (400 mg/d) with 8 weeks of treatment after initial treatment with amphotericin B 0.7 mg/kg/d ± flucytosine x 14 days (NEJM 1997;337:15). • Elevated intracranial pressure: remove fluid to reduce pressure to <200 mm H₂O; repeat LP daily if elevated pressure persists.
Maintenance therapy	• Fluconazole 200 mg/d po	• Amphotericin B 0.6-1 mg/kg 1-3 x/wk • Fluconazole: May increase maintenance dose to 400 mg/d • Itraconazole 400 mg po or 200 mg oral ysuspension/day	• Life-long maintenance treatment required; studies of immune reconstitution may change this recommendation, but guidelines are lacking, and the reported experience is nil. • Itraconazole in dose of 200 mg/d is inadequate (ICAAC 9/95, Abstract 1218); trial with 400 mg/d is ongoing.

			Comments
Prophylaxis (see Comments)	• Not generally recommended	• Fluconazole 200 mg po/d • Itraconazole 200 mg/po/day or 100 mg oral suspension/day	• Immune reconstitution: One study of 6 patients with HAART >16 wks with CD4 >150 showed no recurrences with no antifungal therapy for >8 months (7th CROI, Abstract 250). • **Indications:** Consider with high risk patients — those who work with soil and have CD4 counts <100/mm³. (JID 1999;179:449). • Efficacy has been shown for all patients with CD4 counts <50/mm³, but cryptococcosis is infrequent (8-10%), and there is the potential for azole-resistant candidiasis and drug interactions. • Cost of primary cryptococcosis is $213,000/quality of life saved (JAMA 1998;279:13).
Cryptococcosis without meningitis (pulmonary, disseminated or antigenemia)	• Fluconazole 200-400 mg/d po indefinitely unless immune reconstitution achieved	• Itraconazole 200 mg po bid or 100 mg oral suspension/day indefinitely unless immune reconstitution achieved	• All patients with cryptococcosis should have lumbar puncture to exclude meningitis. • Non-meningeal sites for cryptococcal infection include pulmonary, skin, joints, eye, adrenal gland, GI tract, liver, pancreas, prostate, and urinary tract. • Antigenemia: Obtain chest x-ray, LP, urine and blood culture. If no focus identified and antigenemia persists: treat with fluconazole (CID 1996;23:827).
Maintenance (See comment)	• Fluconazole 200 mg/d po	• Itraconazole 200 mg/d or 100 mg oral suspension/d • Amphotericin B 0.6-1 mg/kg IV weekly or 2x/wk	• Need for maintenance therapy with non-meningeal cryptococcosis is not established.

V. Opportunistic Infections

	Preferred regimen(s)	Alternative regimen(s)	Comment
Histoplasmosis Disseminated Initial treatment	• Amphotericin B 0.7–1.0 mg/kg/day IV ≥ 3–14 days • AmBisome 3 mg/kg/d IV • Itraconazole 200 mg po tid x 3 days, then 200 mg po bid or 100 mg oral suspension bid x 12 wks (mild–moderately severe disease)	• Fluconazole	• Itraconazole may be used for initial treatment of mild to moderate histoplasmosis without CNS involvement or it may be used for maintenance after induction with amphotericin B (Am J Med 1995;98:336). • Therapeutic trial of amphotericin B vs. AmBisome in AIDS patients with histoplasmosis showed more rapid defervesence and fewer adverse reactions in the AmBisome group (7th CROI, Abstract 232). The cost is $750/day (AWP 3/2000) vs. $40/day for amphotericin B. • Verify itraconazole levels of >1 μg/mL after >5 days of itraconazole (San Antonio Lab (210) 567-4131 or Indianapolis Lab (317) 630-2515). • Fluconazole is less active than itraconazole, but a therapeutic trial comparing the two regimens showed equal efficacy in rates of antigen clearance from blood and urine (7th CROI, Abstract 261).
Maintenance	• After amphotericin: Itraconazole 200 mg po tid x 3 days; then 200 mg bid x 12 wks, then 200–400 mg q d indefinitely	• Amphotericin B 1.0 mg/kg 1x/wk • Fluconazole 800 mg po/d	• Efficacy of itraconazole is established (Ann Intern Med 1993;118:610). • Itraconazole is superior to fluconazole (Am J Med 1997;103:223). Fluconazole should be used if itraconazole levels are undetectable, itraconazole is not tolerated, if there is meningeal involvement or if rifamycin therapy is necessary. • Itraconazole plasma levels should be ≥1 μg /mL. Tablets require acidic conditions for absorption. Use liquid formulation, give with acidic drink, and avoid concurrent drugs that

	Preferred	Alternative	Comments
Prophylaxis	• Not generally recommended	• Itraconazole 200 mg po/d • Fluconazole 200 mg po/d	increase gastric pH if levels are inadequate; Itraconazole induces the P450 3A enzyme system, altering levels of some PIs and NNRTIs. • Data are inadequate to provide guidelines for discontinuation of maintenance therapy due to immune reconstitution. • **Indication:** Consider in endemic area with CD4 <100/mm^3, especially if at high risk due to occupation (work with soil) or hyperendemic rate (>10 cases/100 pt-yrs) (CID 1999;28 in press).
Coccidioidomycosis Initial Treatment	• Amphotericin B 1.0 mg/kg/day IV • Fluconazole or itraconazole 400-800 mg/d		• Fluconazole preferred for meningitis (Ann Intern Med 1993;119:28). • Intrathecal amphotericin B should be added for coccidioidomycosis meningitis that fails to respond to fluconazole • Diffuse pneumonia - amphotericin B; other forms - oral fluconazole or itraconazole, 400 mg/day
Maintenance	• Fluconazole 400 mg/day • Itraconazole 400 mg/d		• Fluconazole usually preferred due to better absorption and fewer drug interactions (AAC 1995;39:1907).
Prophylaxis	• Not generally recommended	• Fluconazole or intraconazole 400 mg/d (see comment)	• **Indication:** Serologic screening is sometimes suggested for those living in endemic areas; if positive consider treatment with itraconazole or fluconazole, 400 mg/day (CID 1995;20:1281).

V. Opportunistic Infections

	Preferred regimen(s)	Alternative regimen(s)	Comment
Penicillium marneffei (Penicilliosis) Initial treatment	• Amphotericin B 0.7-1.0 mg/kg/d • Itraconazole 400 mg po/d		• Fever ± pneumonitis, adenopathy, skin and mucosal lesions (papules, nodules or pustules). • Endemic in Thailand, Hong Kong, China, Vietnam and Indonesia (Emerg Inf Dis 1996;2:109; Lancet 1994; 344:110). • *In vitro* sensitivity tests show good activity for amphotericin B, ketoconazole, itraconazole, miconazole and 5FC (J Mycol Med 1995;5:21; AAC 1993;37:2407).
Maintenance	• Itraconazole 200 mg po/d	• Ketoconazole	• Life-long treatment required. • See NEJM 1998;339:1739.
PARASITIC INFECTIONS			
Toxoplasma gondii encephalitis Acute infection	• Pyrimethamine 100-200 mg loading dose, then 50-100 mg/day po + folinic acid 10 mg/day po + sulfadiazine or trisulfapyrimidine 4-8 gm/day po for at least 6 wks	• Pyrimethamine + folinic acid (see preferred regimen) + clindamycin 900-1200* mg IV q6h or 300-450 mg po q6h for at least 6 wks • Pyrimethamine and folinic acid (see preferred regimen) plus one of the following: Azithromycin 1200-1500 mg/day, clarithromycin 1 gm bid or atovaquone 750 mg with food qid • Azithromycin + 900 mg po x 2 1st day, then 1200 mg/day x 6 wks, then 600 mg/day (patients <50 kg receive half dose) (salvage therapy) • Experimental: Azithromycin, clarithromycin, trimetrexate, doxycycline, atovaquone	• Anticipated response is clinical improvement within one week and improvement by CT scan or MRI within 2 weeks. • Corticosteroids if significant edema/mass effect (Decadron 4 mg po or IV q6h). • Pyrimethamine usually given as a loading dose of 200 mg followed by 50 mg/day plus folinic acid 10 mg/day. • Controlled trial in 340 patients showed pyrimethamine (50 mg/d) plus sulfadiazine (4 mg/d x 8 wks, then 2 gm/day) was superior to pyrimethamine (50 mg/d) plus clindamycin (2.4 mg/d x 8 wks, then 1.2 gm/day) (CID 1996;22:268).

Suppressive therapy	• Pyrimethamine 25-75 mg po qd + folinic acid 10 qd + sulfadiazide 0.5-1.0 gm po qid	• Azithromycin for IV use: 500 mg x 2 1st day, then 500 mg/day x 9 days, then oral regimen • Pyrimethamine 25-75 mg/d po + folinic acid 10-25 mg qd + clindamycin 300-450 mg po q 6-8 hrs • Alternatives without established efficacy: Pyrimethamine 25-75 mg/d po + folinic acid 10-25 mg qd + either atovaquone 750 mg q 8-12 hrs, dapsone 100 mg/d po or azithromycin 600 mg/d po	• Regimens with established efficacy are pyrimethamine plus sulfonamide or clindamycin. • Pyrimethamine-sulfadiazine, TMP-SMX and atovaquone ± pyrimethamine provide effective *P. carinii* prophylaxis; pyrimethamine-clindamycin does not. • Patients who respond to primary therapy should receive lifelong suppressive therapy. The role of immune reconstitution in modifying this rule is unclear. Immune reconstitution: consider discontinuation when CD4 >200/mm³ >3 mo and VL <5000 c/mL (7th CROI, Abstract 230).
Prophylaxis (See comment)	• Trimethoprim-sulfamethoxazole 1 DS po qd	• TMP-SMX 1 SS po/d or 1 DS 3x/wk • Dapsone 50 mg/d + pyrimethamine 50 mg/wk + folinic acid 25 mg/wk • Dapsone 200 mg/wk po + pyrimethamine 75 mg/wk po + folinic acid 25 mg/wk po • Other regimens without established efficacy: pyrimethamine-clindamycin, atovaquone, azithromycin, clarithromycin or pyrimethamine-sulfadoxine (Fansidar)	• **Indications:** Patients with positive toxoplasmosis IgG serology plus CD4 count nadir of <100/mm³. • Immune reconstitution: Discontinuation of primary and secondary prophylaxis is not recommended in the 1999 USPHS/IDSA recommendations, but subsequent reports support discontinuation in patients with CD4 count >200/mm³ >3 mo. and VL <5000 c/mL (7th CROI, Abstract 230). This study showed no cases in 155 patients followed for a mean of 33 months, including 22 with prior toxoplasmosis. • Efficacy for prophylaxis is established for TMP-SMX and dapsone/pyrimethamine. Preliminary data show either dapsone or atovaquone may be effective (CPCRA 034/ACTG 277).

	Preferred regimen(s)	Alternative regimen(s)	Comment
Toxoplasma gondii encephalitis Prophylaxis (continued)			• Pyrimethamine 25 mg 3x/wk is ineffective; efficacy of 25 mg po qd is not established. • Efficacy of TMP/SMX at 1 DS qd may be superior to that of lower dose.
Cryptosporidia (See Clin Microbiol Reviews 1999;12:554)	• Paromomycin 1000 mg po bid with food x 14-28 days, then 500 mg po bid • Paromomycin 1 gm bid + azithromycin 600 mg qd x 4 weeks, then paromomycin alone x 8 weeks • Symptomatic treatment with nutritional supplements and anti-diarrheal agents: Lomotil, Loperamide, paregoric, bismuth subsalicylate (Pepto-Bismol)	• Nitazoxanide, 500 mg po bid • Octreotide (Sandostatin) 50-500 µg tid SC or IV at 1 mcg/hr • Azithromycin 1200 mg x 2 po 1st day, then 1200 mg/day x 27 days, then 600 mg/day • Atovaquone 750 mg po suspension with meal bid	• Trials with paromomycin show only modest improvement and no cures (Am J Med 1996;100:370). • An uncontrolled trial of paromomycin plus azithromycin showed good response in terms of clinical symptoms and oocyst excretion (JID 1998;178:900). Azithromycin alone is ineffective. • Nitazoxanide (Unimed Pharmaceuticals, Buffalo Grove, IL) is not yet approved by the FDA, and clinical trial data including ACTG 192 shows minimal or no benefit. • HAART with immune reconstitution is the most effective treatment (Lancet 1998;351:256). • Nonsteroidal anti-inflammatory agents are sometimes useful. • Nutritional supplements often required for severe cases; Vivonex TEN or parenteral hyperalimentation. • Experimental agents: hyperimmune bovine colostrum Sporidin-G, letrazuril, clarithromycin. • Clarithromycin or rifabutin prophylaxis for MAC prophylaxis may reduce risk of cryptosporidiosis (JAMA 1998;279:384).

Isospora Acute Infection	• Trimethoprim/- sulfamethoxazole po bid (2 DS po bid or 1 DS tid) x 2-4 wks	• Pyrimethamine 50-75 mg po/day + folinic acid 5-10 mg/day x 1 mo • There has been one case report of refractory infection that responded to pyrimethamine plus sulfadiazine (Diag Microbiol Infect Dis 1996;26:87). • Duration of high-dose therapy is not well defined.
Suppressive treatment	• Trimethoprim/ sulfamethoxazole 1-2 DS/d po	• Pyrimethamine 25 mg + sulfadoxine 500 mg po q wk (1 Fansidar/wk) • Pyrimethamine 25 mg + folinic acid 5 mg/day • Duration is not well defined.
Microsporidiosis	• Symptomatic treatment with nutritional supple- ments and anti-diar- rheal agents (Lomotil, Loperamide, paregoric, etc.) • Albendazole 400–800 mg po bid x ≥3 weeks (*S. intestinalis*)	• Metronidazole 500 mg po tid • Atovaquone 750 mg po tid with meals bid (AIDS 1996;10:619) • Thalidomide 100 mg q d (AIDS 1995;9:658) • Efficacy of albendazole is established only for infections involving *Septata intestinalis*, which cause 10–20% of cases. • Anecdotal success reported with itraconazole, fluconazole, atovaquone, and metronidazole (Inf Dis Clin N Amer 1994;8:483). • HAART with immune reconstitution is the best therapy, espe- cially for the 80-90% of cases involving *E. bieneusi* (Lancet 1998;351:256; J Clin Micro 1999;37:3421). • Experimental drugs: Fumagillin, TNP-470, Ovalicin.

V. Opportunistic Infections

TB TREATMENT RECOMMENDATIONS

Mycobacterium tuberculosis Treatment (MMWR 1998; 47[RR-20])

Directly observed therapy (DOT) — 2-3x/wk preferred

	Daily	DOT 2x/wk	DOT 3x/wk
INH	5 mg/kg (300 mg)*	15 mg/kg (900 mg)*	15 mg/kg (900 mg)*
RIF	10 mg/kg (600 mg)*	10 mg/kg (600 mg)*	10 mg/kg (600 mg)*
RFB	150-450 mg**	300-450 mg**	300-450mg**
PZA	15-30 mg/kg (2 gm)*	50-70 mg/kg (4 gm)*	50-70 mg/kg (3 gm)*
EMB	15-25 mg/kg (2.5 gm)*	50 mg/kg (2.5 gm)*	25-30 mg/kg (2.5 gm)*
SM	15 mg/kg (1 gm)*	25-30 mg/kg	25-30 mg/kg (1 gm)*

* Maximum dose

** Rifabutin (RFB) to be used with antiretroviral regimens including PIs or NNRTIs. RBT dose is 150 mg daily or 300 mg 2-3x/week when combined with indinavir, nelfinavir or amprenavir; with Efavirenz the RFB dose is 450 mg daily or 450 mg 2-3x/ week. Rifamycins should not be used with Invirase, ritonavir or delavirdine. For dose adjustments of PIs and NNRTIs, see next page.

Induction	Maintenance	Comment
Rifampin-based therapy (no concurrent use of PIs or NNRTIs)		
1. INH/RIF/PZA/EMB (or SM) daily x 2 mo	INH/RIF daily or 2-3x/wk x 18 wks	RIF-containing regimens preclude concurrent use of Protease inhibitors and NNRTI
2. INH/RIF/PZA/EMB (or SM) daily x 2 wks, then 2-3x/wk x 6 wks	INH/RIF or 2-3x/wk x 18 wks	Assess HIV at 3 mos. intervals to determine need for ART
3. INH/RIF/PZA/EMB (or SM) 3x/wk x 8 wks	INH/RIF/PZA/EMB (or SM) 3x/wk x 4 mos.	A 2 wk wash-out period is required between the last RIF dose and initiation of PI or NNRTIs
Rifabutin-based therapy (concurrent PI or NNRTI)		
1. INH/RFB/PZA/EMB daily x 8 wks	INH/RFB daily or 2x/wk x 18 wks	Monitor for RFB toxicity—arthralgias, uveitis, leukopenia
2. INH/RFB/PZA/EMB daily x 2 wks, then 2x/wk x 6 wks	INH/RFB 2x/wk x 18 wks	Dose modifications of RFB and PIs/NNRTI when given concurrently; see pg XX. RFB should be given with SQV or DLV
Streptomycin-based therapy (concurrent PI or NNRTI)		
1. INH/SM/PZA/EMB daily x 8 wks	INH/SM/PZA 2-3x/wk x 30 wks	SM is contraindicated in pregnant women
2. INH/SM/PZA/EMB daily x 2 wks, then 2-3x/wk x 6 wks	INH/SM/PZA 2-3x/wk x 30 wks	If SM cannot be continued for 9 mos. add EMB and treatment should be extended to 12 mos.

INH = isoniazide, RIF = rifampin, RFB = rifabutin, EMB = ethambutol, PZA = pyrazinamide, SM = streptomycin, IDV = indinavir, NFV = nelfinavir, EFV = efavirenz, APV = amprenavir

TB TREATMENT RECOMMENDATIONS (continued)

Options for antiretroviral therapy:

- Regimen that does not contain a protease inhibitor or NNRTI

- Streptomycin-based therapy with no use of rifamycins (see above)

- Rifabutin-based treatment with dose adjustments

PI or NNRTI	Rifabutin
Indinavir, 1000 mg q 8 h	150 mg/d or 300 mg 2x/wk
Nelfinavir, 1000 mg tid	150 mg/d or 300 mg 2x/wk
Amprenavir, 1200 mg bid	150 mg/d or 300 mg 2x/wk
Efavirenz, 600 mg qd	450 mg/d or 450 mg 2x/wk
Ritonavir, standard	150 mg qod
RTV 400 mg/SQV 400 mg bid	150 mg q 3 d or 150 mg q 7 d

No data: nevirapine and Fortovase
Contraindicated: Invirase, delavirdine

- Recommendation of D. Havlin & P. Barnes (NEJM 1999;340:367): INH, ethambutol and pyrazinamide x 18-24 months

- Possible regimen based on pharmacokinetic studies: Efavirenz 800 mg/day + rifampin 600 mg/day or 600 mg 2x weekly

V. Opportunistic Infections

	Preferred regimen(s)	Alternative regimen(s)	Comment
Mycobacterium tuberculosis (continued) Prophylaxis INH-susceptible strain	• INH 300 mg/day po + pyridoxine 50 mg/day po x 9 mos. • INH 900 mg 2x/wk + pyridoxine 50 mg 2x/wk x 9 mos. (DOT) • Rifampin 600 mg/day + PZA 20 mg/kg/d x 2 mos.	• Rifampin 600 mg po qd x 4 mo • PZA 15-30 mg/kg/day plus Rifabutin in place of rifampin to permit concurrent PI or NNRTI (see page 124 for doses) x 2 mo.	• **Indications:** PPD ≥5 mm induration, high-risk exposure, or prior positive PPD without treatment. • Rifampin containing regimens have drug interactions with protease inhibitors and NNRTIs; the preferred regimens are INH or short course prophylaxis with PZA plus rifabutin using dose adjustments shown on page 124. • Rifampin/PZA is commonly favored since it is as effective as INH for 9 months, and the probability of completing the 2 month course is better (JAMA 2000;283:1445).
INH-resistant strain	• Rifampin 600 mg/day po + pyrazinamide 20 mg/kg x 2 mos.	• Rifabutin 150-450 mg/day (dose based on concurrent PI or NNRTI) + pyrazinamide x 2 mo.	• The choice of rifampin versus rifabutin depends on concurrent HAART.
Multiply-resistant strain	• Fluoroquinolone/ pyrazinamide or ethambutol/pyrazinamide		• Base decision on susceptibility tests and consultation with public health officials.
Mycobacterium avium complex (MAC) bacteremia Treatment	• Clarithromycin 500 mg po bid plus ethambutol 15 mg/kg/day po ± rifabutin 300 mg/day po	• Azithromycin 600 mg/d po in place of clarithromycin + ethambutol ± rifabutin (same doses) • Combination treatment with amikacin 10-15 mg/kg/day IV or ciprofloxacin, 500-700 mg bid	• Duration is indefinite in absence of immune reconstitution. With HAART, initial results suggest that MAC treatment may be discontinued when MAC treatment is >1 yr, CD4 count is >100/mm³ for 3-6 mos. and the patient is asymptomatic (JID 1998;178:1446).

- Clarithromycin levels are increased 50-80% with concurrent administration of indinavir, ritonavir and saquinavir; nelfinavir and amprenavir have no effect on clarithromycin levels (See Table 4-18).

- *In vitro* susceptibility tests are not useful in previously untreated patients (CID 1998;27:1369).

- In a comparative trial of azithromycin vs. clarithromycin for MAC bacteremia clarithromycin was superior in time to negative blood cultures (CID 1998;27:1278; See also AAC 1999;43:2869).

- Rifabutin dose adjustments with concurrent PIs or NNRTIs: 50% reduction – indinavir, nelfinavir, amprenavir; 50% increase – efavirenz; no data or contraindicated – delavirdine, nevirapine, saquinavir or ritonavir. Doses of PI and NNRTI also need adjustment – see page 124.

- ACTG 223 compared clarithro/ethambutol, clarithro/rifabutin and clarithro, ethambutol/ rifabutin. Treatment with clarithro/rifabutin was inferior with respect to relapse rates (24% vs 6-7%). The 3 drug regimen was superior with respect to time to negative blood cultures and survival.

- Drug interaction between clarithromycin and rifabutin results in decreased levels of clarithromycin (NEJM 1996;335:428).

- Rifabutin dose is 300-600 mg/day, but should not exceed 300 mg/day if given with clarithromycin or fluconazole. Note interactions with protease inhibitors and NNRTIs.

- ASA or NSAID often effective for symptom relief.

V. Opportunistic Infections

	Preferred regimen(s)	Alternative regimen(s)	Comment
Mycobacterium avium complex (MAC) bacteremia Treatment (continued)			• Clarithromycin at a dose >1000 mg/day was associated with increased mortality (Ann Intern Med 1994;121:905). • Discontinuation of secondary prophylaxis: The risk of relapse following HAART with CD4 increases to >100/mm³ for >6 mos. is low, but studies are too limited to recommend discontinuation of secondary prophylaxis.
Prophylaxis: Initiation and discontinuation	• Clarithromycin 500 mg po bid • Azithromycin 1200 mg q week	• Rifabutin 300 mg/po qd (adjust dose if given with PI or NNRTI) • Azithromycin 1200 mg qwk plus rifabutin 300 mg po qd	• **Indications:** <50/mm³; rule out MAC bacteremia and active TB. Initial studies support discontinuation of primary prophylaxis in patients who respond to HAART with increases in CD4 counts to >100/mm³ for ≥6 mos. combined with substantial suppression of viral load (NEJM 1996;335:392). • Preliminary data suggests low dose clarithromycin (500 mg/d) may be effective (AIDS 1999;13:1367). • Azithromycin contributes to PCP prophylaxis by further reducing rates of PCP (Lancet 1999;354:891). • Combination of azithromycin plus rifabutin associated with an 85% reduction in the expected number of cases of disseminated MAC (NEJM 1996;335:392). There is no apparent benefit to adding rifabutin to clarithromycin for preventive treatment, possibly due to the drug interaction resulting in reduced levels of clarithromycin (NEJM 1996;335:428). • Prophylaxis failures with rifabutin usually involve clarithromycin sensitive strains; failures with clarithromycin or azithromycin often involve clarithromycin-resistant strains.

Immune recovery lymphadenitis	• Treat for MAC-clarithromycin 500 mg bid + ethambutol 15 mg/kg/d ± rifabutin 300 mg/d po • Azithromycin/ethambutol • Corticosteroids with rapid taper for severe symptoms or draining sinuses.	• Characterized by high fever, leukocytosis, and lymphadenopathy often involving the periaortic and mesenteric nodes. Biopsy shows granulomatous lymphadenitis with AFB in large numbers. Occurs within 1-3 months of HAART (Lancet 1998;351:252; JAIDS 1999;20:122). • Long term follow-up of 12 patients who discontinued anti-MAC therapy after a mean of 19 months showed none had recurrence in ≥9 mo. (7th CROI, Abstract 257). Draining sinuses were associated with a poor prognosis and may require corticosteroids.
Mycobacterium kansasii	• INH 300 mg po/day + rifampin 600 mg/day po + ethambutol 15-25 mg/kg/day po x 18 mo to life-long therapy ± Streptomycin 1 gm IM 2x/wk x 3 mos. • Also consider ciprofloxacin 750 mg po bid and clarithromycin 500 mg po bid	• Experience in HIV-infected patients is limited. (JAIDS 1991;4:516; Ann Intern Med 1991;114:861). • Need *in vitro* sensitivity data. • Duration of treatment is arbitrary - many treat HIV infected patients for life. • Most strains are resistant to INH, but it is usually included in the regimen with little supporting data. • Immune reconstitution: Reports of cervical and mediastinal adenopathy, osteomyelitis and arthritis due to *M. kansasii* during the first 3 months of HAART.
Mycobacterium haemophilum	• INH/rifampin/ethambutol • Clarithromycin, doxycycline, ciprofloxacin, and amikacin are active *in vitro*	• Experience is limited (Eur J Clin Micro Inf Dis 1993;12:114).

V. Opportunistic Infections

	Preferred regimen(s)	Alternative regimen(s)	Comment
Mycobacterium - gordonae	• INH/rifampin/clofazimine or clarithromycin	• Streptomycin may be useful	• Most isolates are contaminants (Dermatology 1993;187:301; AIDS 1992;6:1217; AAC 1992;36:1987).
Mycobacterium genavense	• Clarithromycin/ethambutol/rifampin	• Other possible agents: ciprofloxacin, amikacin and pyrazinamide	• Clarithromycin containing regimens are most effective (AIDS 1993;7:1357).
M. xenopi	INH; rifampin, ethambutol and streptomycin		
M. fortuitum	Amikacin 400 mg q 12 h + cefoxitin 12 gm/d x 2-4 wks, then oral agents based on *in vitro* tests – clarithromycin 1 gm/d, doxycycline 200 mg/d, sulfamethoxazole 1 gm tid, ciprofloxacin 500 mg bid		• Duration of therapy: ≥3 mo for cutaneous lesions and ≥6 mo for bone lesions in non-HIV infected patients.
M. malmoense	Rifampin/INH/ethambutol		• See CID 1993;16:540
M. chelonei	Clarithromycin 500 mg bid x ≥6 mo	Variable activity - cefoxitin, amikacin, doxycycline, imipenem, tobramycin	• Need *in vitro* susceptibility test results • Often need combination therapy

VIRUSES

Herpes simplex Initial treatment		
Mild	• Acyclovir 400 mg po tid or famciclovir 250 mg po tid or valacyclovir 1.0 gm po bid; all given 7-10 days	• Failure to respond: give valacyclovir or give acyclovir IV. • Early treatment shortens duration, reduces viral shedding and reduces systemic symptoms; it does not influence probability of recurrence (Med Letter 1995;37:117).
Severe or refractory	• Foscarnet 40 mg/kg IV q8h or 60 mg/kg q12h x 3 wks • Topical trifluridine as 1% opthalmic solution q8h • Alternative topical agents: cidofovir 3% and foscarnet 1% cream • Cidofovir 5 mg/kg q 2 wks (limited experience) • Acyclovir up to 800 mg po 5x/d 15-30 mg/kg IV/day at least 7 days • Valacyclovir 1 gm po bid - tid	• If fails to respond give valacyclovir 1 gm bid or acyclovir 800 mg 5x/day or 15-30 mg/kg/day IV and test sensitivity of isolate to acyclovir; resistant HSV: IV foscarnet, topical trifluridine, oral valacyclovir, or high-dose IV acyclovir (12-15 mg/kg IV q8h or by continuous infusion). Relapses after treatment of acyclovir-resistant strains often involve acyclovir-sensitive strains (NEJM 1991;325:551). • Topical trifluridine solution (Viroptic 1%) is applied after H_2O_2 cleaning and gentle gauze-debridement; cover with non-absorbent gauze with bacitracin and polymyxin ointment (JADS 1996;12:147). Topical foscarnet is available from Astra, and 3% topical cidofovir may be prepared from the IV preparation (JID 1997;17:862; NEJM 1993;327:968).
Recurrent	• Acyclovir 400 mg po tid or 800 mg po bid or famciclovir 125 mg po bid or valacyclovir 500 mg po bid; all given for 5 days	• Early treatment is much more effective (Arch Intern Med 1996;156:1729).

V. Opportunistic Infections

	Preferred regimen(s)	Alternative regimen(s)	Comment
Herpes simplex (continued) Prophylaxis	• Acyclovir 400 mg po bid or famciclovir 125-250 mg po bid or valacyclovir 500 mg po bid or 1 gm q d		• Alternative is to treat each episode. • Patients receiving ganciclovir, foscarnet or cidofovir do not require acyclovir prophylaxis. • AIDS patients may require higher daily doses
Visceral	• Acyclovir 30 mg/kg IV/day at least 14-21 days	• Foscarnet 40 mg/kg IV q8h x ≥10 days • Valacyclovir 1.0 gm po tid	• Includes esophagitis and encephalitis which may involve acyclovir resistant strains in AIDS patients (JID 1990;161:711)
Herpes zoster Dermatomal	• Acyclovir 800 mg po 5x/day at least 7 days (until lesions crust) or famciclovir 500 mg po tid or valacyclovir 1 gm po tid x ≥7 days	• Acyclovir 30 mg/kg/d IV • Foscarnet 40 mg/kg IV q8h or 60 mg/kg IV q 12 h	• Some authorities recommend corticosteroids (Ann Intern Med 1996;125:376). Prednisone 60 mg x 7 days, 30 mg days 8-14, 15 mg days 15-21. • Postherpetic neuralgia is uncommon in persons <55 years • Foscarnet preferred for acyclovir-resistant cases (NEJM 1993;308:1448). • Comparative trial of acyclovir vs valacyclovir showed slight advantage to valacyclovir (AAC 1995;39:1546). • Treatment can be started as long as new lesions are forming. • Pain control: gabapentin, trycyclics, carbamazepime, lidocaine patch, narcotics (effective and underused)

Disseminated, ophthalmic nerve involvement or visceral	• Acyclovir 30-36 mg/kg IV/day at least 7 days	• Foscarnet 40 mg/kg IV q8h or 60 mg/kg q12h	• Role of maintenance therapy unclear.
Acyclovir-resistant strains	• Foscarnet 40 mg/kg IV q8h or 60 mg/kg q12h	• Cidofovir IV • Topical trifluridine	• Foscarnet is drug of choice (Ann Intern Med 1991;115:9; JAIDS 1993;7:254).
Maintenance (see Comments)	• Acyclovir, famciclovir or valacyclovir po in above doses		• **Indication:** Frequent recurrences.
Prevention	• Varicella Zoster Immune Globulin (ZVIG) 5 vials (6.25 ml) within 96 hrs of exposure	• Acyclovir 800 mg po 5x/day x 3 weeks. (Note: Acyclovir has been removed from the 1999 USPHS/IDSA guidelines for IO prophylaxis due to lack of documented efficacy.)	• **Indication:** Exposure to chicken pox or shingles plus no history of either and, if available, negative VZV serology. Preventive treatment must be initiated within 96 hours of exposure and preferably within 48 hours.

V. Opportunistic Infections

	Preferred regimen(s)	Alternative regimen(s)	Comment
Cytomegalovirus Retinitis Initial Treatment Recommendations of the IAS-USA (Arch Intern Med 1998;158:957)	• Intraocular ganciclovir release device (Vitrasert) q 6 mos. + oral ganciclovir 1.0-1.5 gm po with meal tid. (Some consider this to be the preferred therapy and especially for immediately sight-threatening infection.) • Foscarnet (60 mg/kg IV q8h or 90 mg/kg IV q12h x 14-21 days • Ganciclovir 5 mg/kg IV bid x 14-21 days • Cidofovir 5 mg/kg IV q wk x 2, then 5 mg/kg q 2 wks/plus probenecid, 2 gm po 3 hr before each dose, 1 gm po at 2 and 8 hrs post dose	• Alternating or combining foscarnet and ganciclovir • Intraocular injections of foscarnet 1.2-2.4 mg in 0.1 ml (NEJM 1994;330:868) or ganciclovir 2000 µg in 0.05-0.1 mL (Brit J Opthal 1996;80:214) • Fomivirsen, 330 µg by intravitreal injection day 1 and 15, then monthly	• Median times to progression with initial treatment: Ganciclovir IV 47-104 days, foscarnet IV 53-93 days, ganciclovir/foscarnet IV 129 days, oral ganciclovir 29-53 days, ganciclovir implant 216-226 days, cidofovir IV 64-120 days, fomivirsen intravitreal injection 90-110 days. • Valganciclovir is experimental pro-drug of ganciclovir with 60% bioavailability (7th CROI, Abstract 231). • Oral ganciclovir should not be used as sole induction therapy. Maintenance with oral ganciclovir is nearly as effective as IV ganciclovir, but should be avoided with lesions near the optic nerve or fovea (NEJM 1995;333:615). • Foscarnet requires infusion pump, long infusion time, saline hydration. • Intravitreal ganciclovir by injection (ACTG 085) was disappointing as salvage therapy. • Vitrasert (intraocular ganciclovir release device) was superior to IV ganciclovir in time to relapse (220 days vs 71 days), but there is increased risk of involvement of the other eye and increased risk of extraocular CMV disease (NEJM 1997;337:83). The same concern applies to fomivirsen injections. Any local therapy should be accompanied by systemic anti-CMV therapy such as oral ganciclovir (NEJM 1997;337:105). The Roche Ganciclovir Study showed that Vitrasert + oral ganciclovir (4.5 gm/d) was therapeutically equivalent to IV ganciclovir (NEJM 1999;340:1063).

			• Alternating or combination ganciclovir plus foscarnet appears less toxic and more active vs CMV compared to foscarnet alone (JID 1994;170:189). • IAS-USA revised recommendations for initial treatment – 1999 (Am J Opth 1999;127:329): **for those starting HAART** – systemic anti-CMV therapy preferred with the intra-ocular ganciclovir devise for relapse or zone 1 disease; **non-compliant** patient – ganciclovir implant; **treatment experienced patient** – systemic anti-CMV therapy or ganciclovir implant; **HAART failures** – ganciclovir implant preferred for zone 1 and optional for zones 2 and 3.
Progression or relapse (on maintenance therapy)	• Ganciclovir implant (if not used previously). • Induction dose of same agent (ganciclovir 10 mg/kg/day, or foscarnet 120 mg/kg/day) or switch to alternative drug (induction doses) • Combination treatment with ganciclovir/foscarnet in maintenance doses (JID 1993;168: 144; Am J Ophth 1994;117:776); Arch Ophthal 1996;114:23)	• Cidofovir 5 mg/kg (as above) • Fomivirsen, 330 μg by intravitreal injection day 1 and 15, then monthly • Cidofovir (as above)/oral ganciclovir, 1 gm po tid with meal	• Time to relapse varies with definition, use of retinal photographs, and treatment as summarized above. Subsequent relapses occur more rapidly. • ACTG 228 showed no difference between reinduction with the same drug compared to switching to the alternative drug. With combination treatment, there was the best outcome for time to progression (4.8 months versus 1.6-2.1 months), and the worst for quality of life (presumably due to time required for infusions) (Arch Ophthal 1996;114:23). • Preliminary data for cidofovir/oral ganciclovir shows good response rates and good anti-CMV effect, but high rates of drug-related toxicity (CID 1999;28:528). • IAS-USA revised recommendation – 1999 (Am J Opthal 1999;127:329): Ganciclovir implant; prior exposure to ganciclovir is associated with CMV ganciclovir resistance and failure to respond. If the ganciclovir implant fails consider IV or intravitreal foscarnet.

V. Opportunistic Infections

	Preferred regimen(s)	Alternative regimen(s)	Comment
Cytomegalovirus Retinitis (continued) Maintenance	• Foscarnet 90-120 mg/kg IV/day • Ganciclovir 5-6 mg/k/day IV/day 5-7 days/wk or 1000 mg po tid • Cidofovir 5 mg/kg IV every other week • Intraocular ganciclovir release device q 6 mo + oral ganciclovir 1 gm po tid		• **Indications:** Life-long maintenance therapy required for retinitis in patients without immune recovery. Initial studies with HAART show that discontinuation of CMV maintenance therapy was safe in 30/30 patients with CD4 counts of 100-150/mm³ followed for 3-12 months (CID 1999;28:528; Ophthalmology 1998;105:1259). • Foscarnet maintenance dose is arbitrary; one study showed that 120 mg/kg/day was superior to 90 mg/kg/day in survival and time to progression (JID 1993;167:1184). • See above for median time to relapse for different initial regimens. • **Discontinuation:** Several reports demonstrate safety of discontinuation of maintenance therapy for CMV retinitis when CD4 counts increase to >100-150/mm³, with no relapse in follow-up periods of 30-90 weeks. A report from the NEI showed that discontinuation of anti-CMV drugs when the CD4 was >150/mm³ was uniformly successful in 14 patients (JAMA 1999;282:1633). This decision should be based on the magnitude and duration of the CD4 count increase, the HIV viral load suppression, the anatomic location of retinitis and degree of vision loss. An ophthalmologist should be consulted.

Prophylaxis	• Not generally recommended	• Oral ganciclovir 1 gm po tid with meal	• **Indication:** Positive CMV serology + CD4 count <50 mm[3]. Initial study showed 50% reduction in rate of CMV disease (NEJM 1996;334:1491), but a subsequent CPCRA study failed to confirm any benefit (AIDS 1998;12:269). Many conclude that we need a method to identify risk for CMV disease (e.g. quantitative CMV-PCR) (JID 1997;176:1484). • Concerns: Side effects of oral ganciclovir (anemia, leukopenia), limited clinical benefit, lack of survival benefit, possible risk of ganciclovir resistance, and cost (AWP – $17,500/year).
Immune recovery vitritis	• Systemic or periocular corticosteroids		• Posterior segment inflammation in patients with inactive CMV retinitis and immune recovery associated with HAART (Arch Ophthalmol 1998;116:169). May be complicated by cystoid macular edema, epiretinal membrane and papillitis (7th CROI, Abstract 270). • Incidence is highly variable for reasons that are unclear (JAMA 2000;283:653). • Must exclude other causes of uveitis including TB, syphilis, toxoplasmosis, lymphoma and drug reactions (Am J Ophth 1998;125:292).

	Preferred regimen(s)	Alternative regimen(s)	Comment
Cytomegalovirus Extra-0cular disease			
Gastrointestinal	• Ganciclovir 5 mg/kg IV bid x 3-6 wks • Foscarnet 60 mg/kg q 8 h or 90 mg/kg IV q 12 h x 3-6 wks	• Failure: Ganciclovir/foscarnet	• Ganciclovir and foscarnet are equally effective for CMV colitis (Am J Gastro 1993;88:542). • Maintenance therapy should be considered, especially after re-induction and relapse. • Role of oral ganciclovir is unclear. • Patients should have regular ophthalmoscopic screening. • Foscarnet plus ganciclovir are associated with poor quality of life (JID 1993;167:1184).
Neurologic disease	• As above or ganci-clovir/foscarnet		• Consider combination therapy for patients with prior CMV therapy. • Cidofovir: there is no experience with neurologic disease. • Treatment does not extend survival and irreversible damage is often present when treatment is started (Neurology 1996;46:444). • Maintenance therapy should be given after induction phase.
Pneumonitis	• Ganciclovir 5 mg/kg IV bid ≥21 days • Foscarnet 60 mg/kg q 8 h or 90 mg/kg IV q 12 h ≥21 days		• Minimum diagnostic criteria: 1) pulmonary infiltrates; 2) detection of CMV with culture antigen or nucleic acid studies of pulmonary secretions; 3) characteristic intracellular inclusions in lung tissue or BAL macrophages; and 4) absence of another pulmonary pathogen (Arch Int Med 1998;158:957).

		• Consider therapy if there is a co-pathogen that fails to respond to therapy. • Long term maintenance therapy is usually unnecessary unless there is relapse or extra-pulmonary end organ disease.
JC Virus: **Progressive multi-** **focal leukoencepha-** **lopathy (PML)**	Highly active antiretroviral regimen (HAART)	• Diagnosis: PCR for JCV DNA is not sensitive or specific (JID 1992;16:80; J Virol 1992;66:5726). Positive PCR + typical clinical and MRI findings constitute presumptive PML; if PCR negative consider brain biopsy depending on probability of a treatable alternative diagnosis. Median survival after PML diagnosis is 2-4 months (JAIDS 1992;5:1030; NEJM 1998;338:1345). • Multiple studies confirm potential utility of HAART (5th Retrovirus Conference, Abstracts 463–465; AIDS 1999;13:1881). Nevertheless, the results are inconsistent (CID 1999;28:1152). One report showed that HAART resulted in clearance of positive JCV PCR in 5 of 6 cases (CID 2000;30:95). One preliminary report showed possible benefit with cidofovir (5th Retrovirus Conference, 2/98 Abstract 467). • Failed treatments in clinical trials include amantadine, adenosine arabinoside, cytosine arabinoside and intrathecal cytosine arabinoside (NEJM 1998;338:1345). • Anecdotal reports suggest response to alpha interferon (J Neuroviral 1998;4:324). • Initial trial with cidofovir (ACTG 363) shows no benefit.
	• Cidofovir (?) • Interferon alpha, 3 MU/day (see comment)	

	Preferred regimen(s)	Alternative regimen(s)	Comment
Salmonella Acute	• Ciprofloxacin 500 mg po bid x 2-4 wks	• Ampicillin 8-12 gm IV/day x 1-4 wks; then amoxicillin 500 mg po tid to complete 2-4 wk course • Trimethoprim 5-10 mg/kg/day + sulfamethoxazole IV or po x 2-4 wks • Cephalosporins; 3rd generation	• Relapse is common. Eradication of *Salmonella* has been demonstrated only for ciprofloxacin. • AZT is active vs most *Salmonella* strains and may be effective prophylaxis. • Drug selection requires *in vitro* susceptibility data especially for ampicillin.
Maintenance	• Ciprofloxacin 500 mg po bid x several mos.	• Trimethoprim-sulfamethoxazole 5 mg/kg/day, trimethoprim (1 DS po bid)	• Indications for maintenance therapy, specific regimens and duration not well defined.
Staphylococcus aureus	• Antistaphylococcal penicillin (nafcillin, oxacillin) ± gentamicin 1 mg/kg IV q8h or rifampin 300 mg po bid • Oral agents: Cephalexin 500 mg po qid, dicloxacillin 500 mg po qid, ciprofloxacin 750 mg po bid or clindamycin 300 mg po qid	• Cephalosporin: first generation ± gentamicin or rifampin • Vancomycin 1 gm IV bid ± gentamicin 1 mg/kg IV q 8 h x 3 days or rifampin 300 mg po bid • Linezolid 600 mg IV or po bid	• MRSA strains must be treated with vancomycin. • Use of ciprofloxacin or other quinolone requires *in vitro* sensitivity results. • Regimen and duration depends on site of infection and *in vitro* sensitivity tests. • *In vitro* sensitivity tests required for ciprofloxacin use. • Tricuspid valve endocarditis: oxacillin + gentamicin x 14 days *or* oxacillin x 14-28 days + gentamicin x 3 days *or* ciprofloxacin 750 mg bid + rifampin 300 mg bid x 28 days

| *Treponema pallidum* (MMWR 1998;47 [RR-1]:38) | • Primary secondary syphilis and early latent (<1 year): Benzathine penicillin G 2.4 mil units IM weekly x 1 (see Comments)

• Late latent syphilis: Benzathine penicillin G 2.4 mil units IM weekly x 3

• Neurosyphilis: Aqueous penicillin G, 18-24 mil units/day IV x 10-14 days (3-4 mil units q 4 h) | • No alternative to penicillin considered adequate for HIV-infected patients. With a history of penicillin allergy, perform skin test if reagents available (major and minor). If positive skin test or positive history and no skin test: desensitize. | • Follow-up clinically and serologically at 2, 3, 6, 9, and 12 months.

• A therapeutic trial of penicillin G benzathine 2.4 mil units for primary or secondary syphilis showed HIV infected patients responded less well serologically, but clinical failures were rare (NEJM 1997;337:307).

• Patients with latent syphilis of uncertain duration are considered to have late latent syphilis.

• LP is recommended with neurologic symptoms, treatment failure and late latent syphilis. |

V. Opportunistic Infections

* Patients with severe forms of G-6-PD deficiency are at risk for hemolytic anemia when given oxidant drugs such as dapsone, sulfonamides, and primaquine. Some advocate screening all potential recipients, some restrict screening to persons at greatest risk (African-American men and men of Mediterranean descent, from India or from the Far East); some simply observe for evidence of hemolysis, which usually occurs in first several days of treatment and often resolves with continued administration. Patients with the Mediterranean variant are at risk for severe hemolysis.

‡ Ketoconazole, and to a lesser extent, itraconazole require gastric acid for absorption; absorption with hypochlorhydria may be enhanced by administration with 0.2 N HCl or the following soft drinks: Coca-Cola®, Diet Coke®, Pepsi®, ginger ale and Diet Minute Maid® orange juice (AAC 1995;39:1671). The liquid formulation of itraconazole is preferred to capsules for thrush, for patients with achlorhydria and those with subtherapeutic trough serum levels with capsules (<2 mcg/mL); some consider the liquid formulation to be the preferred form for all oral itraconazole therapy, although all clinical trials except for thrush and candida esophagitis were conducted with the capsule form.

Abbreviations used:

AMB: amphotericin B

Amik: amikacin

AZT: zidovudine

Cipro: ciprofloxacin

CMV: cytomegalovirus

CNS: central nervous system

CT: computed topographic scan

DS: double-strength tablet

EMB: Ethambutol

5-FC: flucytosine (5-fluorocytosine)

FUO: fever of unknown origin

G-CSF: granulocyte colony-stimulating factor

HAART: highly active anti-retroviral therapy

HIV: human immuno-deficiency virus

INH: isoniazid

MRI: magnetic resonance imaging

Oflox: ofloxacin

PAS: paraaminosalicylate

PCP: P. carinii pneumonia

PZA: pyrazinamide

Rif: rifampin

SMX: sulfamethoxazole

SS: single-strength tablet

Strep: streptomycin

TMP: trimethoprim

Treatment of Miscellaneous and Non-Infectious Disease Complications/Classified by Organ System

Condition	Treatment	Comment
Cardiac		
Cardiomyopathy	• ACE inhibitors such as enalapril – 2.5 mg bid titrated to 20 mg/day as tolerated or captopril 6.25 mg tid increasing to 25-50 mg tid. Digitalis and diuretics are often added for symptomatic left ventricular disease. • Some patients respond to antiretroviral therapy (HAART)	• Echocardiograms show dilated cardiomyopathy in up to 8% of HIV infected patients (NEJM 1998;339:1093). In most cases biopsies reveal myocarditis and HIV nucleic acid sequences suggesting a direct effect of HIV. Other possible etiologic mechanisms include immunologically mediated alterations, a role for other cardiotrophic viruses or mitochondrial toxicity due to AZT and other NRTIs (Ann Int Med 1992;116:311). • Subclinical cardiac abnormalities are common and correlated with extent of immune suppression (BMJ 1994;309:1605; NEJM 1998;339:1153).
Pulmonary		
Lymphoid interstitial pneumonitis ornon-specific interstitial pneumonitis	• HAART • Prednisone	• Possibly due to HIV infection of the lung. • Clinical presentation and X-ray resemble PCP, but CD4 is often 200-500. Many patients respond when inadvertently treated for PCP (Am J Resp Crit Care Med 1997;156:912). • Indications and optimal dose of corticosteroid treatment not established; most initiate this treatment after initial observation shows progression; maintenance prednisone sometimes required. Some patients become oxygen dependent.
Pneumothorax	• Consider empiric treatment for *P. carinii* • Tube thoracostomy ± pleurodesis	• PCP in 75-95% of cases (Chest 1991;100:1224; Chest 1994;108:946).

V. Opportunistic Infections

Condition	Treatment	Comment
Neurologic HIV-associated dementia (HAD) (continued)		• Dementia staging 0 Normal 0.5 Equivocal symptoms of cognitive or motor dysfunction 1 Evidence of intellectual or motor impairment but able to perform most aspects of work or ADL 2 Cannot work but can do self-care 3 Major intellectual or motor disability; cannot walk unassisted 4 Nearly vegetative
Hematologic Idiopathic thrombocytopenic purpura (ITP) Asymptomatic	• HAART • Discontinue any drugs potentially responsible	• Anecdotal experience with HAART is good (NEJM 1999;341:1239; CID 2000;30:504) • Note: Standard treatments (prednisone, IVIG, splenectomy, etc.) show response rates of 40-90%; main problem is lack of a durable response (See CID 1995;21:415). • Response to AZT may be dose-related; usually responds within 2-4 wks. Utility of other nucleoside analogs is unknown.
Severe hemorrhage	• Packed red cell/platelet transfusions **plus** prednisone 60-100 mg/d or IVIG 1 gm/kg on days 1, 2, 14, and then q 2-3 weeks	

Persistent symptomatic ITP	• AZT 600-1200 mg/day (in combination regimen) and HAART	• Usual AZT dose is 500-600 mg/day; doses of 1000-1200 mg/day are reserved for non-responders. Response is noted in 2-4 wks. Initial results with HAART shows good response (NEJM 1999;341:1239).
	• Discontinue drugs potentially responsible and avoid nonsteroidal anti-inflammatory agents	
	• Prednisone 30-60 mg/day with rapid taper to 5-10 mg/day	• Prednisone may be complicated by opportunistic infections, esp. thrush and herpes, and decreased CD4 count; only 10-20% have persistent response.
	• IVIG 400 mg/kg days 1, 2, 14 then q 2-3 wks or WinRho 25-50 µg/kg IV over 3-5 min, repeat at day 3-4 prn; may need maintenance therapy at 3-4 wk intervals using 6-25 µg/kg	• IVIG is highly effective in raising platelet count within 4 days, but is very expensive and median duration of response is only 3 weeks.
		• WinRho is an alternative to IVIG in Rh positive ITP patients. Advantages are 3-5 minute infusions, good safety profile and low cost (Blood 1991;77:1884).
	• Splenectomy	• Experience with splenectomy is variable; durability of response is variable, some claim risk of HIV progression is increased (Lancet 1987;2:342), and others claim good long-term results (Arch Surg 1989;124:625).
	• Splenic irradiation, danazol, vincristine, interferon	• Experimental or experience limited with all four.
Anemia	Treatment based on cause HIV: HAART	• Decreased production: Marrow infiltrating tumor (lymphoma, KS), infection (MAC, TB, CMV, parvovirus, B19, fungal-esp histoplasmosis), drugs (AZT, amphotericin, ganciclovir hydroxurea, pyrimethamine, interferon), anemia of chronic disease, deficiency states (Fe, folic acid, B12), HIV inhibition of precursors (see CID 2000;30:504).
		• Increased destruction (hemolysis) TTP, drugs (sulfonamides, dapsone or primaquine plus G6PD deficiency).
	Parvovirus B19: IVIG	• Parvovirus B19 - Marrow shows giant pronormoblasts with clumped basophilic chromatin and clear cytoplasmic vacuoles - diagnosis by in situ hybridization or PCR

V. Opportunistic Infections

Condition	Treatment	Comment
Hematologic Anemia (continued)	Guidelines for EPO therapy	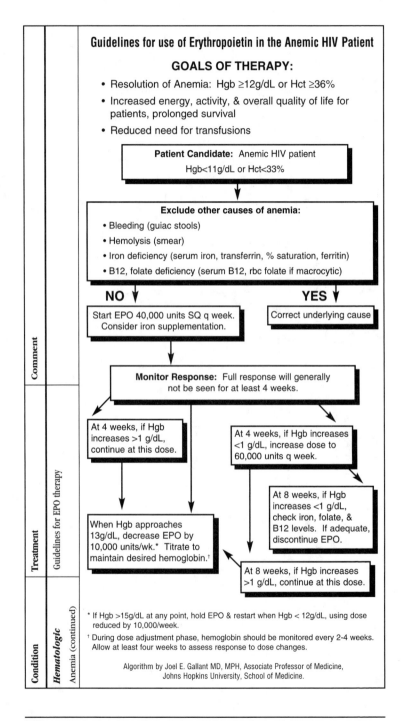

Guidelines for use of Erythropoietin in the Anemic HIV Patient

GOALS OF THERAPY:

- Resolution of Anemia: Hgb ≥12g/dL or Hct ≥36%
- Increased energy, activity, & overall quality of life for patients, prolonged survival
- Reduced need for transfusions

Patient Candidate: Anemic HIV patient
Hgb<11g/dL or Hct<33%

Exclude other causes of anemia:
- Bleeding (guiac stools)
- Hemolysis (smear)
- Iron deficiency (serum iron, transferrin, % saturation, ferritin)
- B12, folate deficiency (serum B12, rbc folate if macrocytic)

NO

Start EPO 40,000 units SQ q week. Consider iron supplementation.

YES

Correct underlying cause

Monitor Response: Full response will generally not be seen for at least 4 weeks.

At 4 weeks, if Hgb increases >1 g/dL, continue at this dose.

At 4 weeks, if Hgb increases <1 g/dL, increase dose to 60,000 units q week.

At 8 weeks, if Hgb increases <1 g/dL, check iron, folate, & B12 levels. If adequate, discontinue EPO.

When Hgb approaches 13g/dL, decrease EPO by 10,000 units/wk.* Titrate to maintain desired hemoglobin.†

At 8 weeks, if Hgb increases >1 g/dL, continue at this dose.

* If Hgb >15g/dL at any point, hold EPO & restart when Hgb < 12g/dL, using dose reduced by 10,000/week.

† During dose adjustment phase, hemoglobin should be monitored every 2-4 weeks. Allow at least four weeks to assess response to dose changes.

Algorithm by Joel E. Gallant MD, MPH, Associate Professor of Medicine, Johns Hopkins University, School of Medicine.

Neutropenia	• G-CSF (Neupogen) or GM-CSF (Prokine) 1-10 µg/kg/day SC; usual initial dose for G-CSF is 1 µg/kg/day with increases of 1 µg/kg/day at 5-7 day intervals to maintain ANC at 1000-2000/mm³, usual maintenance dose is 300 mg given 3-7x/week • HAART	• Drugs associated with neutropenia: AZT and ganciclovir; less common – 3TC, ddI, d4T, foscarnet, ribavirin, flucytosine, amphotericin, sulfonamides, pyrimethamine, pentamidine, anti-neoplastic agents and interferon. Discontinue implicated drug(s) when feasible. • HIV may cause neutropenia by inhibition of precursors (CID 2000;30:504) • Reported risk of infectious complications is variable; largest analysis showed higher risk for hospitalization with ANC <500 (Arch Intern Med 1997;157:1825). • G-CSF therapy: Monitor with CBC and diff 2x/wk and titrate up by 1 µg/kg/day or reduce dose 50% q week for maintenance to keep ANC >1000-2000/mL. Efficacy of G-CSF is established for elevating neutrophil count (NEJM 1987;317:593). • Concern with GM-CSF is possible increased HIV replication, but this is not substantiated in ≥3 trials. Dose recommendations are identical to those given for G-CSF but starting dose is 5 µg/kg/day.
Thrombotic thrombo-cytopenic purpura	• Prednisone 60-100 mg/day plus plasmapheresis	

V. Opportunistic Infections

Condition	Treatment	Comment
Tumors (JAIDS 1999;21:566) Kaposi's sarcoma **ACTG classification** (See Mayo Clin Proc 1995;70:869) *Good prognosis:* Lesions confined to skin and/or nodes; CD4 >150, no "B symptoms" *Poor prognosis:* Lesion associated edema, severe oral KS, visceral KS, CD4 <150, hx of OI, or "B symptoms"	*Local Therapy* • Topical liquid nitrogen • Intralesional vinblastine (0.01-0.002 mg/lesion) q 2 wks x 3 • Radiation (low dose, eg 400 rads q wk x 6 wks) • Laser *Systemic Therapy* • Liposomal daunorubicin (DaunoXome) 40-60 mg/m² IV q 2 wks or liposomal doxorubicin (Doxil) x 10-20 mg/m² • Taxol 100-135 mg/m² q 2-3 weeks • Adriamycin, bleomycin and either vincristine or vinblastine (ABV) • Vincristine/vinblastine • Bleomycin/vinca alkaloids • Alpha interferon (18-36 million IU/day) IM or SC x 10-12 wks then 18 million units/day – 36 million units 3x/wk • Experimental: Foscarnet (Scand J Infect Dis 1994;26:749); thalidomide (CID 1996;23:501); HAART; Intralesional B-human chorionic gonadotropin 2,000 U per lesion; retinoic acid isomers	• Restrict to few lesions that are small. • Restrict to few lesions that may be larger (>1 cm). • Skin - well tolerated; oral lesion - mucositis common. Best with localized lesions. • Laser, radiation, or vinblastine injection preferred for oral lesions. • Liposomal anthracyclines are alternatives to ABV chemotherapy that shows comparable clinical efficacy and reduced toxicity (AIDS 1996;10:515). • Systemic therapy is preferred for patients with widespread skin involvement (>25 lesions), extensive cutaneous KS that is nonresponsive to local treatment extensive edema, and/or symptomatic visceral organ involvement (especially lung KS) (Lancet 1995;346:26). Taxol is FDA-approved for KS. • Treatment is often limited by drug intolerance or myelosuppression. • Response rates better for patients with CD4 count >100/mm³; neutropenia common with AZT: Use G-CSF and/or discontinue AZT. • HHV-8 is susceptible to foscarnet, ganciclovir and cidofovir (J Clin Invest 1997;99:2082); role of antiviral agents in therapy is unclear. A retrospective analysis of patients with CMV disease showed foscarnet therapy was associated with a significant delay in progression of KS (JAIDS 1999;20:34); oral or IV ganciclovir given for CMV retinitis significantly reduced the frequency of KS (NEJM 1999;340:1063).

Condition	Treatment	Comments
Non-Hodgkin's lymphoma (NHL)	• Regimens containing methotrexate, bleomycin, doxorubicin, cyclophosphamide, adriamycin, vincristine and corticosteroids ± cranial radiation; standard regimens are CHOP and mBACOD + GM-CSF	• Low dose chemotherapy is as effective as standard dose (ACTG 142): methotrexate 200 mg/m², bleomycin 4 U/m², doxorubicin 25 mg/m², cyclophosphamide 300 mg/m², vincristine 1.4 mg/m², dexamethasone 3 mg/m² + GM-CSF 5 mcg/kg for ≥4 cycles. The AIDS Malignancy Consortium recommends low dose CHOP or low dose mBACOD based on this ACTG study (NEJM 1997;336:1641).
CNS lymphoma	• CNS lymphoma - cranial radiation plus high dose corticosteroids ± chemotherapy	• Many respond to radiation (J Neurosurg 1990;73:206), but average survival is only 2-5 months (Cancer 1994;73:2570).
Dermatologic complications Bacillary angiomatosis	• Erythromycin 500 mg po qid or doxycycline 200 mg/d x ≥3 mo	• See Bartonella pg. 129
Molluscum contagiosum	• Cryotherapy; electrosurgery; curettage, topical cantharidin or cidofovir • HAART	• Cidofovir appears to work when given IV or topically (Lancet 1999;353:2042).
Eosinophilic folliculitis	• Astemizole 10 mg qd + topical steroids • Ultraviolet light • Antihistamine	• Limited experience with oral agents: itraconazole 200 mg/d x 14-21 days, dapsone 100-200 mg/day, isotretinoin 1 mg/kg/day or metronidazole (Arch Derm 1995;131:1047; Arch Derm 1995;131:359). • Efficacy of UV light established (NEJM 1988;318:1183). • Only sedating antihistamines are useful.

V. Opportunistic Infections

Condition	Treatment	Comment
Staphylococcal folliculitis	Cephalexin or dicloxacillin 500 mg po qid x 7-21 days	• Add rifampin 600 mg/day x 7 days if severe or refractory. • Recurrent disease: chronic antibiotic (clindamycin 150 mg q d or TMP-SMX 1 DS q d) and/or nasal mupirocin.
Dermatophytic fungi	• Skin — Topical miconazole or clotrimazole. Refractory cases: ketoconazole 200 mg po/day x 1-3 mos. or itraconazole 100 mg/day • Nails — Griseofulvin 660 mg/day x 6-15 mos. or itraconazole 200 mg bid x 1 week/mo x 2 (fingernails) or 3-4 mos. (toenails) or terbinafine 250 mg/d x 6 weeks (fingernails) or 12 weeks (toenails)	• Ointments (micronazole and clotrimazole) are over the counter.
Scabies	• Permethrin cream 5% x 12 hrs. Repeat 3-7 days later. • Topical lindane (Kwell) • Ivermectin 200 mg x 1	• Must apply permethrin cream or Kwell to all skin surfaces.
Seborrhea	• Skin — Steroid cream (hydrocortisone 1%) ± precipitated sulfur (desonide cream) or topical ketoconazole applied bid • Scalp — Shampoos containing selenium sulfide, zinc pyrithiore, salicylic acid or coal tar applied 1x/day or ketoconazole shampoo 2x/week	• Use topical hydrocortisone (2.5%) until lesions resolve, then 1% for maintenance.

Gastrointestinal		
Anorexia	• Megace 400-800 mg qd • Dronabinol (Marinol) 2.5 mg po bid	• Weight gain is mostly fat. May lower testosterone levels leading to muscle wasting. • Synthetic THC, an active ingredient in marijuana. Weight gain is mostly fat.
Nausea/vomiting	• Compazine 5-10 mg po q 6-8h; Tigan 250 mg po q 6-8h; Dramamine 50 mg po q 6-8h; Ativan 0.025-0.05 mg/kg IV or IM; Haloperidol 1-5 mg bid po or IM; Ondansetron (Zofran) 0.2 mg/kg IV or IM; Dronabinol, 2.5-5 mg po bid	• Phenothiazines (Compazine, etc.), haloperidol, (Haldol), trimethobenzamide (Tigan), and metoclopramide (Reglan) may cause dystonia. • Consider medications as cause of nausea.

V. Opportunistic Infections

Condition	Treatment	Comment
Mouth		
Aphthous ulcers	• Mouth rinses with Mile's solution, dex-amethasone (0.5 mg/mL), Dyclone (10%), Benadryl or viscous lidocaine (2%)	• Mile's solution - 60 mg hydrocortisone, 20 cc mycostatin, 2 gm tetracycline, and 120 cc viscous lidocaine.
	• Topical fluocinonide (Lidex) 0.05% ointment mixed 1:1 with Orobase	• Lesions are considered major or minor on basis of size, depth and duration. Major lesions are >1 cm, deep, usually painful, usually persistent and often recur.
	• Decadron 0.5 mg/5 mL elixir mouth rinse 1-3x/day (multiple lesions)	
	• Thalidomide 200 mg po/day x 4-6 wks, then 100 mg 2x/wk	• Thalidomide is experimental for this indication, and there are strict restrictions for use in women, but initial results are good (NEJM 1997;337:1086; CID 1995;20:250; JID 1999;180:61).
	• Colchicine 1.5 mg/day (J Am Acad Derm 1994;31:459)	
	• Prednisone 40 mg po/day x 1-2 wks, then taper (severe or refractory cases)	
Oral hairy leukoplakia	• Acyclovir 800 mg po 5x/day x 2-3 wks, then 1.2-2 gm /day	• Most relapse and may require maintenance high-dose acyclovir.
	• Tretinoin (Retin A) .025-0.05% solution applied 2-3 x/day	• Famciclovir, valacyclovir, foscarnet, ganciclovir should be as effective as acyclovir.
		• Most lesions are asymptomatic and do not require treatment; relapses are common when acyclovir is discontinued.
Salivary gland enlargement	• Xerostomia: Sugarless gum and artificial saliva; pilocarpine for refractory cases	• CT scan will distinguish cystic and solid lesions (Laryngoscope 1988;98:772). Biopsy if malignancy is suspected. (Most are benign cystic lesions.)
	• Painful cystic lesions: Needle aspiration	• Fine needle aspirate permits microbiologic analysis and decompression.

Mouth (continued) Gingivitis/periodontitis	• Curettage and debridement of involved tissue + topical antiseptic such as povidine—iodine solution and chlorhexidine (Peridex) mouth rinses • Metronidazole 250 mg tid or 500 mg po bid x 7-14 days or clindamycin 300 mg tid x 7-14 days in selected cases	• Four phases: gingival erythema, necrotizing gingivitis, necrotizing peridontitis, and necrotizing stomatitis (Ann Intern Med 1996;125:485). • Usual presenting complaints are oral pain and bleeding.
Esophagitis *Candida*	• Fluconazole 200 mg po/d x 14-21 days	• Alternatives: Ketoconazole (less effective) (Ann Intern Med 1992;117:655); itraconazole (some fluconazole-resistant *Candida sp.* are sensitive) (ACC 1994;38:1530); amphotericin B systemically for refractory cases.
Cytomegalovirus	• Ganciclovir 5 mg/kg IV bid x 14-21 days or foscarnet 60 mg/kg/IV q 8h x 14-21 days	• For patients with complete response, discontinue after induction therapy and use maintenance only if there is relapse.
Herpes simplex	• Acyclovir 400-800 mg po 5x/day or 5 mg/kg IV tid x 7-10 days or Valacyclovir or Famciclovir	• Relatively rare cause of esophagitis
Aphthous ulcer	• Prednisone 40 mg/day po x 2 wks, then slow taper • Intralesional steroids • Thalidomide 200 mg po/day	• Thalidomide is considered experimental and there are strict restrictions for use in women, but efficacy is documented (BMJ 1989;289:432; NEJM 1997;337:1086; AIDS Res Human Retroviruses 1997;13:301; CID 1995;20:250; JID 1999;180:61).

V. Opportunistic Infections

Condition	Treatment	Comment
Diarrhea		
Specific microbial agent	See comment	*E. coli:* Travelers diarrhea – ciprofloxacin 500 mg po bid x 3 days
		C. jejuni: Ciprofloxacin 500 mg po bid x 3-5 days Erythromycin 250-500 mg po qid x 5 days
		C. difficile: Metronidazole 500 mg tid x 10-14 days Vancomycin 125 mg po qid x 10-14 days
		Salmonella: Ciprofloxacin 500 mg po bid x 14 days Cefotaxime 4-8 gm/day IV x 14 days
		E. histolytica: Metronidazole 500-750 mg IV or po tid x 5-10 days
		Giardia: Metronidazole 250 mg po tid x 5-10 days
	Salmonella	Cryptosporidia, isospora, microsporidia: See Table 5, pg. 110-111
Bacterial overgrowth	• Doxycycline (100 mg po bid), metronidazole (500-750 mg po bid) or amoxicillin-clavulanate (500 mg po qid)	• Diagnosis requires quantitative culture of small bowel aspirate or hydrogen breath test.
Symptomatic treatment	• Lomotil/loperamide/paregoric, etc. • Diet modification: low fat, no caffeine, no milk or milk products	• Utility of bismuth salts (Pepto-Bismol), indomethacin, and octreotide not known. • Protease inhibitors commonly cause diarrhea, especially nelfinavir - presumed mechanism is secretory (7th CROI, Abstract 62).

Cholangiopathy *Papillary stenosis*	• ERCP with sphincterotomy	• Presentation: RUQ pain, LFTs show cholestasis; diagnosis is established with ERCP. Sensitivity of ultrasound is 75-95%. • Usual causes are cryptosporidium (most common), microsporidia, CMV and cyclospora. About 20% are idiopathic. • Treatment directed against microbial pathogen is unsuccessful for cholangitis. • Improvement with ursodeoxycholic acid is reported in a small number of patients (Am J Med 1997;103:70).
Cholangiopathy without papillary stenosis	• Ursodeoxycholic acid 300 mg po tid (experience limited)	
Isolated bile duct stricture	• Endoscopic stenting	
Hepatitis C - HIV co-infection	• Hepatitis A vaccine if HAV seronegative • HCV therapy: alpha interferon, 3 million units SC 3x/week plus ribavirin, 1000-12000 mg po q d x 24-48 wks (Lancet 1999;351:1426).	• Diagnostic evaluation: See page 38 • Indications to treat: NIH Consensus (MMWR 1998;47[RR-19]: 1) Elevated ALT, 2) detectable HCV RNA and 3) biopsy showing bridging fibrosis or moderate inflammation and necrosis. Due to limited experience with HCV treatment of co-infected patients, these patients should participate in a clinical trial. • HIV promotes accelerated progression of HCV-associated liver disease (CID 1999;29:75).
Hepatitis B co-infection	• 3TC 150 mg bid (HIV) or 100 mg/day (HBV) • Interferon 30-35 mil units/wk x 4 mo.	• Efficacy of 3TC is well established and it is FDA approved for this indication (NEJM 1998;339:61). • HBV control may be achieved with HAART containing no agents with anti-HBV agents (NEJM 1999;340:1765). • 3TC + famciclovir (500 mg bid or tid) is sometimes used to decrease 3 TC resistance and is considered experimental.

V. Opportunistic Infections

Condition	Treatment	Comment
Pancreatitis		
Drug associated	D/C implicated drug	Most common – ddI, possible enhanced rate when ddI is combined with hydroxyurea. Others: pentamidine, sulfonamides and corticosteroids. Possible causes: INH, 3TC, rifampin, erythromycin, paromomycin, d4T and other NRTIs as a component of mitochondrial toxicity.
Infection (OIs)	Treat implicated agent	CMV; less common: MAI, TB, cryptosporidium; toxoplasmosis.
General causes	Tailor to cause	ETOH, hypertriglyceridemia, ERCP, morbid obesity, cholelithiasis.
Wasting (See pp. 362-364)	*Enteral feedings* • Polymeric formulas: Ensure, Sustecal, Enrich, Megnacal, etc. • Elemental formulas: Vivonex TEN	• Polymeric formulas: Non-prescription about $1.50/can; 10 cans/day required for total caloric needs. Usually not effective in wasting. • Elemental diet for severe malabsorption states; often due to cryptosporidia, microsporidia, or severe CMV infection. • Parenteral hyperalimentation: Rarely indicated except for devastating diarrhea due to cryptosporidiosis. • Caloric supplements in patients with stable weight do not lead to weight gain (JAIDS 1999;22:253).

Appetite Stimulants • Megace 400-800 mg/day • Dronabinol (Marinol) 2.5 mg po bid	• Recommended only if weight loss is due to reduced intake. • Megace: Weight gain is mostly fat. May lower testosterone levels, leading to impotence. • Dronabinol: Weight gain is mostly fat.
Anabolic steroids • Nandrolone 100-200 mg IM q 1-2 wks • Oxandrolone 20-40 mg/d po • Anadrol 100-150 mg/d po, up to 300 mg/d	• High anabolic effect and low androgenic effect. Most wt. gain is lean body mass. • Safety of nandrolone in women is established by experience with treatment of post-menopausal osteoporosis. • Oxandrolone shows highest weight gain of all treatments. • May reverse fat accumulation seen with protease inhibitors.
Testosterone • Testoderm scrotal patch 4 or 6 mg/day • Androderm patch 5 mg/d • Testoderm TTS patch 5 mg/d • Testerone enanthate or testerone cypionate 200-400 mg IM q 2 wks or 100-200 mg IM q week by self injection	• Testosterone is available for oral, injectable, or transdermal use. Oral compounds have been associated with liver toxicity and should be avoided; IM injections consist of an ester in oil that extend half-life to permit weekly or biweekly administration; the transdermal scrotal patch is changed daily and worn 22 hours/day. • Serum testosterone levels <450 ng/dL are associated with decreased libido. Drugs associated with decreased testosterone levels are megesterol, ketoconazole, and cimetidine. • High androgenic and anabolic effect with improved mood; increased libido, energy, appetite and lean body mass. • About 50% of men with AIDS have hypogonadism (J Clin 1996;81:4051). Testosterone is most effective in these cases (NEJM 1999;340:1740). Optimal results are achieved when testosterone is combined with a resistance exercise program (JAMA 2000;283:763).

V. Opportunistic Infections

Condition	Treatment	Comment
Wasting (continued)	• Resistance exercise: 20-120 min/d x 3/wk	• Effective in increasing lean body mass; preliminary results suggest efficacy reversing the fat accumulation syndrome ascribed to protease inhibitors (AIDS 1999;13:1373).
	Cytokine suppression • Thalidomide (Thalomid) 100 mg po/day, up to 300 mg/day • Pentoxifyline (Trentol)	• Experimental; interest is based on possible suppression of TNF; efficacy established for tuberculosis and promising in three unpublished controlled trials for AIDS patients. • Pentoxifyline: Usually not effective.
	• Growth hormone (Serostim) 6 mg SC qd x 12 wks	• Most weight gain is lean body mass. • Disadvantages are high cost ($1,750/wk), need for injection and side effects. • Alternative regimen is for administration for 2 weeks at the time of OIs (AIDS 1999;13:1195). • May reverse fat accumulation (may make fat loss worse) seen with protease inhibitors (AIDS 1999;13:2099).

Pain (See Medical Letter 1993;35:1-6)	• ASA, acetaminophen, 325-650 mg q 4h • Nosteroidal anti-inflammatory agents (Motrin 200-400 mg q 6h; Naprosyn 230-375 q 6-8 h) • Codeine 30-60 mg q 4-6h po SC or IM • Meperidine 50-150 mg q 3-4h po, SC, IM, IV • Methadone 2.5-10 mg q 6-8 h po, 10 mg IM • Dilaudid 2-8 mg q 4-8h po or rectal; 20-60 mg po • MS Contin 15-60 mg po bid • Nortriptyline 25-75 mg qd hs • Fentanyl patch 25-100 mcg/hr • Ultram (tramadol) 50-100 mg q 4-6 h, up to 400 mg/day	• Severe pain is best relieved with opioids. • Chronic pain is best treated with nonopioid initially (ASA, acetaminophen, ibuprofen, nortriptyline). • Dependence liability for opioids. • Side effects of opioids: sedation, constipation, respiratory depression, nausea and vomiting. • Oral codeine, propoxyphene (Darvon) and pentazocine in usual doses are no more effective than ASA. Morphine, dilaudid, methadone, levorphanol, fentanyl and large doses of oxycodone are needed for severe pain. • Morphine and other full agonists have no limit on analgesic effectiveness except for the limit ascribed to side effects.
Psychiatric & Sleep Disorders Anxiety	• Buspirone (BuSpar) 5 mg tid	• Nonbenzodiazepine-nonbarbiturate; dependence liability negligible; increase dose 5 mg q 2-4 days to effective daily dose of 15-30 mg. • Major side effects are nausea, nervousness, insomnia, weight loss, dry mouth, constipation; insomnia may be treated with Desyrel 25-50 mg hs. • Nortriptyline: Titrate level (70-125 mg/dL) promotes sleep Desipramine (<125 ng/dL); promotes sleep

V. Opportunistic Infections

Condition	Treatment	Comment
Psychiatric & Sleep Disorders (continued))		
Depression	• Fluoxetine (Prozac) 10 mg increasing to ave. 20 mg qd	• Major side effects are nausea, nervousness, insomnia, weight loss, dry mouth, constipation; insomnia may be treated with Desyrel 25-50 mg hs.
	• Nortriptyline (Pamelor) 10-25 mg hs increasing to 50-150 mg hs or desipramine (Norpramin) 10-25 mg hs increasing to 50-200 mg hs	• Nortriptyline: Titrate level (70-125 mg/dL) promotes sleep Desipramine (<125 ng/dL); promotes sleep
	• Sertraline (Zoloft) 25-50 mg qd increasing to 50-150 mg/d	• Side effects are similar to those noted for Prozac, but are less severe due to shorter half-life
	• Paroxetine (Paxil) 20-50 mg po/d	• Promotes sleep: initial dose is 20 mg/d; increase by 10 mg increments
	• Bupropion (Wellbutrin) 150 mg bid of SR formulation	• Initial dose is 150 mg bid; increase to 300 mg/day after 3 days, as necessary
	• Nefazodone (Serzone) 100 mg bid increasing to 300-600 mg/d	• Promotes sleep
Delirium	• Haldol (0.5-1 mg) hs	
Insomnia	• Diphenhydramine (Benadryl) 25-50 mg hs	• Non-prescription.
	• Trazodone (Desyrel) 25-100 mg po hs	
	• Chloral hydrate 500-1000 mg po hs	• Class IV, but often considered one of the safest and least habit-forming sedatives
	• Ambien 5-10 mg hs	
	• Nortriptyline or amitriptyline 25-50 mg hs	

Apathy	• Ritalin 5-10 mg tid	• Utility is not well confirmed
Substance Abuse	1. Detoxification: Sometimes with long acting benzodiazepines 2. Treatment of co-morbid conditions: mental health (depression, bipolar disorder, schizophrenia, personality disorders, etc.), medical conditions, and chronic pain syndromes. 3. Maintenance treatment and relapse prevention: Individualized to patient need	
Terminal Illness	• Morphine or other opioids orally or parenterally; • MS Contin (continuous release morphine) po 15, 30, 60 or 100 mg; usual dose is 15-60 mg po q 12h • Patient-controlled analgesia (PCA) for morphine • Methadone (above doses) • Fentanyl Patch	• Patients given opioids for acute pain or cancer pain rarely experience euphoria and rarely develop psychic dependence; clinically significant physical dependence develops after several weeks with large doses.

V. Opportunistic Infections

VI. Drugs: Guide To Information

Listings are alphabetical by generic name.

Trade name and pharmaceutical company source are provided unless there are multiple providers.

Cost is based on average wholesale price according to Medi Span, Hospital Formulary Pricing Guide, February 1999. Prices are often provided for generic and trade-name products for comparison.

Pharmacology, side effects, and drug interactions: Data are from Drug Information - 1998, American Hospital Formulary Service, Bethesda, MD, pp. 37-612, 1998; PDR-1998; and Drug Evaluations Subscription (three volumes), AMA, Chicago, IL 1996.

Creatinine clearance

> Males: Weight (kg) x (140-age in years)/
>   72x serum creatinine (mg/dL)

> Females: Determination for males x 0.85

Note:

1. Obese patients - use lean body weight.

2. Formula assumes stable renal function. Assume CrCl of 5-8 mL/min for patients with anuria or oliguria.

3. Pregnancy and volume expansion: GFR may be increased in third trimester of pregnancy and with massive parenteral fluids.

Classification of controlled substance:

Category	Interpretation
I	**High potential for abuse and no current accepted medical use.** Examples are heroin and LSD.
II	**High potential for abuse.** Use may lead to severe physical or psychological dependence. Examples are opioids, amphetamines, short-acting barbiturates, and preparations containing small quantities of codeine. Prescriptions must be written in ink or typewritten and signed by the practitioner. Verbal prescriptions must be confirmed in writing within 72 hours and may be given only in a genuine emergency. No renewals are permitted.
III	**Some potential for abuse.** Use may lead to low-to-moderate physical dependence or high psychological dependence. Examples are barbiturates and preparations containing small quantities of codeine. Prescriptions may be oral or written. Up to five renewals are permitted within six months.
IV	**Low potential for abuse.** Examples include chloral hydrate, phenobarbital, and benzodiazepines. Use may lead to limited physical or psychological dependence. Prescriptions may be oral or written. Up to five renewals are permitted within six months.
V	**Subject to state and local regulation.** Abuse potential is low; a prescription may not be required. Examples are antitussive and antidiarrheal meds containing limited quantities of opioids.

Classification for use in pregnancy based on FDA categories: Ratings range from "A" for drugs that have been tested for teratogenicity under controlled conditions without showing evidence of damage to the fetus, to "D" and "X" for drugs that are definitely teratogenic. The "D" rating is generally reserved for drugs with no safer alternatives. The "X" rating means there is absolutely no reason to risk using the drug in pregnancy.

Category	Interpretation
A	**Controlled studies show no risk.** Adequate, well-controlled studies in pregnant women have failed to demonstrate risk to the fetus.
B	**No evidence or risk in humans.** Either animal findings show risk, but human findings do not; or, if no adequate human studies have been done, animal findings are negative.
C	**Risk cannot be ruled out.** Human studies are lacking, and animal studies are either positive for fetal risk, or lacking as well. However, potential benefits may justify the potential risk.
D	**Positive evidence of risk.** Investigational or post-marketing data show risk to the fetus. Nevertheless, potential benefits may outweigh the potential risk.
X	**Contraindicated in pregnancy.** Studies in animals or humans, or investigational or post-marketing reports, have shown fetal risk which clearly outweighs any possible benefit to the patient.

Pregnancy registry for antiretroviral drugs: This is a joint project sponsored by staff from pharmaceutical companies with an advisory panel with representatives from the CDC, NIH obstetrical practitioners and pediatricians. The registry allows anonymity of patients and birth outcome follow-up is obtained by registry staff. Healthcare professionals should report prenatal exposures to antiretroviral agents to: Antiretroviral Pregnancy Registry, 155 N. Third Street, Suite 306, Wilmington, NC 28401; (800) 258-4263; fax (800) 800-1052.

Patient assistance programs: Usual requirements are lack of a prescription drug plan (including state plans and Ryan White funds) plus income/asset criteria.

VI. Drugs

ABACAVIR (ABC)

Trade name: Ziagen (Glaxo Wellcome)

Form and price: 300 mg tabs @$4.65/tab or $3,540/year, oral suspension with 20 mg/mL

Usual regimen: 300 mg tabs po bid (no food restrictions)

Class: Nucleoside analog

Trials: With monotherapy, abacavir reduced viral load 1.5-2 logs—significantly more than other nucleosides.

The first major comparative trial was CNA 3003 (ABC/AZT/3TC vs. AZT/3TC) in 173 treatment naïve patients with CD4 >100/mm[3]. At 24 weeks 70% of those in the three drug arm had VL <400 c/mL, and the average increase in CD4 count was 86/mm[3]. This was significantly better than results in the AZT/3TC arm. The response at 48 weeks was sustained; however, a subset analysis of participants with baseline viral loads of >100,000/mL demonstrated that only 33% achieved undetectable virus (Fischl M et al, 6th Conference on Retroviruses and Opportunistic Infections, Chicago, 1999, Abstract #16).

CNA 3005 compared the triple NRTI regimen (ABC/AZT/3TC) with indinavir/AZT/3TC in 562 treatment naïve patients. At 48 weeks 51% in both groups had achieved VL <400 c/mL by intent-to-treat analysis. Only 31% receiving the ABC regimen with a baseline VL >100,000 c/mL had reduction to <400 c/mL compared to 45% in the IDV arm (S. Staszewski, ICAAC 9/99, Abstract 505). There was comparable immune restoration in the two groups with median CD4 count increases of about 140/mm[3]. Genotypic resistance analysis of HIV strains from failures usually showed wild-type virus or the RT codon 184 mutation (7th CROI, Abstract 331).

In nucleoside experienced patients, the efficacy of ABC has been disappointing. In the expanded access program that included 2,200 patients who failed standard therapy with two nucleosides plus a PI and had CD4 counts <100/mm[3] and viral loads >30,000 c/mL, only 25% experienced a reduction in viral load of ≥0.5 log with the addition of abacavir. In study 3002 patients receiving any prior regimen with VL 500-50,000 c/mL had their regimens "intensified" with ABC. At eight weeks 39% of ABC recipients had VL <400 c/mL. There was no difference between those with or without prior 3TC experience or the M184V mutation.

CNA 2006 was a non-randomized study of ABC/APV in treatment-naïve patients with CD4 counts >400/mm[3]. By intent-to-treat analysis at 72 wks, 68% had VL <50 c/mL and 40% had VL <5 c/mL. The mean CD4 count increase was 239/mm[3] (7th CROI, Abstract 336).

CNA 2007 involved the use of ABC/amprenavir (APV)/efavirenz (EFV) as a salvage regimen for patients with VL >500 despite PI containing regimens for >20 weeks. At 16 weeks 26% achieved VL <400 by intent-to-treat analysis. The best results were seen in patients with low VL at entry and in patients naïve to NNRTIs.

The Swiss Cohort Study examined patients who responded to PI containing regimens and were then randomized to continue the PI regimen or switch to a triple NRTI regimen with ABC/AZT/3TC. At 48 wks VL and CD4 count responses were comparable in both groups, and blood lipid profiles were better in the triple NRTI group (7th CROI, Abstract 457).

In summary, ABC is a potent NRTI, although experience with combination treatment using antiretroviral drugs other than AZT/3TC is limited. The "triple nuke" regimen is an appropriate option for initial therapy in selected patients, with the advantages of preserved options, probable reduction in lipodystrophy and convenient dosing regimen. A possible disadvantage is reduced potency in patients with high baseline viral loads. ABC does not appear to be effective as a component of salvage therapy in patients with extensive NRTI experience. Some authorities advocate the addition of ABC to the regimens containing AZT + 3TC, sine this increases potency with minimal risk of increased resistance. Others would advocate reserving ABC for early intensification in the event of viral rebound.

In vitro activity: The IC_{50} vs. HIV-1 is 0.07-1.0 μM. There is synergy when ABC is combined with amprenavir, nevirapine and AZT; activity is additive when ABC is combined with ddI, 3TC, d4T and ddC.

Resistance: Mutations at the following codons on the RT gene confer resistance: 65, 74, 115, and 184. There is one-way cross resistance with 3TC, ddI and ddC. Each of these mutations results in a 2-4 fold decrease in susceptibility; significant resistance requires ≥2 mutations. Clinical trials indicate that AZT resistance with ≥3 mutations predicts ABC failure. These trials also show that the M184V mutation does not preclude response to ABC *per se*, but mutations at codon 184 combined with mutations at 65, 74 or ≥3 AZT resistance mutations are associated with high rates of failure.

Indications: See Chapter 4

Pharmacology

> **Bioavailability:** 83%; alcohol increases ABC levels 41%.

> **T½:** 1.5 hours (serum); intercellular T½–3.3 hrs. CSF levels: 27-33% serum levels

> **Elimination:** 81% metabolized by alcohol dehydrogenase and glucuronyl transferase with renal excretion of metabolites; 16% recovered in stool and 1% unchanged in urine. (Metabolism does not involve the P450 pathway).

> **Dose modification in renal failure:** None

Side effects: Hypersensitivity reaction: A serious and potentially lethal side effect is noted in 2-3% of patients. Clinical features include fever (usually 39-40°C), skin rash (maculopapular or urticarial), fatigue, malaise, GI symptoms (nausea, vomiting, diarrhea, abdominal pain), arthralgias cough and/or dyspnea. Some patients do not develop the rash. Laboratory changes may include increased CPK, elevated liver function tests and lymphopenia. These clinical and laboratory findings usually occur within the first 6 weeks of therapy. Possibly drug-related lethal hypersensitivity reactions were reported in up to 8 of 13,000 recipients for a mortality of ≤0.05%. Rechallenge has been associated with definite drug-associated mortality in two patients. Hypersensitivity reactions should be reported to the Abacavir Hypersensitivity Registry at (800) 270-0425. Patients should be warned to stop ABC if they note skin rash + fever, typical GI symptoms, cough, dyspnea or constitutional symptoms. A warning sheet is available from pharmacists. Other side effects include nausea, vomiting, malaise, headache, diarrhea, or anorexia. Rare patients may develop lactic acidoses with or without steatosis.

Drug interactions: Alcohol increases ABC levels 41%; no effect on alcohol levels.

Pregnancy: Class C. Rodent teratogen test showed skeletal malformations and anasarea at 35x the comparable human dose. Placental passage positive in rats.

ACYCLOVIR

Generic

Trade name: Zovirax (Glaxo Wellcome)

Forms and price:

> 200 mg caps – $0.34/cap
> 400 mg tabs – $0.62/tab
> 800 mg tabs – $1.26/tab
> 200 mg/5 cc suspension – $93.55/473 mL or $0.82/200 mg
> 500 mg and 1 gm vials (IV) – $52.80/500 mg
> 5% ointment, 3 gm – $20.43; 15 gm – $47.33 (utility limited)

Class: Synthetic nucleoside analog derived from guanine

Annual cost cap: Eligible patients whose use exceeds 552 gm in <1 year may receive free drug up to additional 620 gm; call (800) 722-9294.

Patient assistance program: (800) 722-9294. Eligibility based on lack of third party drug coverage, monthly income criteria using Medicaid guidelines, and asset information; forms are reviewed on an individual case basis.

Indications and dose: (Regimens suggested are based on PDR 1998; MMWR 1993;42 [RR-14]: 1; Strauss S, Whitely R. Inf Dis Clin Pract 1992;2:100; and clinical trials - JAMA 1991;264:747; NEJM 1983;308:916; NEJM 1986;314:144; NEJM 1989;320:293; NEJM 1991;325:551; Ann Intern Med 1992;117:358):

HSV* **First episode genital** 400 mg po q 8 h x 10-14 days or 5 mg/kg IV q 8 h x 5-7 days. Up to 800 mg 5x/day po or 15 mg/kg/day IV for severe or retractory cases.

> **Recurrent:** 400 mg po tid or 800 mg po bid x 5 days; AIDS patients may require higher doses.

Perirectal: 400 mg po 5x/day x 10 days

Progressive mucocutaneous: 5-10 mg/kg IV q 8 h x 7-14 days

Prophylaxis: 400 mg po bid (this is standard dose in immunocompetent patients); 400 mg po 3-5x/day may be required by AIDS patients. Prophylaxis is contraindicated in pregnancy.

Acyclovir-resistant: Doses up 800 mg 5x/day po or 10 mg/kg IV q 8 h or by constant infusion (or foscarnet, 40 mg/kg IV q8h)

> **Note:** There is a good correlation between *in vitro* activity and *in vivo* response. Probability of failure with acyclovir-resistant strains using standard doses of acyclovir is 95% (AAC 1994;38:1246). Valacyclovir or famciclovir are frequently preferred agents for oral treatment of HSV or VZV.

VZV* **Chickenpox:** 800 mg po 5x/day x 7- 10 days

Dermatomal zoster: 10 mg/kg IV q 8 h x 7 days or 800 mg po 5x/ day x 7 days. (Famciclovir or valacyclovir are preferred for oral therapy of shingles due to better efficacy or levels.)

Disseminated zoster: 10 mg/kg IV q 8 h x 7 days

Acyclovir-resistant: Foscarnet (40 mg/kg IV q 8 h)

> **Note:** Varicella vaccine is a live-virus vaccine and is contraindicated in HIV-infected people.

EBV **Oral hairy leukoplakia:** 800 mg po 5x/day x 2-3 weeks, then 1.2-2.0 gm/day. (Most cases are not treated and those that are usually relapse after treatment. Ganciclovir is also effective.)

* Acyclovir or other antiviral agent should be started within 24 hours of the exanthem with HSV and within four days or while new lesions are still forming with dermatomal zoster.

Pharmacology

Bioavailability: 15-20% with oral administration

T½: 2.5-3.3 hours, CSF levels: 50% serum levels

Elimination: Renal

Table 6-1: Acyclovir - Dose Modification In Renal Failure:

Usual dose	Creatinine clearance	Adjusted dose
200 mg 5x/day	>10 mL/min <10 mL/min	200 mg 5x/day 200 mg q 12 h
800 mg 5x/day	>50 mL/min 10-50 mL/min <10 mL/min	800 mg 5x/day 800 mg q 8 h 800 mg q 12 h
5-10 mg/kg IV q 8 h	>50 mL/min 10-50 mL/min <10 mL/min	5-10 mg/kg IV q 8 h 5-10 mg/kg q 12-24 h 5-10 mg/kg q 24 h

Side effects (Infrequent and rarely severe): irritation at infusion site, rash, nausea and vomiting, diarrhea, renal toxicity (especially with rapid IV infusion, prior renal disease, and concurrent nephrotoxic drugs), dizziness, abnormal liver function tests, itching, and headache. Rare complications include: CNS toxicity with encephalopathy, disorientation, seizures, hallucinations, anemia, neutropenia, thrombocytopenia, and hypotension.

Pregnancy: Category C: Not teratogenic, but potential to cause chromosomal damage at high doses. Burroughs Wellcome CDC Registry shows no increased incidence of fetal abnormalities among 601 women for whom pregnancy outcome data were available (MMWR 1993;42:806). The Registry may be reached at (800) 258-4263. The CDC recommends use of acyclovir during pregnancy only for life-threatening disease.

Drug interactions: Increased meperidine effect; probenecid prolongs half-life of acyclovir.

Table 6-2: Comparison of Drugs for Infections Caused by Herpes Simplex and Varicella Zoster (see NEJM 1999;340:1255)

	Duration	Acyclovir	Valacyclovir	Famciclovir	Other
Herpes simplex					
Genital					
First episode	7-10 days	400 mg tid	1 gm bid	250 mg tid	—
Recurrent	5 days	400 mg tid	500 mg bid	125 mg bid	—
Suppression	years	400 mg bid	500 mg qd or 500 mg bid	125-250 mg bid	—
Severe disease	≥5 days	5-10 mg/kg/d q 8h IV	1 gm tid	—	—
Perirectal	7-10 days	800 mg tid	—	—	—
Oral lesions					
Treatment	5 days	200 mg 5x/day	—	—	Penciclovir topical
Prophylaxis	—	400 mg bid	—	—	—
Mucocutaneous progressive	7-14 d	400 mg 5x/d 5 mg/kg q 8h IV	1 gm tid	—	—
Acyclovir-resistant	—	—	—	—	Cidofovir,* Foscarnet,* Topical trifluridine*
Varicella zoster					
Zoster-dermatomal	7 days	800 mg 5x/d 10 mg/kg q 8h IV	1 gm tid	500 mg tid	—
Zoster-disseminated	7 days	10 mg/kg q 8h IV	—	—	—
Acyclovir-resistant	—	—	—	—	Foscarnet

* HSV resistant or refractory to treatment with acyclovir may be treated with topical or intravenous cidofovir (JID 1997;176:892; AAC 1995;39:2120; CID 1994;18:570), topical trifluridine (JAIDS 1996;12:147) or foscarnet (NEJM 1991;325:551).

ALBENDAZOLE

Trade name: Albenza (SmithKline Beecham)

Form: 200 mg tablets; $1.00/200 mg tab available from SmithKline (800) 877-7074

Dose: 400-800 mg po bid x ≥3 weeks, usually 400 mg po/d x 3 weeks

Clinical Trials: Albendazole (400 mg bid x 3 weeks) is highly effective with microsporidiosis involving *Encephalitozoon (Septata) intestinalis*, but is less effective or not effective for *Enterocytozoon bienusi*.

Indication: Microsporidiosis

Pharmacology

> **Bioavailability:** Low, but absorption is increased 5-fold if taken with a fatty meal versus administration in a fasting state. Should be taken with fatty meal.

> **T½:** 8 hours

> **Elimination:** Metabolized in liver to albendazole sulfoxide, then excreted by enterophepatic circulation.

> **Dose modification in renal failure:** None

Side effects: Hepatotoxicity and reversible pancytopenia or neutropenia- monitor CBC and liver function tests at least every two weeks.

Pregnancy: Category C. Albendazole is teratogenic and embryotoxic in rodents.

ALPRAZOLAM

Trade name: Xanax (Upjohn)

Forms and price (Generic form): 0.25 mg tab – $0.06; 0.5 mg tab – $0.06; 1 mg tab – $0.09; 2 mg tab - $0.15

Class: Benzodiazepine, controlled substance category IV

Indications and dose regimen:

> **Anxiety:** 0.25-0.5 mg tid; increase if necessary at intervals of 3-4 days to maximum of 4 mg/day.

> **Panic disorder:** 0.5 mg tid with increase at increments of ≥1 mg/day to maximum of 6-10 mg/day

> **Dose reduction or withdrawal:** Decrease by ≥0.5 mg q 3 days; some suggest decrease by 0.25 mg at 3-7 intervals

Pharmacology

> **Bioavailability:** >90%

T½: 11 hours, prolonged with obesity and hepatic dysfunction

Elimination: Metabolized and renally excreted

Side effects: See Benzodiazepines (page 175). Seizures, delirium, and withdrawal symptoms with rapid dose reduction or abrupt discontinuation. Withdrawal symptoms at 18 hours to three days after abrupt discontinuation. Seizures usually occur at 24-72 hours after abrupt withdrawal.

Pregnancy: Category D; fetal harm – contraindicated; possible role in cleft lip and heart abnormalities.

Drug interactions: Additive CNS depression with other CNS depressants including alcohol. Disulfiram and cimetidine prolong the half-life of alprazolam. Levels of apra-zolam are increased by some protease inhibitors, but concurrent use is not indicated.

Relative contraindications: History of serious mental illness, drug abuse, alcoholism, open-angle glaucoma, seizure disorder, severe liver disease.

AMPHOTERICIN B

Trade name: Fungizone (Bristol-Myers Squibb—oral form); Parental form—generic

Forms and price: 50 mg vials at $38.55/vial; Amphotericin B oral suspension with 100 mg/mL in 24 mL bottles at $25.20/24 mL bottle (1 wk supply)

Class: Amphoteric polyene macrolide with activity against nearly all pathogenic and opportunistic fungi.

Indications and regimens:

Oral suspension for thrush: 1-5 mL qid; use calibrated dropper to place directly on tongue, then swish "as long as reasonably possible," then swallow.

Pharmacology

Bioavailability: Absorption is nil - serum levels of 0.05 µg/mL with 400-600 mg po/d; CSF levels - 3% of serum concentrations

T½: 24 hours, detected in blood and urine up to four weeks after discontinuation

Elimination: Serum levels in urine; metabolic pathways are unknown.

Dose adjustment in renal failure: None

Table 6-3: Systemic (intravenous) Amphotericin B

Condition	Daily dose	Total dose	Comment
Aspergillus	0.5-1.5 mg/kg	30-40 mg/kg	±Flucytosine
Candida stomatitis esophagitis line sepsis disseminated	0.3-0.5 mg/kg 0.3-0.5 mg/kg 0.3-0.5 mg/kg 0.3-0.8 mg/kg	200-500 mg 200-500 mg 200-500 mg 20-40 mg/kg	Reserved for refractory cases
Coccidioidomycosis	0.5-1.0 mg/kg	30-40 mg/kg	Maintenance with fluconazole, itraconazole, ketoconazole, or Ampho B 1 mg/kg weekly
Cryptococcosis	0.5-1.0 mg/kg usually 0.7 mg/kg	500-1000 mg	Maintenance with fluconazole, itraconazole, or Ampho B 0.6-1 mg/kg once or twice weekly
Histoplasmosis	0.5-1.0 mg/kg	30-40 mg/kg	Maintenance with itraconazole or Ampho B 1 mg/kg weekly

Administration: Oral form-see above. IV form - Slow infusion; first dose is 1 mg in 350 mL 5% dextrose given over 2-4 hours with monitoring of vital signs q 30 min x 4 hours. Subsequent dose may be increased to 0.3 mg/kg at four hours after test dose and given over 2-6 hours; then daily maintenance doses are given. Alternatively, less serious infections may be treated with daily or periodic increases in dose by 5 mg/day or conversion to double doses on alternative days. The daily dose should never exceed 1.5 mg/kg, and monitoring should include CBC, serum creatinine, and serum electrolytes. There is no reason to protect infusions from sunlight.

Side effects: Oral form: rash, GI intolerance and allergic reactions. Toxicity with IV form is dose-related and less severe with slow administration.

1. Chills, usually 1-3 hours post infusion and lasting up to four hours post infusion. Reduce with hydrocortisone (10-50 mg added to infusion, but only if necessary due to immunosuppression); alternatives that are now often preferred are meperidine, ibuprofen, or napofam prior to infusion. A randomized trial showed nafopam (0.3 mg/kg IV over 60 seconds) was more effective than meperidine (0.7 mg/kg) (Arch Intern Med 1997;157:1589).

2. Hypotension, nausea, vomiting, usually 1-3 hours post infusion - may be reduced with compazine.

3. Nephrotoxicity in 80% ± nephrocalcinosis, potassium wasting, renal tubular acidosis. Reduce with gradual increase in dose, adequate hydration, avoidance of concurrent nephrotoxic drugs, and possibly, sodium loading. Discontinue or reduce dose with BUN >40 mg/dL and creatinine >3 mg/dL.

4. Hypokalemia, hypomagnesemia and hypocalcemia corrected with supplemental K+, Mg++, and Ca++.

5. Normocytic normochromic anemia with average decrease of 9% in hematocrit.

6. Phlebitis and pain at infusion sites—add 1,200-1,600 units of heparin to infusate.

Pregnancy: Category B; harmless in experimental animal studies, but no data for patients.

Drug interactions: Increased nephrotoxicity with concurrent use of nephrotoxic drugs – aminoglycosides, cisplatin, cyclosporine, methoxyflurane, vancomycin; increased hypokalemia with corticosteroids and diuretics.

AMPHOTERICIN B
Alternative Preparations

New preparations of amphotericin B include:

Abelcet (The Liposome Co.): Amphotericin B complexed with 2 phospholipids—DMPC and DMPG

Amphotec (Sequus Pharmaceuticals, Inc.): Amphotericin B colloidal dispersion with cholesterol sulfate

AmBisome Liposomal amphotericin B is a true liposomal delivery system.

Advantages: Compared to amphotericin B in D5W, the newer formulations are advocated primarily to reduce nephrotoxicity and reduce infusion-related reactions (NEJM 1999;340:764). Improved efficacy is demonstrated in some animal models of fungal infections, and three clinical trials of variable quality: one trial with Amphotec for aspergillosis (Blood 1996;88(Suppl 11):302a); one study of Abelcet for aspergillosis (Blood 1995;13:849a) and one double blind trial of AmBisome vs amphotericin B in febrile neutropenic patients that showed higher rates of breakthrough candidemia and aspergillosis in amphotericin recipients (NEJM 1999;340:764). This latter report comparing AmBisome and amphotericin B in 677 patients treated empirically for fever and neutropenia showed a statistically significant reduction in the frequency of chills (38% vs 74%), fever >1°C (17% vs 44%), and nephrotoxicity with creatinine increases to >2x baseline (19% vs 34%) favoring AmBisome. In a therapeutic trial of amphotericin B vs. AmBisome in AIDS patients with histoplasmosis, AmBisome recipients had fewer adverse reactions and more rapid defervescence (7th CROI, Abstract 232). Pharmacokinetic studies show high concentrations of amphotericin B in spleen and liver with Abelcet and Amphotec. Penetration across the blood brain barrier appears reduced due to large size; these drugs should be used with caution in patients with CNS infections. A major deterrent to use is the high price of these drugs compared to conventional amphotericin B.

Table 6-4: Comparision of Amphotericin B Preparations

Comparison	Ampho B	Abelcet	Amphotec	AmBisome
Dose Forms	**50 mg vial**	**100 mg vial**	**50+100 mg vials**	**50 mg vials**
Cost/unit Average dose Cost/dose	$38.55/50 mg 50 mg $38	$194/100 mg $350 mg $776	$160/100 mg 300 mg-400 mg $480-$640	$188.40/50 mg 200-400 mg $750-$1,500
Dose (FDA recommended dose)	0.7-1.0 mg/kg/d	5 mg/kg/day	3-4 mg/kg/d + increase to 6 mg/kg	3-5 mg/kg/d
Infusion rate (infusion duration)	0.2-0.4 mg/kg/hr (2-5 hr)	2.5 mg/kg/hr (2 hr)	1 mg/kg/hr (3-4 hr)	1.5-2.5 mg/kg/hr (2 hr)
ADRs*				
Chills	55%	15-20%	50-70%	18%
Fever >1°C	40%	10-20%	10-20%	7%
Creatinine rise ≥2x baseline	30-40%	15-20%	10-20%	19%
Hypotension	5-10%	5-10%	5-10%	4%
Hypokalemia ≤2.5/mL	12%	5%	10%	7%
Test dose	Advocated	Not Advocated	Advocated	Not advocated

* Frequencies of adverse drug reactions (ADR's) cannot be accurately compared because results are not from comparative trials except for AmBisome vs. amphotericin B (NEJM 1999;340:764).

Conclusions regarding formulations of amphotericin B:

1. *The lipid complex preparations permit delivery of high doses over short periods without serious drug toxicity.* They would be preferred to conventional amphotericin B for virtually all systemic mycoses if the prices were comparable.

2. Many authorities conclude that AmBisome, Abelset, and Amphotec are *comparable to each other in efficacy*; Abelcet may have increased rates of ADRs.

3. Use in hospitalized patients may be regulated due to high cost. *Indications* justifying cost are controversial; some suggest the following criteria for use:

   a. Creatinine clearance decreasing 25-50% with amphotericin B, especially with pre-existing renal failure or concurrent risks of nephrotoxicity-diabetes, aminoglycoside therapy, etc.

   b. Inability to maintain serum K concentration >3.0 mEq/mL.

   c. Intolerable infusion-related adverse reactions.

   d. Therapeutic failure with amphotericin.

4. *Drug distribution* does not appear to be problematic. Studies with Abelcet and AmBisome show these drugs are comparable to amphotericin B in cryptococcal meningitis based on CSF fungal clearance.

5. *Doses:* For empiric therapy, the usual dose is Ampho B – 0.6 mg/kg/d and for lipid preparations is 3 mg/kg/d. For serious infections such as aspergillosis, the recommendation is amphotericin B – 1.0 to 1.4 mg/kg/d and for all lipid preparations is 5 mg/kg/d.

VI. Drugs

AMPRENAVIR (APV)

Trade name: Agenerase, Glaxo Wellcome

Form: 50 mg and 150 mg soft gel capsules; 15 mg/mL oral soln. AWP for 150 mg cap is $1.32 or $10.56/day.

Recommended dose: 1200 mg bid (eight 150 mg caps), given with or without food

Clinical trials: Monotherapy with the currently recommended dose resulted in a median decrease in plasma HIV RNA levels of 1.95 $\log_{10}$ c/mL.

Amprenavir was combined with abacavir, indinavir, ritonavir, saquinavir (Fortovase) or nelfinavir in 17 treatment naïve patients with baseline RNA ≥5,000 c/mL. At 24 weeks 44-60% had RNA <50 c/mL by intent-to-treat analysis [6th Conf. on Retroviruses, 1999, Abstract 625].

In PROAB 3001 amprenavir was combined with AZT/3TC vs. AZT/3TC alone in 332 treatment naïve patients. At 48 weeks viral load was <400 c/mL in 41% in the APV arm vs. 3% in the dual NRTI arm, but the study was marred by the high drop-out rate in both arms (D. Hardy, ICAAC, 9/99, Abstract 509).

ACTG 347 compared amprenavir alone vs. APV/AZT/3TC in 92 patients who were naïve to PIs and 3TC. Virologic failure (RNA >500 c/mL) at 12 weeks occurred in 2% of those on the triple drug combination compared to 28% in those receiving amprenavir alone [5th Conf. on Retroviruses, 1998, Abstract 512].

Bart and colleagues studied amprenavir/abacavir in 41 treatment-naïve patients [6th Conference on Retroviruses, 1999, Abstract 626]. By intent-to-treat analysis and as-treated analysis the proportion with RNA <5 c/mL was 58% and 78%, respectively, at 60 weeks. This was accompanied by a mean CD4 increase of 265/mm^3 including 130/mm^3 naïve cells and 84/mm^3 memory cells.

PROAB 3006 is a randomized multicenter study comparing amprenavir (1200 mg bid) + 2 NRTIs and indinavir (800 mg q8h) in 504 patients. Criteria for inclusion were lack of prior treatment with protease inhibitors and HIV RNA levels >400 c/mL. Interim analysis at 24 weeks showed the number of patients who achieved HIV RNA levels <400 c/mL by intent-to-treat analysis was 43% in the APV group compared to 53% in the IDV group; most of this 10% difference was ascribed to drug discontinuation due to adverse reaction: 16% for APV vs 8% for IDV.

ACTG 398 (7th CROI, Abstract LB7) was a salvage protocol in PI experienced patients who were given APV/ABC/EFZ/ADV + either IDV, NFV or SQV. Among 481 patients only 34% had a VL <200 c/mL at 24 weeks, indicating poor utility of APV for patients with extensive prior PI experience.

QUEST is a multicenter study of therapy of primary HIV infection using AZT/3TC/ABC/APV. Among 98 patients followed to ≥28 weeks the VL decreased from a median of 5.2 $\log_{10}$ c/mL at baseline to <50 c/mL in 87% and <5 c/mL in 58%; the mean CD4 count increase was 249/mm^3 (7th CROI, Abstract 552).

Resistance: At least two mutations, at codons 46, 47 and/or 50, are required to increase phenotypic resistance 10-fold. Mutations at codons 10, 54, 84 and 90 foster cross-resistance to other protease inhibitors. Phenotypic testing shows that 37% of HIV strains that are resistant to all other PIs are susceptible to APV but it is not known if this translates into clinical benefit in salvage regimens (7th CROI, Abstract 726).

Pharmacology

Bioavailability: Estimated at 89%; high fat meal decreases AUC 21% - can be taken with or without meal, but avoid a high fat meal.

T½: 7.1-10.6 hours

Elimination: Hepatic metabolism - most found in stool; 14% in urine. CYP_3A_4 inhibition is RTV>IDV=NFV=APV>SQV.

Hepatic disease: AUC increases 2.5x with liver disease, 4.5x with severe cirrhosis; dose recommendation is 450 mg bid with liver disease and 300 mg bid with severe cirrhosis (ICAAC, 9/99, Abstract 326).

Side Effects: The major side effects in clinical trials were GI intolerance (nausea-15%, diarrhea-14%, vomiting-5%), rash-11%, headache-6%, oral paresthesias-28%, fat redistribution-4 patients. Amprenavir may cause hepatotoxicity. Among patients in phase III trials who discontinued amprenavir temporarily or permanently for side effects, the reason was nausea in 3%, rash in 6%, and paresthesias-0.6%. Therapeutic trials show high rates of drop-out for adverse reactions, primarily nausea, vomiting and rash (D. Hardy, ICAAC, 9/99, Abstract 509). Class side effects: Diabetes, fat redistribution, blood lipid changes and increased bleeding in hemophilia.

The oral solution of amprenavir contains significant quantities of propylene glycol (55%), compared to 5% for the capsules. The oral solution is contraindicated in patients with renal failure, hepatitic failure, in pregnant women, or in patients receiving disulfiram or metronidazole. Patients treated with the oral solution should be monitored for adverse effects of propylene glycol that include seizures, stupor, tachycardia, hyperosmolarity, lactic acidosis, renal failure and hemolysis. Patients taking the oral solution should change to the capsule form when able to do so, and they should avoid alcoholic beverages when taking the oral solution.

Drug interactions:

1. **The following drugs are contraindicated for concurrent use:** Astemazole, bepridil, cisapride, dihydroergotamine, ergotamine, midazolam, terfenadine, triazolam, rifampin, simvastatin, lovastatin

2. **The following drugs should be given concurrently with caution:** amiodarone, clozapine, lidocaine, phenobarbital, phentytoin, carbamazepine, quinidine, tricyclic anti-depressants, warfarin and oral contraceptives (use alternative method of birth control) There are no data on methadone interaction.

Table 6-5: Amprenavir Interactions with other PIs and NNRTIs

Drug	Concurrent drug AUC	AUC APV	Dose*
Indinavir	↓38%	↑33%	IDV-800 mg tid + APV-800 mg tid
Nelfinavir	↑15%	↑1.5x	NFV-750 mg tid + APV-800 mg tid
Saquinavir-sgc	↓19%	↓32%	Inadequate data
Efavirenz	↑15%	↓36%	EFV-600 mg qhs APV-1200 mg tid or APV 1200 mg bid + RTV 200 mg bid + EFV 600 mg hs
Ritonavir	NC	↑2.5x	RTV-200 mg bid + APV 1200 mg bid + EFV 600 mg hs or RTV 100-200 mg bid + APV 600 mg bid or RTV 200 mg qd + APV 1200 mg qd (RTV + APV combination is under study)

* Pharmacokinetic studies show that RTV increases APV peak and trough levels by 238% and 1325% respectively, suggesting feasibility of once daily dosing (7th CROI, Abstracts 77 and 78).

3. **Other drug interactions:** Rifampin decreases APV AUC 82% and should not be used concurrently. Rifabutin decreases APV AUC 15% and APV increases rifabutin AUC 193%; use standard APV dose and rifabutin at half dose (150 mg/d). Clarithromycin increases APV AUC 18%; use standard doses of both drugs. Ketoconazole increases APV AUC 32% and ketoconazole AUC increases 44%; there are no available recommendations for concurrent use.

APV increases sildenafil AUC by 2-11x. Do not exceed 25 mg/48 hrs.

Pregnancy: C. Rat teratogen test shows incomplete ossification, thymic elongation, and low birth weight. Placental passage is unknown.

ANCOBON – See Flucytosine (p. 206)

ATIVAN – See Lorazepam (p. 234)

ATOVAQUONE

Trade name: Mepron (Glaxo Wellcome)

Form and price: 750 mg/5 mL bottle: $612.59/210 mL bottle (21 day supply).

Cost cap program for patients without third party coverage with use >271 gms in ≤1 year may receive free drug: call (800) 722-9294.

Patient assistance program: (800) 722-9294. Eligibility based on lack of third party drug coverage, monthly income criteria using Medicaid guidelines, and asset information; forms are reviewed on an individual case basis.

Indications: Oral treatment of mild to moderate PCP (A-a 02 gradient <45 mm Hg and Pa02 >60 mm Hg) in patients who are intolerant of trimethoprim-sulfamethoxazole (TMP-SMX)

Dose: 750 mg (5 mL) twice daily with meals x 21 days

Efficacy: In a comparative trial with TMP-SMX for mild-moderate PCP, TMP-SMX was associated with fewer failures (6% vs 17%) and more adverse effects requiring drug discontinuation (20% vs 7%) (NEJM 1993;328:1521). Decreased efficacy of atovaquone compared to TMP-SMX may be due to reduced bioavailability of the tablet form used previously and/or lack of activity vs common bacterial pathogens (some advocate use with antibacterial agent when used empirically). In a comparative trial of atovaquone vs IV pentamidine, there were fewer failures in the pentamidine arm (17 vs 29%, not statistically significant) and fewer adverse effects with atovaquone (4% vs 36%). The tablet form, which was used in the trials cited above, has been replaced by the suspension, which has a twofold increase in bioavailability. Atovaquone (750 mg po bid) is as effective as dapsone for PCP prophylaxis (NEJM 1998;339:1889), but the cost is $10,600/year compared to <$100/year for dapsone.

Pharmacology

> **Bioavailability:** Absorption of suspension averages 47% in fed state (with meals) compared to 23% with the tablet. Concurrent administration of fatty food increases absorption by two-fold. There is significant individual variation in absorption. Administration with fatty food needs emphasis.

> **T½:** 2.2-2.9 days

> **Elimination:** Enterohepatic circulation with fecal elimination; <1% in urine

> **CSF/plasma ratio:** <1%

> **Effect of hepatic or renal disease:** No data

Side effects: Rash (20%), GI intolerance (20%), diarrhea (20%); possibly related - headache, fever, insomnia; life-threatening side effects: none; number requiring discontinuation due to side effects: 7-9% (rash - 4%)

Pregnancy: Category C. Not teratogenic in animals; no studies in humans.

Drug interactions: Rifampin reduces atovaquone levels by 50%; rifabutin probably has a similar effect. Avoid combination or increase dose of atovaquone (MMWR 1999;48[RR-10]:47).

AVENTYL – See Nortriptyline (p. 244)

AZITHROMYCIN

Trade name: Zithromax (Pfizer)

Forms and price: 250 mg caps - $6.53; 600 mg tab-$15.73/tab. Z-Pak with 6 tabs (500 mg, then 250 mg/d x 4 days) - $39.33; powder packets (1 gm) $20.33; IV formulation as 500 mg vial - $23.71/500 mg vial

Class: Macrolide

Patient assistance program: (800) 646-4455 or (800) 438-1985. Physician must write letter stating: 1) The drug desired; 2) the diagnosis, and 3) confirm patient is indigent with no third party payor including ineligibility for Medicaid. A three-month supply will be provided.

Activity (*in vitro*): *S. pneumoniae* (about 10-15% of *S. pneumoniae* strains are resistant to azithromycin and other macrolides), streptococci (not Enterococcus), erythromycin-sensitive *S. aureus, H. influenzae, Legionella, Chlamydia pneumoniae, Mycoplasma pneumoniae, C trachomatis, M. avium,* and *T. gondii.* Azithromycin appears to reduce risk of *P. carinii* pneumonia (Lancet 1999;354:891).

Table 6-6: Azithromycin Regimens by Conditions

Indications	Dose
M. avium prophylaxis*	1.2 gm (two 600 mg tabs) each as 1 dose/wk or 1 gm (powder packet)
Sinusitis, bronchitis, and pneumonia*	500 mg IV qd 500 mg x 1, then 250 mg po/day x 4 (6 tabs)
*Chlamydia trachomatis**	1 gm po x 1
Toxoplasmosis†	900 mg po x 2 on day 1, then 1200 mg/d as single dose x 6 wks, then 600 mg/dy (patients <50 kg receive half dose)
Cryptosporidiosis†	1200 mg x 2 po on day 1, then 1200 mg/d x 27 days, then 600 mg/d
M. avium treatment†	600 mg po/day

* FDA-approved indications

† Treatment IND has been discontinued

Pharmacology

Bioavailability: Absorption is ~30-40%. The 250 mg caps should be taken one hour before or 2 hours after meals; the 600 mg tabs and the 1 gm powder packet may be taken without regard to food, but food improves tolerance (Note: Food reduces absorption of capsules and promotes absorption of the tablet form).

T½: 68 hrs; detectable levels in urine at 7-14 days; with the 1200 mg weekly dose, the azithromycin levels in peripheral leukocytes remains above 32 µg/mL for 60 hrs.

Distribution: High tissue levels; low CSF levels (<0.01 µg/mL)

Excretion: Primarily biliary; 6% in urine

Dose modification in renal or hepatic failure: "Use with caution"

Side effects: GI intolerance (nausea, vomiting, pain); diarrhea – 4%. With 1,200 mg dose weekly, major side effects are diarrhea, abdominal pain and nausea. Frequency of discontinuation in non-AIDS patients receiving standard dose – 0.7%. Frequency of discontinuation in AIDS patients receiving high doses – 6%, primarily GI intolerance and reversible ototoxicity (2%); rare – erythema multiforme, increased transaminases.

Contradications: Hypersensitivity to erythromycin

Drug interactions: Al- and Mg-containing antacids and food reduce absorption; increases levels of theophylline and coumadin. Concurrent use with antiretroviral agents, rifampin and rifabutin is safe. Concurrent use with pimozide may cause fatal arrythmias and must be avoided.

Pregnancy: Category B (safe in animal studies; no data in humans)

Warnings:

1. Should be taken one hour before meals or two hours after meals.

2. Use with caution in patients with hepatic disease, especially with prolonged course and high doses.

AZT – See Zidovudine (p. 283)

BACTRIM – See Trimethoprim-Sulfamethoxazole (p. 276)

BENZODIAZEPINES

Benzodiazepines are commonly used for anxiety and insomnia. They are also commonly abused, with some studies showing up to 25% of AIDS patients taking these drugs. The decision to use these drugs requires careful consideration of side effects and discussion with the patient:

1. Dependency (larger than usual doses or prolonged daily use of therapeutic doses).

2. Abuse potential (most common in those with abuse of alcohol and other psychiatric drugs).

3. Tolerance (primarily to sedation and ataxia; minimal to antianxiety effects).

4. Withdrawal symptoms, related to duration of use, dose, rate of tapering, and drug half-life. Features are: a) recurrence of pretreatment symptoms developing over days or weeks; b) rebound with symptoms that are similar to but more severe than pretreatment symptoms occurring within hours or days (self-limited); and c) the benzodiazepine withdrawal syndrome with autonomic symptoms, disturbances in equilibrium, sensory disturbances, etc.

5. Daytime sedation, dizziness, incoordination, ataxia, and hangover: Use small doses initially and gradually increase. Patient must be warned that activities requiring mental alertness, judgment and coordination require special caution; concomitant use with alcohol or other sedating drugs is unusually hazardous.

6. Drug interactions: Sedative effects are antagonized by caffeine and theophylline. Erythromycin, clarithromycin, fluoroquinolones, protease inhibitors (indinavir, nelfinavir, saquinavir, ritonavir), cimetidine, omeprazole, and INH may reduce hepatic metabolism and prolong half-life. Rifampin and oral contraceptives increase hepatic clearance and reduce half-life.

7. Miscellaneous side effects: Blurred vision, diplopia, confusion, memory disturbance, amnesia, fatigue, incontinence, constipation, hypotension, disinhibition, bizarre behavior.

8. Antiretroviral agents: Concurrent use of triazolam and midazolam with protease inhibitors and delavirdine is contraindicated.

Selection of agent and regimen: Drug selection is based largely on indication and pharmacokinetic properties (See table on next page). Drugs with rapid onset are desired when temporary relief of anxiety is needed. The smallest dose for the shortest time is recommended, and patients need frequent re-evaluation for continued use. Short-term use is advised in patients with a history of abuse of alcohol or other sedative-hypnotic drugs. Dose adjustments are usually required to achieve the desired effect with acceptable side effects. Long-term use (more than several weeks) may require an extended tapering schedule over 6-8 weeks (20-30% dose reduction weekly) adjusted by symptoms and sometimes facilitated by antidepressants or hypnotics.

VI. Drugs

ANXIETY AND INSOMNIA

Table 6-7: Comparison of Benzodiazepines

Agent	Trade Name	Anxiety	Insomnia	Tmax (hrs)	Mean half-life (hrs)	Dose forms	Regimens
BENZODIAZEPINES							
Chlordiazepine	Librium	+	–	0.5-4	10	5, 10, 25 mg tabs	15-100 mg/d hs or 3-4 doses
Clorazepate*	Tranxene	+	–	1-2	73	3.75, 7.5, 15, 11.25+22.5 mg tabs	15-60 mg/d hs or 2-4 doses
Diazepam*	Valium	+	+	1.5-2	73	2, 4, 5, 10 mg tabs	15-60 mg/d hs or 2-4 doses
Flurazepam*	Dalmane	–	+	0.5-2	74	15, 30 mg caps	4-40 mg/d, 2-4 doses
Quazepam	Doral	–	+	2	74	7.5, 15 mg tabs	30 mg hs
Alprazolam	Xanax	+	–	1-2	11	0.25, 0.5, 1, 2 mg tabs	15 mg hs
Lorazepam	Ativan	+	+	2	14	0.5, 1, 2 mg tabs	0.25-0.5 mg tid up to 4 mg/d
Oxazepam	Serax	+	+	1-4	7	10, 15, 30 mg caps	2-6 mg/d in 2-3 doses
Temazepam	Restoril	–	+	1-1.5	13	15, 30 mg caps	30-120 mg/d in 3-4 doses
Triazolam* **	Halcion	–	+	1-2	3	0.125, 0.25 mg tabs	0.25 mg hs

*Concurrent use with ritonavir is contraindicated.

**Concurrent use with protease inhibitors or delavirdine is contraindicated.

BIAXIN – See Clarithromycin (p. 182)

BUPROPION

Trade name: Wellbutrin, Wellbutrin SR, and Zyban (Glaxo Wellcome)

Forms and price: 75 mg tab – $0.79; 100 mg – $1.06, 150 mg – $1.40, 150 mg sustained release tabs – $1.38

Class: Atypical antidepressant

Indications: Depression: 150 mg qd x 4 days then 150 mg bid (SR formulation); antidepressant effect may require 4 weeks.

Pharmacology

Bioavailability: 5-20%

T½: 8-24 hrs

Eliminations: Extensive hepatic metabolism to ≥6 metabolites including two with antidepressant activity; metabolites excreted in urine.

Dose modification in renal or hepatic failure: Not known, but dose reduction may be required.

Side effects: Seizures – dose dependent and minimized by gradual increase in dose, dose not to exceed 450 mg/day, maximum single dose of 150 mg. Use with caution in seizure-prone patients and with concurrent use of alcohol and other antidepressants.

Other side effects: Agitation, insomnia, restlessness; GI - anorexia, nausea, vomiting; weight loss - noted in up to 25%; rare cases of psychosis, paranoia, depersonalization.

BUSPAR – See Buspirone (below)

BUSPIRONE

Trade name: BuSpar (Mead Johnson)

Forms and price: 5 mg tab – $0.72; 10 mg tab – $1.25

Class: Nonbenzodiazepine-nonbarbiturate antianxiety agent; not a controlled substance

Indications and dose regimens:

Anxiety: 5 mg po tid; increase by 5 mg/day every 2-4 days. Usual effective dose is 15-30 mg/day in 2-3 divided doses. Onset of response requires one week and full effect requires four weeks. Total daily dose should not exceed 60 mg/day.

VI. Drugs

Pharmacology

> **Bioavailability:** >90% absorbed when taken with food.

> **T½:** 2.5 hours

> **Elimination:** Rapid hepatic metabolism to partially active metabolites; <0.1 % of parent compound excreted in urine.

> **Dose adjustment in renal disease:** Dose reduction of 25-50% in patients with anuria.

> **Hepatic disease:** May decrease clearance and must use with caution.

Side effects: Sleep disturbance, nervousness, headache, nausea, diarrhea, paresthesias, depression, increased or decreased libido, headache, dizziness, and excitement. Compared to benzodiazepines, dependency liability of buspirone is nil, it does not potentiate CNS depressants including alcohol, it is usually well tolerated by elderly, and there is no hypnotic effect, no muscle relaxant effect, less fatigue, less confusion, and less decreased libido, but nearly comparable efficiency for anxiety. Nevertheless, the CNS effects are somewhat unpredictable, and there is substantial individual variation; patients should be warned that buspirone may impair ability to perform activities requiring mental alertness and physical coordination such as driving.

Pregnancy: Category B

CHLORAL HYDRATE

Trade name: Noctet (Apothecon), Aquachloral Suppretes (Apothecon) (suppositories), and generic

Forms and price: 325, 500, and 650 mg caps; 500 mg - $0.17/cap; suppositories - $.19/325 mg; syrup with 250 and 500 mg/5 mL syrup - $.32/500 mg

Class: Nonbenzodiazepine-nonbarbiturate hypnotic, controlled substance category IV

Indications and dose regimens:

> **Insomnia:** 500 mg – 1 gm po hs; usually produces sleep in 30 minutes which lasts 4-8 hours.

> **Sedation:** 250 mg po tid

Note: Tolerance develops within five weeks.

Pharmacology

> **Bioavailability:** >90%

> **T½:** Hepatic metabolism to achieve metabolite (trichlorethanol) with a half-life of 4-9.5 hours

> **Elimination:** Renal excretion of trichloroethanol

Hepatic or renal disease: Contraindicated

Side effects: Gastric intolerance; dependence and tolerance with long-term use

Pregnancy: Category C

Drug interactions: Potentiates action of oral anticoagulants

CIDOFOVIR

Trade name: Vistide (Gilead Sciences)

Forms and Price: 375 mg in 5 mL vial; $727.09/375 mg vial

Patient assistance program and reimbursment hotline: (800) 445-3235

Activity: Active *in vitro* versus CMV, VZV and EBV; less active versus HSV (Exp Med Biol 1996;394:105). CMV strains resistant to ganciclovir are usually sensitive to cidofovir; cidofovir-resistant strains are usually resistant to ganciclovir and sensitive to foscarnet. HSV resistant to acyclovir are often sensitive to cidofovir.

Indications: CMV retinitis; efficacy in other forms of CMV disease has not been established.

Clinical trials: A SOCA trial comparing cidofovir vs. deferred treatment of patients with CMV retinitis demonstrated a median time to progression of 120 days in the treated group compared to 22 days in the deferred group (Ann Intern Med 1997;126:257). Dose-limiting nephrotoxicity was noted in 24% and dose-limiting toxicity to probenecid was noted in 7%.

Regimen: Induction dose – 5 mg/kg IV over 1 hr* weekly x 2
Maintenance dose – 5 mg/kg IV over 1 hr q 2 wks*

* Probenecid, 2 gm given 3 hrs prior to cidofovir and 1 gm given at 2 and 8 hrs after infusion (total of 4 gm). Patients must receive >1 L 0.95 N (normal) saline infused over 1-2 hrs immediately before cidofovir infusion

Note:

1. Cidofovir is diluted in 100 mL 0.9% saline.

2. Renal failure: Cidofovir is contraindicated in patients with preexisting renal failure (serum creatinine >1.5 mg/dL, creatinine clearance ≤55 mL/min or urine protein >100 mg/dL or 2+ proteinuria).

3. Co-administration of nephrotoxic drugs in contraindicated, including non-steroidal anti-inflammatory agents, amphotericin B, aminoglycosides, and IV pentamidine; there should be a 7 day "washout" following use of these drugs.

4. Dose adjustment for renal failure during cidofovir treatment:

    a) serum creatinine increase 0.3-0.4 mg/dL: reduce dose to 3 mg/kg

        b) serum creatinine increase ≥0.5 mg/dL or ≥3 + proteinuria: discontinue therapy.

5. Gastrointestinal tolerance of probenecid may be improved with food ingestion or an antiemetic prior to administration. Antihistamines or acetaminophen may be used for probenecid hypersensitivity reactions.

6. Cases of nephrotoxicity should be reported to Gilead Sciences, Inc. (800) GILEAD-5, or to the FDA's Medwatch (800) FDA-1088.

Phamacokinetics

Bioavailability: Requires IV administration; probenecid increases AUC by 40-60% presumably by blocking tubular secretion. CSF levels are undetectable.

T½: The elimination half-life of the active intracellular metabolite is 17 to 65 hours permitting long intervals between doses.

Excretion: 70-85% excreted in urine

Side Effects: The major side effect is dose-dependent nephrotoxicity. Proteinuria is an early indicator. IV saline and probenecid must be used to reduce nephrotoxicity. Monitor renal function with serum creatinine and urine protein within 48 hrs prior to each dose. About 25% will develop ≥2 + proteinuria or a serum creatinine >2-3 mg/dL and these changes are reversible if treatment is discontinued (Ann Intern Med 1997;126:257 and 264). Cases of nephrotoxicity should be reported to (800) GILEAD-5.

Other side effects: Neutropenia in about 15% (monitor neutrophil count) and metabolic acidosis with Fanconi's syndrome and decreased serum bicarbonate indicating renal tubule damage. Probenecid causes side effects in about 50% of patients including fever, chills, headache, rash, or nausea, usually after 3-4 treatments. Side effects usually resolved within 12 hours. Dose-limiting side effects are usually GI intolerance. These side effects may be reduced with food before probenecid, antiemetics, antipyretics, or antihistamines (Ann Intern Med 1997;126:257).

Drug interactions: Must avoid concurrent nephrotoxic drugs including aminoglycosides, amphotericin B, foscarnet, IV pentamidine and non-steroidal anti-inflammatory agents. Patients receiving these drugs should have a ≥7 day "wash-out" prior to treatment with cidofovir. Probenecid prolongs the half-life of acetaminophen, acyclovir, aminosalicylic acid, barbituates, betalactam antibiotics, benzodiazepines, bumetanide, clofibrate, methotrexate, famotidine, furosemide, non-steroidal anti-inflammatory agents, theophylline and AZT.

Pregnancy: Category C – use only if potential benefit justifies the risk.

CIPRO – See Ciprofloxacin (below)

CIPROFLOXACIN (See "Fluoroquinolones" for comparisons - pg 207)

Trade name: Cipro (Miles)

Forms: 250, 500, and 750 mg tabs; IV-200 and 400 mg vials

Price: $3.41/250 mg tab; $3.99/500 mg tab; $4.13/750 mg tab; $28.80/400 mg vial (for IV use)

Patient assistant program: (800) 998-9180

Class: Fluoroquinolone

Spectrum: Active vs most strains of *Enterobacteriaceae, P. aeruginosa, H. influenzae*, Legionella, *C. pneumoniae, M. pneumoniae, Mycobacterium tuberculosis, M. avium*, most bacterial enteric pathogens other than *C. difficile*. Somewhat less active vs *S. pneumoniae* than levofloxacin, grepafloxacin and trovafloxacin; the clinical significance of this difference is debated. There is increasing and substantial resistance by *S. aureus* (primarily MRSA) and *C. jejuni*.

Indications and dose:
Respiratory infections: 500-750 mg po bid x 7-14 days
Gonorrhea: 500 mg x 1
Tuberculosis: 500-750 mg po bid
Salmonellosis: 500-750 mg po bid 2-4 wks
UTI: 250-500 mg po bid x 3-7 days

Pharmacology

Bioavailability: 60-70%

T½: 3.3 hours

Excretion: Metabolized and excreted (parent compound and metabolites) in urine

Dose reduction in renal failure: CrCl>50 mL/min - 250-750 mg q 12 h; 10-50 mL/min - 250-500 mg q 12 h; <10 mL/min - 250-500 mg q 18 h

Side effects: Usually well tolerated; most common - GI intolerance with nausea - 1.2% diarrhea - 1.2%; CNS toxicity - malaise, drowsiness, insomnia, headache, dizziness, agitation, psychosis (rare), seizures (rare), hallucinations (rare); tendon rupture-about 25 cases reported involving fluoroquinolones; Candida vaginitis; contraindicated in persons <18 years due to concern for arthropathy (seen in animals).

Drug interactions: Increased levels of theophylline and caffeine; reduced absorption with cations (Al, Mg, Ca) in antacids, sucralfate, ddI; gastric achlorhydria does not influence absorption

Pregnancy: Category C. Arthropathy in immature animals with erosions in joint cartilages; relevance to patients is not known. Medical Letter consultants and CDC consider use in pregnant women and person <18 years contraindicated. This admonition applies to all quinolones.

VI. Drugs

CLARITHROMYCIN

Trade name: Biaxin (Abbott Laboratories)

Forms and price:

> 250 mg tab = $3.45
>
> 500 mg tab = $3.45
>
> 250 mg/5 mL; 100 mL = $56.85

Patient assistance program: (800) 688-9118. Patient must have financial need and indication for *M. avium* treatment or prophylaxis.

Class: Macrolide

Spectrum: *S. pneumoniae* (10-15% of strains and 40% of penicillin-resistant strains are resistant in most areas of the U.S.), erythromycin-sensitive *S. aureus, S. pyogenes, M. catarrhalis, H. influenzae, M. pneumoniae, C. pneumoniae, Legionella, M. avium, T. gondii, C. trachomatis, U. urealyticum*

Trials: Clarithromycin is highly effective in the treatment and prevention of MAC disease (NEJM 1996;335:385; CID 1998;27:1278). Clarithromycin has proven superior to azithromycin in the treatment of MAC bacteremia in terms of median time to negative blood cultures 4.4 wks vs >16 wks [CID 1998;27:1278]). There is no evidence that it is superior to azithromycin for MAC prophylaxis.

Table 6-8: Clarithromycin Indications and Regimens

Indication	Dose regimen*
Pharyngitis, sinusitis, otitis, pneumonitis, skin and soft tissue infection**	250-500 mg po bid
M. avium prophylaxis**	500 mg po bid (MMWR 1995;44[RR-8]:1)
M. avium treatment** (plus ethambutol ± rifabutin or ciprofloxacin)	500 mg po bid
Toxoplasmosis (plus pyrimethamine)	500 mg po bid

*Doses of ≥2 gm/day are associated with excessive mortality (CID 1999;29:125)

**FDA-approved for this indication

Pharmacology

Bioavailability: 50-55%

T½: 4-7 hours

Elimination: Rapid first pass hepatic metabolism plus renal clearance to 14-hydroxyclarithromycin

Dose modification in renal failure: CrCl >30/mL - 250-500 mg po bid; CrCl <30/mL - 250 mg po bid

Side effects: GI intolerance - 4% (compared to 17% with erythromycin); transaminase elevation - 1%, headache - 2%, PMC - rare

Pregnancy: Category C; teratogenic in animal studies and no adequate studies in humans

Drug interactions: Clarithromycin increases levels of rifabutin (4-fold), theophylline, carbamazepine (Tegretol), cisapride (Propulsid), pimozide (Orap) and Seldane; increased levels of Seldane, pimozide and Propulsid may cause fatal arrhythmias. Azithromycin has no substantial interaction. Nelfinavir induces clarithromycin metabolism to reduce AUC 35% - monitor closely (MMWR 1999;48[RR-10]:47). Ritonavir and indinavir increase clarithromycin levels 50-77%. Reduce dose of clarithromycin when combined with ritonavir in patients with a creatinine clearance <30 mL/min (MMWR 1999;48[RR-10]:47). Rifabutin and rifampin reduce clarithromycin by 50% and 120%, respectively.

CLINDAMYCIN

Trade name: Cleocin (Pharmacia & Upjohn) and generic

Forms and price: Clindamycin HCl 75 mg, 150, 300 mg caps; 150 mg tab=$0.52; Clindamycin PO4 with 150 mg/mL in 2, 4 and 6 mL vials; 600 mg vial=$13.84

Patient assistant program: (800) 242-7014; (800) 253-8600 x36004

Activity: Most gram-positive cocci are susceptible except *Enterococcus* and some *Staphylococci*, most anaerobic bacteria

Indications: PCP: Clindamycin 600-900 mg q 6-8 h IV or 300-450 mg q 6 h po/primaquine 15 mg (base): Toxoplasmosis: Clindamycin 600 mg IV q 6 h or 300-450 mg po q 6 h/pyrimethamine 100-200 loading dose, then 50-100 mg/day po/leukovorin, 10-25 mg day; Other infections: 600-900 mg q 8 h IV or 150-300 mg po q 6-8 h

Pharmacology

Bioavailability: 90%

T½: 2-3 hours

CNS penetration: Poor

Elimination: Metabolized; 10% in urine

Dose modification in renal failure: None

Side effects: GI - diarrhea in 10-30%. Six percent of patients develop *C. difficile*-associated diarrhea; most respond well to discontinuation of the drug; small subset develop pseudomembranous colitis. Other GI side effects include nausea, vomiting, and anorexia. **Rash** – generalized morbilliform is most common; less common is urticaria, pruritis, Stevens-Johnson syndrome.

Drug interactions: Loperamide or Lomotil increases risk of diarrhea and *C. difficile*-associated colitis.

CLOFAZIMINE

This drug is no longer used for *M. avium* infections because it does not improve outcome and is associated with high rates of side effects and increased mortality (NEJM 1996;335:377).

CLOTRIMAZOLE

Source: Lotrimin (Schering), Mycelex (Alza), Gyne-Lotrimin (Schering), FemCare (Schering)

Forms and price:
Troche 10 mg – $0.82; bottles of 70 and 140
Topical cream (1%) 15 gm – $9.67; 30 gm – $16.53
Topical solution/lotion (1%) 10 mL – $10.80; 30 mL – $22.47
Vaginal cream (1%) 45 gm – $12.00
Vaginal tablets 100 mg – $1.71 (x 7 days) = $12.00
Vaginal tablets 500 mg – $13.88 (single dose) = $13.88

Class: Imidazole (related to miconazole)

Spectrum: Active against *Candida albicans* and dermatophytes

Indications and regimens:

Thrush: 10 mg troche 5x/day; must be dissolved in the mouth.

Dermatophytic infections and cutaneous candidiasis: Topical application of 1% cream, lotion, or solution to affected area bid x 2-8 wks; if no improvement – reevaluate diagnosis.

Candidal vaginitis: Intravaginal 100 mg tab bid x 3 days (preferred); alternatives: 100 mg tabs qd x 7; 500 mg tab x 1. Vaginal cream: One applicator (about 5 gm) intravaginally at hs x 7-14 days.

Pharmacology

> **Bioavailability:** Lozenge (troche) dissolves in 15-30 min; administration at three-hour intervals maintains constant salivary concentrations above MIC of most *Candida* strains. Topical application of 500 mg tab intravaginally achieves local therapeutic levels for 48-72 hours. Small amounts of drug are absorbed with oral, vaginal, or skin applications.

Side effects: Topical to skin – (rare) erythema, blistering, pruritis, pain, peeling, urticaria; Topical to vagina – (rare) rash, pruritis, dyspareunia, dysuria, burning, erythema; Lozenges – elevated AST (up to 15% – monitor LFTs); nausea and vomiting (5%)

Pregnancy: Category C. Avoid during first trimester

CRIXIVAN – See Indinavir (p. 219)

CYTOVENE – See Ganciclovir (p. 212)

DALMANE – See Benzodiazapines (p. 176)

DAPSONE

Generic

Forms and price: 25 mg tab – $0.19; 100 mg tabs – $0.20

> Comparison prices for PCP prophylaxis:
>
> Dapsone (100 mg/day) = $6.00/mo
>
> TMP-SMX (1 DS/day) = $2.00/mo
>
> Aerosolized pentamidine = $100/mo (plus administration costs)

Class: Synthetic sulfone with mechanism of action similar to sulfonamides – inhibition of folic acid synthesis by inhibition of dihydropteroate synthetase.

VI. Drugs

Table 6-9: Dapsone Indications and Dose Regimens

Indication	Dose regimen
PCP prophylaxis	100 mg po qd or 50 mg po bid
PCP treatment	100 mg po qd (plus trimethoprim 15 mg/kg/d po or IV) x 3 wks
PCP + Toxoplasmosis prophylaxis	50 mg po qd (plus pyrimethamine 50 mg/wk plus folinic acid 25 mg/wk) or dapsone 200 mg (+ pyrimethamine 75 mg + leukovorin 25 mg) once weekly

Efficacy: For PCP prophylaxis, a review of 40 published studies found dapsone (100 mg/day) to be less effective than TMP-SMX and comparable to aerosolized pentamidine. Nevertheless, it appears to be cost-effective (CID 1998;27:191). For PCP treatment, dapsone/trimethoprim is as effective as TMP-SMX for patients with mild or moderately severe disease (Ann Intern Med 1996;124:792).

Pharmacology

> **Bioavailability:** Nearly completely absorbed except with gastric achlorhydria (Dapsone is insoluble at neutral pH)
>
> **T½:** 10-56 hours, average – 28 hours
>
> **Elimination:** Hepatic concentration, enterohepatic circulation, maintains tissue three weeks after treatment is discontinued.
>
> **Dose modification in renal failure:** None

Side effects: Most common in AIDS patients – rash, pruritis, hepatitis, anemia, and/or neutropenia in 20-40% receiving dapsone prophylaxis for PCP in a dose of 100 mg/day.

Most serious reaction – dose dependent hemolytic anemia, with or without G-6-PD deficiency and methemoglobinemia; rare cases of agranulocytosis and aplastic anemia. Suggested monitoring includes screening for G-6-PD deficiency prior to treatment, especially in high risk patients including African-American men and men of Mediterranean extraction. Some suggest monthly CBC to detect marrow suppression and hemolytic anemia. G-6-PD deficiency is not a contraindication to dapsone in the case of the African variant, but enhances need for monitoring; dapsone should not be used with the Mediterranean variant of G6PD deficiency. Hemolysis and Heinz body formation are exaggerated in patients with a G-6-PD deficiency, methemoglobinreductase deficiency, or hemoglobin M. Asymptomatic methemoglobinemia independent of G-6-PD deficiency has been found in up to two thirds of patients receiving 100 mg dapsone/day plus trimethoprim (NEJM 1990;373:776). Acute methemoglobinemia is uncommon, but the usual features are dyspnea, fatigue, cyanosis, deceptively high pulse oximetry and chocolate-colored blood (JAIDS 1996;12:477). Methemoglobinemia levels are related to the dose and duration of dapsone; TMP increases dapsone levels, so TMP may precipitate methemoglobinemia; they are usually <25% which is generally tolerated except for patients with lung disease. TMP increases dapsone levels, so TMP-dapsone may precipitate methemoglobinemia. Patients with glutathione or G-6-PD deficiency are at increased risk. Treatment consists of oxygen supplementation, packed cell transfusions for anemia and discontinuation of the implicated drug. This is usually adequate if the methemoglobin level is <30%. Activated charcoal (20 mg qid) may be given to reduce dapsone levels. Treatment for severe cases in the absence of G-6-PD deficiency is IV methylene blue (1-2 mg/kg by slow IV infusion). In less emergent situations methylene blue may be given orally (3-5 mg/kg q 4-6 h); methylene blue should not be given with G-6-PD deficiency since methylene blue reduction requires G-6-PD; hemodialysis also enhances elimination.

GI intolerance – common; may reduce by taking with meals.

Infrequent – nausea, vomiting, headache, dizziness, peripheral neuropathy. Rare side effect is "sulfone syndrome" after 1-4 weeks of treatment consisting of fever, malaise, exfoliative dermatitis, hepatic necrosis, lymphadenopathy, and anemia with methemoglobinemia (Arch Derm 1981;1217-38).

Pregnancy: Category C. No data in animals; limited experience in pregnant patients with Hansen's disease shows no toxicity. Hemolytic anemia with passage in breast milk reported (CID 1995;21 suppl 1:S24).

Drug interactions: Decreased dapsone absorption - ddI, H2 blockers, antacids, omeprazole; decreased levels of dapsone - rifampin and rifabutin; trimethoprim - increased levels of both drugs; coumadin - increased hyppoprothrombinemia; pyrimethamine - increased marrow toxicity (monitor CBC); probenecid - increased dapsone levels; primaquine - hemolysis due to G-6-PD deficiency.

Relative contraindications: G-6-PD deficiency - monitor hematocrit and methemoglobin levels if anemia develops.

DARAPRIM – See Pyrimethamine (p. 252)

DAUNORUBICIN CITRATE LIPOSOME INJECTION

Trade name: DaunoXome (NeXstar)

Form and price: Vials containing equivalent of 50 mg daunorubicin; $311.50/50 mg

Patient assistance program: (800) 226-2056

Class: Daunorubicin encapsulated within lipid vesicles or liposomes

Indication (FDA labeling): First line cytotoxic therapy for advanced HIV-associated Kaposi's sarcoma

Clinical trial results: A prospective controlled trial compared liposomal daunorubicin (40 mg/m^2) with doxorubicin (10 mg/m^2) bleomycin (15 U) and vincristine (1 mg)

given IV q 2 wks in 227 patients with advanced KS (>25 mucocutaneous lesions, visceral KS or lymphedema). Clinical response and survival were similar. Recipients of ABV experienced significantly more alopecia and neuropathy. Recipients of DaunoXome had more neutropenia. No patients had cardiotoxicity (J Clin Oncol 1996;14:2353).

Regimen: Administer IV over 60 minutes in dose of 40 mg/m2; repeat q 2 wks. CBC should be obtained before each infusion and therapy withheld if absolute leukocyte count is <750/mL. Treatment is continued until there is evidence of tumor progression with new visceral lesions, progressive visceral disease, >10 new cutaneous lesions, or 25% increase in the number of lesions compared to baseline.

Pharmacology: Mechanism of selectively targeting tumor cells is unknown. Once at the tumor, daunorubicin is released over time.

Side effects:

1. Granulocytopenia is the most common toxicity requiring monitoring of the CBC.

2. Cardiotoxicity is the most serious side effect. It is most common in patients who have previously received anthracyclines or who have preexisting heart disease. Common features of cardiomyopathy are decreased left ventricular ejection fraction (LVEF) and usual clinical features of congestive heart failure. Cardiac function (history and physical exam) should be evaluated before each infusion and LVEF should be monitored when the total dose is 320 mg/m^2, 480 mg/m^2, and every 2240 mg/m^2 thereafter.

3. The triad of back pain, flushing, and chest tightness is reported in 14%; this usually occurs in the first 5 minutes of treatment, resolves with discontinuation of the infusion, and does not recur with resumption of infusion at a slower rate.

4. Care should be exercised to avoid drug extravasation which can cause tissue necrosis.

Drug interactions: None established

Pregnancy: Category D - Studies in rats showed severe maternal toxicity, embryolethality, fetal malformations, and embryotoxicity.

ddC – See Zalcitabine (p. 281)

ddI – See Didanosine (p. 191)

DELAVIRDINE (DLV)

Trade name: Rescriptor (Agouron)

Forms and price: 200 mg tabs at $1.22/tab ($7.06/day) (Note: Delavirdine is now produced by Agouron, and the formulation has changed from a large 100 mg tab that had to be mixed with water to produce a slurry to a new formulation that is a smaller 200 mg tab that is taken intact.)

Patient assistance program: (800) 711-0807; information: (800) 432-4702; reimbursement issues (800) 711-0807.

Dose: 400 mg po tid. Take without regard to meals, but separate dosing of ddI or antacids by 1 hour.

Class: Non-nucleoside reverse transcriptase inhibitor

Efficacy: Study 0021 demonstrated a modest benefit for delavirdine plus AZT vs AZT alone in viral load. Study 0071 demonstrated equivalence between delavirdine plus ddI vs ddI monotherapy in CD4 response and viral load. In ACTG 261 the following three regimens were equivalent in terms of viral load and CD4 count: delavirdine/AZT, delavirdine/ddI and AZT/ddI. In an as-treated analysis of protocol 0021-2 at 52 weeks, 70% of patients receiving delavirdine/AZT/3TC had viral loads <400/mL accompanied by CD4 count increases of 49-135/mm³. The viral load results were significantly superior to those achieved with AZT/3TC or delavirdine/AZT. Delavirdine has drug interactions that produce increased blood levels of saquinavir, indinavir, and nelfinavir. In Protocol 0063 DLV + IDV (400-600 mg bid) + AZT produced increased IDV peak levels compared to IDV 800 mg tid, and viral load response at 24 weeks that was comparable to results with IDV, AZT + 3TC. In Protocol 0073, a limited clinical trial comparing DLV (600 mg bid) + NFV (1,250 mg bid) + ddI ± d4T, a good virologic response was seen at 40 weeks. Delavirdine appears to resensitize HIV to AZT.

Resistance: Monotherapy results in 50-500-fold reduction in susceptibility in most patients within eight weeks. The major mutation change associated with resistance is at codon 103 of the RT gene; less common are mutations at codones 100, 101, 106, 181 and 188. Most of these lead to cross resistance with nevirapine; mutations at 106 and 181 do not show cross resistance with efavirenz.

Indications: See Chapter 4

Pharmacology

Bioavailability: Absorption is 85%; there are no food restrictions. Food reduces absorption by 20%. Antacids, ddI and gastric achlorhydria decrease absorption.

Distribution: CSF: plasma ratio=0.02

T½: 5.8 hours

Elimination: Primarily metabolized by hepatic cytochrome P450 (CYP 3A) enzymes. Delavirdine inhibits P450 CYP 3A indicating it inhibits its own metabolism as well as that of indinavir, nelfinavir, ritonavir and saquinavir.

VI. Drugs

> **Dose reduction in renal or hepatic failure:** None; consider empiric dose reduction with severe liver disease.

Side effects: Rash noted in about 18%; 4% require drug discontinuation. Rash is diffuse, maculopapular, red and predominantly on upper body and proximal arms. Erythema multiforme and Stevens-Johnson syndrome are rare. Duration of rash averages two weeks and usually does not require dose reduction or discontinuation (after interrupted treatment). Rash accompanied by fever, mucous membrane involvement, swelling or arthralgias should prompt discontinuation of treatment. Other side effects are headaches and increased transaminases.

Drug interaction: Inhibits P450 enzymes — the following drugs should not be used concurrently: terfenadine (Seldane), rifampin, rifabutin, ergot derivatives, astemizole, cisapride, midazolam, triazolam, simvastatin, lovastatin, H_2 blockers, and proton pump inhibitors. Other drugs that have increased half-life and potential toxicity when given with delavirdine: clarithromycin, dapsone, quinidine, wafarin and rifabutin. Delavirdine probably increases concentrations of sildenafil, so dosing should not exceed 25 mg/48 hours. There are no data on interactions with ketoconazole, oral contraceptives, or methadone. Drugs that decrease levels of delavirdine: carbamazepine, phenobarbital, phenytoin, rifabutin and rifampin. Absorption of delavirdine is decreased with antacids, ddI (administer $\geq$ one hour apart) and H_2 blockers.

Table 6-10. Delavirdine Combined with Protease Inhibitors

Drug	AUC	Regimen
Indinavir	IDV ↑ >40% DLV no change	IDV 600 mg q8h DLV 400 mg tid
Ritonavir	RTV ↑ 70% DLV no change	No data
Saquinavir (Fortovase)	SQV ↑ 5x DLV no change	Fortovase 800 mg tid DLV 400 mg tid
Nelfinavir	NFV ↑ 2x DLV ↓ 50%	NFV 1250 mg bid DLV 600 mg bid
Amprenavir	—	No data

Pregnancy: Category C. Ventricular septal defects in rodent teratogenicity assay; placental passage studies show a newborn : maternal drug ratio of 0.15.

d4T – See Stavudine (p. 266)

DESYREL – See Trazodone (p. 273)

DIDANOSINE (ddI)

Trade name: Videx (Bristol-Myers Squibb)

Forms: 25 mg, 50 mg, 100 mg, and 150 mg wintergreen-flavored tabs; 100 mg, 167 mg, and 250 mg buffered powder packets; pediatric powder for oral solution in 4- and 8-ounce bottle containing 2 gm or 4 gm ddI, respectively. New 200 mg tabs for once daily dosing (400 mg qd) became available in 12/99 when the FDA approved the once daily dosing regimen (AIDS 1999;13:F87). This is the preferred preparation because it has the appropriate buffering for the 400 mg dose. The 200 mg tab should not be used bid because there is insufficient buffering unless two tabs are given together.

Price: 100 mg tab = $1.72; cost/wk (200 mg bid) = $48.16/wk; 250 mg powder = $4.30

Class: Nucleoside analog

Financial assistance: (800) 272-4878. For patients without insurance coverage plus financial need.

Indications: In ACTG 116/117, ACTG 175, and the Delta Trial, ddI was found to be effective alone and in combination with AZT for patients with CD4 counts <500/mm³. ddI or ddI/AZT was superior to AZT monotherapy in CD4 cell count response, viral load response, delaying AIDS-defining complications, and prolonging survival. There is extensive experience with ddI plus d4T. Hydroxyurea (1 gm/day) magnifies the antiviral effect of ddI; in ACTG 307 ddI monotherapy decreased VL 1.2 logs compared to 1.8 logs for ddI/hydroxyurea.

Resistance: Mutations at codon 74 are most important; less common are codons 65 and 184. The 184 mutation confers high-level resistance to 3TC and may cause partial loss of susceptibility to ddI, ddC, and abacavir. 5-10% of recipients of AZT plus ddI develop mutations that confer resistance to all nucleoside RT inhibitors; some are due to SSS-69 insertions and some show codon 151 mutations.

Table 6-11: Didanosine Dose Regimen

Dose	Tabs*	Powder
Wt ≥60 kg	200 mg po bid or 400 mg qd	250 mg po bid
Wt <60 kg	125 mg po bid or 250 mg qd	167 mg po bid

* Tabs: Must be taken as two tabs in above dose that are chewed thoroughly or crushed or dispersed in ≥1 ounce of water for use within one hour and given on an empty stomach (≥30 minutes before meal or ≥2 hours after a meal). The buffered powder form is citrus-flavored and usually used if the tablet form is not tolerated; the contents of one packet are dissolved in four ounces of water. An alternative is administration of pediatric powder with Mylanta or Maalox (see side effects #3 next page).

VI. Drugs

Pharmacology

Bioavailability: Tablet - 40%; powder - 30%

T½: 1.6 hours; **Intracellular T½:** 25-40 hours

CNS penetration: CSF levels are 20% of serum levels (CSF: plasma ratio = 0.16–0.19)

Elimination: Renal excretion - 50%

Renal or hepatic failure:

Table 6-12: Creatinine Clearance (mL/min)

Weight	>50	26–49	10–25	<10
>60 kg	200 mg bid	200 mg qd	100 mg qd	100 mg qd
<60 kg	125 mg bid	125 mg qd	50 mg qd	100 mg qd

With hemodialysis the suggested dose is 100 mg q 24 h after dialysis. Mg++ load may be a problem with renal failure, and sodium load may be problematic for patients requiring sodium restriction. There are no clear guidelines for dose adjustment with severe liver disease; some advocate an empiric dose reduction.

Side effects:

1. Pancreatitis: Reported in 1-9% and is fatal in 6% of those with pancreatitis (JID 1997;175:255). Frequency is increased in patients with alcoholism, a history of pancreatitis, advanced stage HIV disease, and concurrent meds that cause pancreatitis. Concurrent drugs that increase the risk of pancreatitis include d4T and hydroxyurea (see below). Some advocate monitoring amylase levels at 1- to 2-month intervals, although the value in predicting or preventing pancreatitis is not established. Most reduce dose or discontinue ddI if serum amylase level is >1.5-2x the upper limit of normal. The drug should be discontinued if there is clinical evidence of pancreatitis until laboratory studies are available. In November 1999, Bristol-Myers Squibb issued a warning about pancreatitis as a result of four deaths ascribed to this complication is an ACTG trial. Analysis of these cases and those reported to the FDA MedWatch showed most cases were associated with ddI/d4T with or without hydroxyurea. Many or most patients have other risk factors for pancreatitis including: alcohol abuse, morbid obesity, history of pancreatitis, hypertriglyceridemia, cholelithiasis, ERCP, other drugs that cause pancreatitis (pentamidine), or medications known to increase exposure to ddI (hydroxyurea, allopurinol etc).

2. Peripheral neuropathy with pain and/or paresthesias in extremities. Frequency is 5-12%; it is increased significantly when ddI is given with d4T or hydroxy-

urea or both (AIDS 2000;14:273). Onset usually occurs at 2-6 months of ddI therapy and may be persistent and debilitating if ddI is continued despite symptoms.

3. Gastrointestinal intolerance and difficulty with tablets are common. An alternative is ddI pediatric powder reconstituted with 200 mL water and mixed with 200 mL Mylanta DS or Maalox extra strength with anti-gas suspension in patient's choice of flavor. The final concentration is 10 mg/mL and the usual dose is 25 mL. GI intolerance also includes diarrhea (from buffer) and mouth sores.

4. Hepatitis with increased transaminase levels.

5. Miscellaneous: Rash, marrow suppression, hyperuricemia, hypokalemia, hypocalcemia, hypomagnesemia, optic neuritis

6. Sodium load: 11.5 mEq/tab and 60 mEq/powder packet. Mg++ load: 8.6 mEq/tab (may be problematic in renal failure).

7. Class adverse effect: Lactic acidosis and hepatic steatosis.

Drug interactions: Drugs that require gastric acidity for absorption should be given 1-2 hours before or after ddI. These include dapsone, indinavir, ritonavir, delavirdine, ketoconazole, tetracyclines, and fluoroquinolones. (This limitation does not apply to nelfinavir, amprenavir, saquinavir, efavirenz, or nevirapine.) Drugs that cause pancreatitis (ethambutol or pentamidine) should be avoided; alcohol should be taken with caution. Drugs that cause peripheral neuropathy should be used with caution or avoided: ethambutol, INH, vincristine, gold, disulfiram, or cisplatin. Methadone reduces AUC by 60%; ddI has no effect on methadone levels. Consider ddI dose increase. Concurrent use with ddC is contraindicated. Ganciclovir increases ddI AUC by 100%, but clinical significance is not known - monitor for ddI toxicity.

Pregnancy: Category B. No lifetime harm in rodent teratogen and carcinogenicity studies; placental passage in humans shows newborn: maternal drug ratio of 0.5; no controlled studies in humans.

DIFLUCAN – See Fluconazole (p. 204)

DOXYCYCLINE

Generic

Trade names: Vibramycin (Pfizer), Doryx, Doxychel, Vivox

Forms and price: 50 mg cap and 100 mg tab; $0.11/100 mg tab; IV form $21.00/100 mg

Dose: 100 mg po bid

Class: Tetracycline

Indications:

> ***Chlamydia trachomatis*** - 100 mg po bid x 7 days. Common respiratory tract
> infections (sinusitis, otitis, bronchitis) - 100 mg po bid x 7-14 days

> **Bacillary angiomatosis** - 100 mg po bid x 6 wks

Pharmacology

> **Bioavailability:** 93%; complexes with bivalent cations (Ca++, Mg++, Fe++,
> Al++, etc.) So milk, mineral preps, cathartics, and antacids with metal salts
> should not be given concurrently.

> **T½:** 18 hours

> **Elimination:** Excreted in stool as chelated inactive agent independent of renal
> and hepatic function

> **Dose modification with renal or hepatic failure:** None

Side effects: GI intolerance (10% and dose-related, reduced with food), diarrhea;
deposited in developing teeth - contraindicated from mid-pregnancy to term and in
children <8 years of age (Committee on Drugs, American Academy of Pediatrics);
photosensitivity (exaggerated sunburn); Candida vaginitis; "black tongue"; rash.

Pregnancy: Category D; use in pregnant women and infants may cause retardation of
skeletal development and bone growth; tetracyclines localize in dentin and enamel of
developing teeth to cause enamel hypoplasia and yellow-brown discoloration.
Tetracyclines should be avoided in pregnant women and children <8 years unless
benefits outweigh these risks.

Drug interactions: Chelation with cations to reduce oral absorption; half-life of doxycycline decreased by carbamazepine (Tegretol), cimetidine, phenytoin, barbiturates;
may interfere with oral contraceptives; potentiates oral hypoglycemics, digoxin, and
lithium.

DRONABINOL

Trade name: Marinol (Roxane Labs)

Forms: Gelatin capsules of 2.5, 5, and 10 mg

Costs: $3.17/2.5 mg cap; $6.27/5 mg cap; $13.03/10 mg cap

Patient Assistance Program: (800) 274-8651

Indication: Anorexia associated with weight loss (also used in higher doses as antiemetic in cancer patients). Long-term therapy has led to significant improvement in
appetite, but minimal weight gain; when weight gain is achieved, it is primarily fat
(J Pain Sympt Man. 1997;14:7).

Class: Psychoactive component of marijuana

Dose: 2.5 mg bid (before lunch and before dinner)

CNS symptoms (dose-related mood high, confusion, dizziness, somnolence) usually resolve in 1-3 days with continued use. If these symptoms are severe or persist: reduce to 2.5 mg before dinner and/or administer at hs. If tolerated and additional therapeutic effect desired: increase dose to 5 mg bid; occasionally patients require 10 mg bid.

Pharmacology

Bioavailability: 90-95%

T½: 25-36 hours

Elimination: First pass hepatic metabolism and biliary excretion; 10-15% in urine.

Biologic effects post dose:
Onset of action: 0.5-1 hr, peak 24 hrs
Duration psychoactive effect 4-6 h; appetite effect: ≥24 hours

Side effects (dose-related): CNS with "high"-euphoria (3-10%), paranoia (3-10%), somnolence (3-10%), depersonalization, confusion, visual difficulties; GI intolerance (3-10%); central sympathomimetic effects - dizziness (3-10%), hypotension, palpitations, vasodilation, tachycardia; asthenia

Pregnancy: Category C

Drug interactions: Sympathomimetic agents (amphetamines, cocaine, etc.) – increased hypertension and tachycardia; anticholinergic drugs (atropine, scopolamine), amitriptyline, amoxapine, and other tricyclic antidepressants – tachycardia, drowsiness.

Warnings: Dronabinol is a psychoactive component of *Cannabis sativa* – marijuana

Schedule II (CII) – potential for abuse; use with caution in: a) substance abuse; b) patients with psychiatric illness (mania, depression, schizophrenia); c) patients concurrently receiving sedatives, hypnotics, etc.; d) elderly patients (experience limited); e) cardiac disorder (hypotension).

Warn patient: a) of CNS depression with concurrent use of alcohol, benzodiazepines, barbiturates, etc.; b) to avoid driving, operating machinery, etc. until safety and tolerance is established; c) of mood and behavior changes.

EFAVIRENZ (EFV)

Trade name: Sustiva (DuPont)

Form and price: 50, 100 and 200 mg capsules; $4.39/200 mg capsule or $394.22/month

Patient assistance program: (800) 344-4486

Class: Non-nucleoside reverse transcriptase inhibitor

Indication (FDA labeling): Recommended for treatment of HIV-1 infection in combination with other antiretroviral agents.

Dose: 600 mg/day, usually as three 200 mg capsules taken in the evening to reduce the CNS side effects that are common in the first 2–3 weeks. Patients should be warned of these side effects and of the possibility of rash. When changing from a PI containing regimen to efavirenz, overlap the PI and EFV by one week, since this is the time required to reach therapeutic levels.

Resistance: Mutations at the RT position 103 cause high level resistance to this as well as to other NNRTIs, including nevirapine (NVP) and delavirdine (DLV). Due to this relatively frequent one-step mutation that reduces susceptibility 10-fold, patients must be counseled about the importance of compliance. Other mutations associated with reduced susceptibility are at RT codons 100, 101, 108, 179 and 225. Mutations at codons 106 and 181 confer resistance to NVP and DLV, but EFV retains activity. Some patients failing therapy with NVP or DLV may not have the codon 103 mutation, and may respond to EFV. Genotypic resistance testing of early EFV virologic failures failed to show characteristic resistance mutations in 11/32 patients; these failures did not appear to be related to non-adherence and are unexplained (7th CROI, Abstract 752).

Clinical trial results: DuPont 006 included 750 participants with CD4 counts >50/mm³ and viral loads >10,000 and who had not received NNRTIs, protease inhibitors or 3TC. Participants were randomized to receive EFV/AZT/3TC, EFV/indinavir (IDV), or IDV/AZT/3TC. By intent-to-treat analysis at 48 weeks, 64% of those given EFV + 2 NRTIs had VL <50 c/mL compared to 43% given IDV + 2 NRTIs, and 47% given IDV/EFV (p<0.01) (NEJM 1999;341:1865). The mean increase in CD4 counts was 180-201/mm³ in these 3 groups. Subset analysis showed that EFV was as effective in patients with a baseline viral load >100,000 c/mL as in those with VL <100,000 c/mL. A subsequent ITT analysis at 72 weeks continued to show that significantly more patients in the EFV + 2 NRTI arm achieved HIV RNA levels <50 c/mL (60% vs. 40%), and again showed superiority of EFV in patients with baseline VL >100,000 c/mL (S. Staszewski, ICAAC 9/99, Abstract 507).

DuPont trial 020 included 282 patients with a CD4 cell count >50/mm³, viral load >10,000 c/mL and no prior treatment with NNRTIs or PIs. Participants were randomized to receive EFV + IDV + 1-2 NNRTIs versus IDV + 1-2 NRTIs. At 24 weeks 60% in the EFV arm had no detectable virus (<400 c/mL) compared to 50% in the IDV arm without EFV. ACTG 364 compared EFV and nelvinavir (NFV) in patients who had prolonged NRTI experience and who were naïve to NNRTIs and PIs, and had a baseline viral load >500 c/mL. EFV and/or NFV were added along with open label changes in NRTIs. By 40–48 weeks, the proportions with viral loads <500 c/mL were: EFV–60%, NFV–35% and NFV/EFV–74%. The superior response with EFV vs. NFV was statistically significant (6th Retrovirus Conf, 2/99, Chicago, Abstract 489).

ACTG 368 enrolled 195 patients who failed treatment with NRTIs but were naïve to PIs and NNRTIs. Participants received 1-2 NRTIs + NFV, EFV, or NFV + EFV. Results at 40-48 wks showed VL <50 c/mL in 22%, 44%, and 67%, respectively.

EFV is a favored agent for salvage or rescue therapy in patients who have failed PI-containing regimens and do not have prior NNRTI exposures or the RT 103 codon mutation.

Regimen: 600 mg/day in a single daily dose preferably in the evening (in combination with 2 nucleosides)

Combination with PIs: The combination most extensively studied is EFV (600 mg qd) + indinavir (1,000 mg q 8 h). In trial DMP-003, 74% had <50 c/mL at 48 weeks; in trial DMP-024, 53% had <50 c/mL at 24 weeks. These results are inferior to those achieved with EFV + 2 NRTIs; therefore, NRTIs should be included. Many authorities are reluctant to use this combination in treatment naïve patients due to the potential problem of resistance to both PIs and NNRTIs.

Indications: See Chapter 4

Pharmacology

> **Oral bioavailability:** 40–45% with or without food; high fat meals increase absorption 50% and should be avoided.

> **Half-life:** 40-55 hours

> **Distribution:** Highly protein-bound (>99%); CSF levels are 0.25-1.2% plasma levels which is above the IC_{95} for wild-type HIV (JID 1999;180:862).

> **Elimination:** Metabolized by cytochrome P450 (3A); 14-34% excreted in the urine as glucuronide metabolites and 16-61% in stool.

> **Dose modification with renal or hepatic disease:** No dose modification is advocated.

Side effects:

> **Rash:** Approximately 15-27% develop a rash, which is usually morbilliform and does not require discontinuation of the drug. More serious rash reactions that require discontinuation are blistering, and desquamating rashes, noted in about 1-2% of patients, and Stevens-Johnson syndrome, which has been reported in one of 2,200 recipients of EFV. The median time of onset of the rash is 11 days, and the duration with continued treatment is 14 days. The frequency with which the rash requires discontinuation of efavirenz is 1.7% compared to 7% given nevirapine and 4.3% given delavirdine.

> **CNS** side effects have been noted in up to 52% of patients, but are sufficiently severe to require discontinuation in only 2-5%. Symptoms are noted on day one and usually resolve after 2-4 weeks. They include confusion, abnormal thinking, impaired concentration, depersonalization, abnormal dreams, and

dizziness. Other side effects include somnolence, insomnia, amnesia, hallucinations and euphoria. Patients need to be warned of these side effects and also told that symptoms should resolve in 2-4 weeks. It is recommended that the drug be given in the evening during the initial weeks of treatment. This reduces side effects, but does not eliminate them because of the long half-life of efavirenz. There is a potential additive effect with acohol or other psychoactive drugs. Patients need to be cautioned to avoid driving or other potentially dangerous activities if they experience these symptoms.

Hyperlipidemia with increased cholesterol (including an *increase* in HDC) levels has been noted and should be monitored.

False positive cannabinoid test (marijuana) (screening test only, and only 1 brand.)

Increased aminotransferase levels: Levels >5 x ULN in 2-3%. Frequency is increased with hepatitis C or with concurrent hepatotoxic drugs.

Teratogenic in non-human primates. The drug should be avoided in pregnant women, and females should be warned to take adequate measures of contraception, including both barrier and other methods. Women of childbearing potential should have a negative pregnancy test prior to initiating efavirenz. (It should be noted that other antiretroviral agents have not been tested in primates, and the FDA has assigned a pregnancy category of C which is similar to most other antiretroviral drugs.)

Drug interactions: Efavirenz both induces and inhibits the cytochrome P450 3A4 enzymes, giving a variable effect on concentrations of concurrently administered drugs that utilize this pathway.

Contraindicated drugs for concurrent use: Astemizole, midazolam, trazolam, cisapride, and ergot alkaloids.

Other drugs with significant interactions: Rifabutin, rifampin, ethinyl estradiol, warfarin, and clarithromycin: There is a 46% incidence of rash reactions when combining efavirenz and clarithromycin, and levels of clarithromycin are decreased 39%; a clarithromycin, alternative should be used. EFV may reduce concentrations of phenobarbital, phenytoin and carbamazepine; monitor levels of anticonvulsant. Rifampin decreases efazirenz levels 25%; RIF levels are unchanged. Use standard doses. Rifabutin has no effect on EFV levels, but EFV reduces levels of rifabutin by 35%; with concurrent use the recommended dose of rifabutin is 450 mg/day plus the standard EFV dose. Concurrent use with ethinyl estradiol increases levels of the contraceptive by 37%; implications are unclear. EFV reduces methadone levels; titrate methadone levels to avoid opiate withdrawal. There are no data on interactions between EFV and the lipid lowering agents simvastatin and lovastatin. Monitor warfarin when used with EFV. Interactions and dose recommendations for EFV in combination with protease inhibitors are the following:

Table 6-13: Protease Inhibitors Interactions and Dose Recommendations

PI	PI AUC	EFV AUC	Recommendation
Indinavir	↓ 31%	No change	IDV 1,000 mg q 8 h + EFV 600 mg/d
Ritonavir	↑ 18%	↑ 21%	RTV 500-600 mg bid + EFV 600 mg/d
Nelfinavir	↑ 20%	No change	NFV 750 mg tid or 1,250 mg bid + EFV 600 mg/d
Saquinavir	↓ 62%	↓ 12%	Not recommended
Amprenavir	↓ 36%	No change	APV 1200 mg tid as single PI *or* APV 1200 mg bid + RTV 200 mg bid + EFV 600 mg/d
Saquinavir/ Ritonavir	SQV/RTV no change	No change	Standard dose

Combination of 2 PIs/EFV:

- EFV 600 mg qd/SQV 400 mg bid/RTV 400 mg bid

- EFV 600 mg qd/APV 1200 mg bid/RTV 200 mg bid

- EFV 600 mg qd/APV 1200 mg bid/NFV 1250 mg bid

- EFV/RTV/IDV combination is under study

Pregnancy: Class C. This drug causes birth defects (anencephaly, anophthalmia and microophthalmia) in cynomolgus monkeys. Other antiretroviral drugs have not been studied for safety in non-human primates, and the FDA has assigned FDA pregnancy category C which is the same as with AZT, d4T, 3TC, ABC, IDV, APV, NVP, and DLV. The current recommendation is to carefully avoid efavirenz during pregnancy, to warn potentially pregnant women of this complication, and to assure adequate contraceptive protection.

ENOXACIN – See Ciprofloxacin (Fluoroquinolone Summary, page 207)

EPIVIR – See Lamivudine (3TC) (p. 229)

EPOGEN – See Erythropoietin (p. 199)

ERYTHROPOIETIN (EPO)

Trade name: Procrit (Ortho Biotech)

AWP/vial: 2,000 units = $24; 3,000 units = $36; 4,000 units = $48;
10,000 units = $120
Usual dose: 10,000 units 3x/week = $360/wk

Patient assistance program: Procrit – Reimbursement and financial assistance (800) 553-3851. Patient must have no insurance coverage (or denial after reimbursement appeal) plus physician contact to qualify for financial assistance.

Product Information: EPO is a hormone produced by recombinant DNA technology. It has the same amino acid sequence and biologic effects as endogenous erythropoietin, which is produced primarily by the kidneys in response to hypoxia and anemia. Both forms act by stimulating the proliferation of red blood cells from progenitor cells found in the bone marrow.

Indications: Serum EPO level <500 milliunits/mL plus: 1) anemia ascribed to HIV infection, and 2) anemia ascribed to AZT treatment in doses <600 mg/d (Ann Intern Med 1992;117:739; JAIDS 1992;5:847).

Efficacy: A U.S. trial using recombinant human erythropoietin (rHU EPO) was initiated in July 1989, with 1,943 evaluable patients. Participants had serum EPO levels of <500 U/L and hematocrits <30%; 75% were receiving AZT at entry or at some point during the study period. The initial dose was 4,000 U SQ 6 days/week; mean weekly doses ranged from 22,700-32,500 U/week (340-490 U/kg/week). Response to treatment, defined as an increase in baseline hematocrit by six percentage points (eg, 30%-36%) with no transfusions within 28 days, was achieved in 44%; transfusion requirements decreased from 40% of participants in six weeks pretreatment to 18% at weeks 18-24. The average hematocrit among participants was 28% at entry and 35% at one year. To determine if the effects of rHu EPO therapy would be comparable for patients not receiving AZT, Balfour and colleagues performed a retrospective analysis of a subgroup of patients who were AZT naïve or received AZT previously but not at the time of the study. Response to treatment was similar for all groups and was independent of AZT administration (Internat J Antimicrob Ag 1997;8:189).

Dose recommendations: Initial dose is 40,000 units subcutaneously weekly (see page 138). Onset of action is within 1-2 weeks, reticulocytosis is noted at 7-10 days, increases in hematocrit are noted in 2-6 weeks, and desired hematocrit is usually attained in 8-12 weeks. Response is dependent on the degree of initial anemia, baseline EPO level, dose of EPO, and available iron stores. Response will usually not be seen for ≥2 weeks. Transferrin saturation should be ≥20%; serum ferritin should be ≥100 ng/mL. If levels are suboptimal, supplement with iron. (Some experts advocate routine iron supplementation in all patients taking EPO.) If after 4 weeks of therapy the Hb rise is <1 g/dL, dose may be increased to 60,000 U SQ weekly. After an additional 4 weeks, if Hb does not increase by at least 1 g/dL from baseline value, discontinue EPO therapy. After achieving the desired response (i.e., increased Hb/Hct level or reduction in transfusion requirements), titrate the dose for maintenance. If Hb >13 g/dL or Hct >40% decrease EPO by 10,000 units/wk. When Hb is >15 g/dL, discontinue EPO, reducing dose by 10,000 units/week. With failure to respond or suboptimal response, consider iron deficiency, occult blood loss, folic acid or B12 deficiency or hemolysis.

Pharmacology

> **Bioavailability:** EPO is a 165-amino acid glycoprotein that is not absorbed with oral administration. IV or SC administration is required; SC is preferred.
>
> **T½:** 4-16 hours
>
> **Elimination:** Poorly understood but minimally affected by renal failure.
>
> **Dose adjustment in renal or hepatic failure:** None

Side effects: Generally well tolerated; serious reactions have not been described. Headache and arthralgias are most common; less common – flu-like symptoms, GI intolerance, diarrhea, edema, fatigue. Hypertension is an uncommon complication that has been noted more frequently in patients with renal failure. EPO is contra-indicated in patients with hypertension that is uncontrolled. The most common reactions noted in the therapeutic trial with 1,943 AIDS patients were rash, medication site reaction, nausea, hypertension, and seizures; relationship to EPO was often unclear.

Pregnancy: Class C. Teratogenic in animals; no studies in humans

ETHAMBUTOL

Trade name: Myambutol (Lederle; Wyeth-Ayerst)

Forms and price: 100 and 400 mg tabs at $1.85/400 mg tab

Patient assistant program (Wyeth): (800) 568-9938

Indication: Active tuberculosis or infections with *M. avium* complex or *M. kansasii*

Dose: For tuberculosis: 15 mg-25 mg/kg po given as one daily dose, usually 25 mg/kg/day x 1-2 months, then 15 mg/kg/day; maximum dose: 2.5 gm/day. Twice weekly treatment: 50 mg/kg; thrice weekly treatment: 25-30 mg/kg. Dose for *M. avium*: 15 mg/kg/day (800-1200 mg/day).

Pharmacology

> **Bioavailability:** 77%
>
> **T½:** 3.1 hours
>
> **Elimination:** Renal
>
> **Dose modification in renal failure:** CrCl >50 mL/min – 15-25 mg/kg q 24 h; 10-50 mL/min – 15-25 mg/kg q 24-36 h; <10 mL/min – 15-25 mg/kg q 48 h

Side effects: Dose-related ocular toxicity (decreased acuity, restricted fields, scotomata, and loss of color discrimination) with 25 mg/kg dose (0.8%), hypersensitivity (0.1%); peripheral neuropathy (rare); GI intolerance

Pregnancy: Category C. Teratogenic in animals; no reported adverse effects in women; "use with caution."

Warnings: Patients to receive ethambutol should undergo a baseline screening for visual acquity and red-green color perception; this exam should be repeated at monthly intervals during treatment (MMWR 1998;47[RR20]:31).

Drug interactions: Al++ containing antacids may decrease absorption.

FAMCICLOVIR – See Acyclovir (p. 160)

FENTANYL

Trade name: Duragesic (Janssen), Fentanyl Orlet (Abbott)

Forms: Injection-Fentanyl citrate, 50 µg/mL; Buccal (transmucosal) lozenge – 200, 300, 400 µg

> Transdermal
> | | | | |
> |---|---|---|---|
> | 25 µg/hr (2.5 mg/cm²) Duragesic .... | 25: | $11.80 |
> | 50 µg/hr (5 mg/cm²) Duragesic .... | 50: | $17.60 |
> | 75 µg/hr (7.5 mg/cm²) Duragesic .... | 75: | $28.20 |
> | 100 µg/hr (40 mg/cm²) Duragesic................ | 100: | $35.00 |

Class: Opiate; Schedule II controlled substance

Indications: Chronic pain requiring opiate analgesia

Note: Buccal (transmucosal) form should be used only with monitoring in the hospital (OR, ICU, EW) due to life-threatening respiratory depression. Use in AIDS is primarily restricted to management of chronic pain in late-stage disease using the transdermal form. This drug should not be used for the management of acute pain.

Pharmacology: Transdermal fentanyl systems deliver an average of 25 µg/hr/10 cm² at a constant rate. Serum levels increase slowly, plateau at 12-24 hours and then remain constant for up to 72 hours. The labeling indicates the amount of fentanyl delivered/hr. Peak serum levels for the different systems are the following: fentanyl – 25: 0.3-1.2 ng/mL, 50: 0.6-1.8 ng/mL, 75: 1.1-2.6 ng/mL, and 100: 1.9-3.8 ng/mL. After discontinuation, serum levels decline with a mean half-life of 17 hours. Absorption depends on skin temperature and theoretically increases by one-third when the body temperature is 40°C. In acute pain models, the 100 µg/hr form provided analgesia equivalent to 60 mg of morphine IM.

Dosing recommendations: Dose depends on desired therapeutic effect, patient weight, and most importantly, existing opiate tolerance. The initial dose in opiate-naive patients is a system delivering 25 µg/hr.

Cachectic patients should not receive a higher initial dose unless they have been receiving the equivalent of 135 mg of oral morphine. Most patients are maintained with patch applications at 72-hour intervals. Adequacy of analgesia should be evaluated at 72 hours. The dose should be increased to maintain the 72-hour interval if possible, but application q 48 hrs is another option. Supplemental opiates may be required with initial use to control pain and to determine optimal fentanyl dose. The suggested conversion ratio is 90 mg of oral morphine/24 hours to each 25 µg/hr labeled delivery. To convert patients who currently receive opiate therapy, the following daily doses are considered equivalent to 30-60 mg of oral morphine sulfate: Morphine sulfate, 10 mg IM; codeine 200 mg po, heroin 5 mg im or 60 mg po, meperidine 75 mg IM, methadone 20 mg po, and oxycodone 15 mg IM or 30 mg po. The equivalent doses of fentanyl patches are:

Tables 6-14: Equivalence of Fentanyl Patches and Oral Morphine Sulfate

Oral MS/day	Fentanyl (µg/hr)	Oral MS	Fentanyl (µg/hr)
45-134 mg	25	495-584 mg	150
135-224 mg	50	675-764 mg	200
225-314 mg	75	55-994 mg	250
315-404 mg	100	1035-1124 mg	300

Side effects: Respiratory depression with hypoventilation. This occurs throughout the therapeutic range of fentanyl concentration, but increases at concentrations >2 ng/mL in opiate-naive patients and in patients with pulmonary disease. **CNS depression** is seen with concentrations >3 ng/mL in opiate-naive patients. At levels of 10-20 ng/mL there is anesthesia and profound respiratory depression. **Tolerance** occurs with extended courses, but there is considerable individual variation. **Local effects** include erythema, papules, pruritis, and edema at the site of application. **Drug interactions** include increased Fentanyl levels with protease inhibitors given concurrently.

Application instructions: The protective liner-cover should be peeled just prior to use. Application is to a dry nonirritated flat surface of the upper torso by firm pressing for 30 seconds. Hair should be clipped, not shaven, and the skin cleansed with water (not soaps or alcohol that could irritate skin) prior to application. Avoid external heat to the site since absorption is temperature-dependent. Use different sites with sequential use. After removal, the used system should be folded so the adhesive side adheres to itself, and flushed in the toilet.

FILGRASTIM – See G-CSF (p. 214)

FLAGYL – See Metronidazole (p. 237)

FLOXIN – See Ciprofloxacin (Fluoroquinolone Summary, page 207)

FLUCONAZOLE

Trade name: Diflucan (Pfizer)

Forms and price: 50 mg tab – $4.60; 100 mg tab – $7.24; 150 mg tab – $11.50; 200 mg tab – $11.83; IV vials of 200 mg – $85.50; IV vials of 400 mg – $125

Patient assistance program: (800) 869-9979 or (800) 646-4455. Patients must have no insurance coverage, including Medicaid, and meet income criteria (<$25,000/yr for single person and <$40,000 for married couple). Up to three-month supply provided.

Class: Triazole related to other imidazoles – ketoconazole, clotrimazole, miconazole; tri-azoles (fluconazole and itraconazole) have three nitrogens in the azole ring.

Pharmacology

> **Bioavailability:** >90%
>
> **CSF levels:** 50-94% serum levels
>
> **T½:** 30 hours
>
> **Elimination:** Renal, 60-80% of administered dose excreted unchanged in the urine
>
> **Dose modification in renal failure:** CrCl >50 mL/min – usual dose; 10-50 mL/min half dose; <10 mL/min – quarter dose.

Resistance: Major concern with long-term use of fluconazole is azole resistant *Candida sp.* Resistance correlates with azole exposure and CD4 count <50/mm^3. All azoles predispose to resistance. *In vitro* sensitivity testing is not usually helpful.

Table 6-15: Dose Recommendations for Fluconazole

Indications	Dose regimen*	Comment
Candida:		
Thrush	50-100 mg po/d x 14 days	Response rate 80-100%. Maintenance therapy often required.
Esophagitis	200 mg po/d x 2-3 weeks	Superior to ketoconazole. (Ann Intern Med 1992;117:655)
Vaginitis	150 mg x 1 or 50 mg/d x 3 or 200 mg weekly	Response rate 90-100% in absence of HIV infection.
Cryptococcosis:		
Non-meningeal	200-400 mg po/d	Usual initial dose is 400 mg/day x 8 wks, then 200 mg/d.
Meningitis	200 mg po/d (maintenance)	Initial treatment with amphotericin B usually preferred; if fluconazole used initially, the standard dose is 400 mg/day x 8 weeks, then 200 mg/day.
Prophylaxis	100-200 mg po/d	Efficacy established for preventing thrush, candida esophagitis, and cryptococcosis; concerns are cost, drug interactions, and promotion of azole-resistant candida infections (NEJM 1995;332-700). Not advocated in CDC-IDSA recommendations for prophylaxis (MMWR 1995;44[RR-8]:1).
Coccidioidomycosis:		
Maintenance	200 mg/po/d	Drug of choice.
Prophylaxis	200 mg po/d	Prophylaxis is not generally recommended.

*Note: Many use double dose the first day (200-400 mg) when treating established infections.

Side effects: GI intolerance (1.5-8%, usually does not require discontinuation); rash (5%); transient increases in hepatic enzymes (5%), increases of ALT or AST to >8x upper limit of normal requires discontinuation (1%); dizziness, hypokalemia, and headache (2%). Reversible alopecia in 10-20% receiving ≥400 mg/day at median time of three months after starting treatment (Ann Intern Med 1995;123:354).

Pregnancy: Category C. Animal studies show reduced maternal weight gain and embryolethality with dose >20x comparable doses in humans; no studies in humans.

Drug interactions: Inhibits cytochrome P450 hepatic enzymes to cause increased levels of atovaquone, benzodiazepines, clarithromycin, opiate analgesics, coumadin, saquinavir, phenytoin, oral hypoglycemics, rifabutin, and cyclosporine; increased levels of terfenadine (Seldane) and Propulsid may cause life-threatening arrhythmias. Fluconazole levels are reduced with rifampin and rifabutin; fluconazole increases levels of rifabutin with increased risk of uveitis.

FLUCYTOSINE (5-FC)

Generic

Trade name: Ancobon (Roche)

Forms and price: 250 & 500 mg caps; $2.52/500 mg caps

Class: Fluorinated pyrimidien structurally related to fluorouracil

Indication: Used with amphotericin B to treat serious infections caused by *Candida sp.* and cryptococcosis. ACTG 159 showed there was no advantage from addition of 5-FC (100 mg/kg/day) in AIDS patients with cryptococcal meningitis compared to amphotericin B alone (ICAAC, 9/95 Abstract 12/6). A subsequent report suggested benefit with the addition of 5-FC; many advocate its use for the first two weeks of treatment.

Dose: 25-37.5 mg/kg po q 6 h (100-150 mg/kg/d)

Pharmacology

> **Bioavailability:** >80%
>
> **T½:** 2.4-4.8 hours
>
> **Elimination:** 63-84% unchanged in urine
>
> **CNS penetration:** 80% serum levels
>
> **Dose modification in renal failure:** CrCl >50 mL/min – 25-37.6 mg/ kg q 6 h; 10-50 min/mL – 25-37 mg/kg q 12-24 h; <10 mL/min – not recommended.
>
> **Therapeutic monitoring:** Measure serum concentration two hours post oral dose with goal of peak level of 50-100 mcg/mL.

Side effects: Dose related leukopenia and thrombocytopenia, especially with renal failure (often secondary to concurrent amphotericin B), levels >100 mcg/mL and concurrent use of other marrow suppressing agents; GI intolerance; rash; hepatitis; peripheral neuropathy.

Pregnancy: Category C. Teratogenic in animals; no studies in patients. Contraindicated in pregnancy unless benefits outweigh potential risks.

Table 6-16: FLUOROQUINOLONE SUMMARY

	Ciprofloxacin Cipro	Levofloxacin Levaquin	Gatifloxacin Tequin	Moxifloxacin Avelox
Oral Forms	+	+	+	+
IV form	+	+	+	—
Price (Avg wholesale)	$4.29/500 mg	$8.53/500 mg	$7.00/400 mg	$8.71/400 mg
T½	3.3 hrs	6.3 hrs.	8 hrs	12 hrs
T½ renal failure	8 hrs	35 hrs.	16 hrs	12 hrs
Oral bioavailability	65%	99%	96%	90%
Activity *in vitro*				
P. aeruginosa	++(90%)	++	+	+
S. pneumoniae	+	++	++	++
Mycobacteria	++	++	++	++
Anaerobes	—	+	++	++
Regimens (oral)*	250-750 mg bid	500mg qd	400 mg qd	400 mg qd

All fluoroquinolones are active against most *Enterobacteriaceae*, enteric bacterial pathogens (except *C. difficile*), methicillin-sensitive *S. aureus*, *Neisseria sp.*, and pulmonary pathogens including *S. pneumoniae*, *H. influenzae*, *C. pneumoniae*, *H. influenzae*, *C. pneumoniae*, Legionella and *Mycoplasma pneumoniae*. Major advantages of newer fluoroquinolones are once daily dosing, good tolerance and activity vs. *S. pneumoniae*, including >98% of penicillin-resistant strains. Class side effects include prolongation of QT interval when given to persons predisposed primarily by concurrent meds, tendon rupture, and CNS toxicity including seizures. All are contraindicated in persons <18 years and in pregnant women. Divalent cations reduce absorption – avoid concurrent antacids with Mg++ or Al++, sucralfate, Fe++, Zn++, and ddl.

VI. Drugs

FLUOXETINE

Trade name: Prozac (Lilly-Dista)

Forms and price: 10, 20 mg caps, solution 20 mg/5 mL; 10 mg cap – $2.43; 20 mg cap – $2.50

Class: SSRI (serotonin reuptake inhibitor) antidepressant; not a controlled substance. Other drugs in this class include Paxil, Zoloft, and Serzone.

Indications and dose

> Major depression: 10-40 mg/day usually given once daily in the morning. Onset of response requires 2-6 wks. Doses of 5-10 mg/day may be adequate in debilitated patients.

> Obsessive compulsive disorder: 20-80 mg/day

Pharmacology

> **Bioavailability:** 60-80%

> **T½:** 7-9 days for norfluoxetine (active metabolite)

> **Elimination:** Metabolized by liver to norfluoxetine; fluoxetine eliminated in urine

> **Dose modification in renal failure:** None

> **Dose modification in cirrhosis:** Half-life prolonged – reduce dose

Side effects: Toxicity may not be apparent for 2-6 weeks. GI intolerance (anorexia, weight loss, nausea) – 20%; anxiety, agitation, insomnia – 20%; less common – headache, tremor, drowsiness, dry mouth, sweating, diarrhea, sexual dysfunction (anorgasmia or delayed orgasm), acute dystonia, akathisia (sensation of motor restlessness).

Note: Case reports suggested an association with suicidal preoccupation; reanalysis of data showed no significant difference compared to treatment with other antidepressants or placebo (J Clin Psychopharm 1991;11:166), and the FDA concluded there was no unreasonable or unexpected risk.

Drug interactions: MAO inhibitors – avoid initiation of treatment with fluoxetine until ≥14 days after discontinuing MAO inhibitor; avoid starting MAO inhibitor until ≥5 wks after discontinuing fluoxetine (risk is "serotonergic syndrome").

Inhibits P450 cytochrome: Increased levels of tricyclic agents (desipramine, nortriptyline, etc.), phenytoin, digoxin, coumadin, terfenadine (ventricular arrhythmias), saquinavir, astemizole, theophylline, haloperidol, carbamazepine.

FLURAZEPAM – See Benzodiazapines (p. 176)

FOMIVIRSEN

Trade name: Vitravene (Isis Pharmaceuticals)

Form: 2 mL intravitreal injection

Cost: $880/dose ($1,760 1ˢᵗ month, then $880/month)

Indication: CMV retinitis

Class: Antisense phosphorothioate oligonucleotide. This is a 21 nucleotide with a sequence that is complementary to mRNA transcribed from the major immediate-early transcriptional unit of CMV (AAC 1998;42:971; AAC 1996;40:2004).

FDA labeling: Local treatment of CMV retinitis in patients with AIDS who are intolerant of or have a contraindication to alternative treatments (Package insert).

Activity: Potent activity vs. CMV including strains resistant to ganciclovir, foscarnet and cidofovir. Activity is 30 fold greater than ganciclovir (Antiviral Res 1995;28:101).

Dose: 330 mcg (0.05 mL) intravitreal injection day 1 and day 15, then once monthly

Efficacy: Median time to response is 7-10 days, and median time to progression is 90-110 days

Pharmacology

> **T½ in vitreous humor:** 60–80 hrs

> **Elimination:** Exonucleases

Side effects: 1) Ocular inflammation (uvcitis) with iritis and vitritis in 25% – usually responds to topical corticosteroids. 2) Increased intraocular pressure – usually transient, but should be monitored.

Pregnancy: Category C

FORTOVASE – See Saquinavir (p. 262)

FOSCARNET

Trade name: Foscavir (Astra)

Forms: Vials of 6,000 mg and 12,000 mg with 24 mg/mL

Cost: $73.25/6,000 mg (70 kg patient): induction – $146/day; maintenance – $73/day. Ganciclovir comparison: induction – $52/day; maintenance – $26/ day

Patient assistance program: (800) 488-3247

Activity: Active against herpes viruses including CMV, HSV-1, HSV-2, EBV (oral hairy leukoplakia), VZV, HHV-6, HHV-8 (Kaposi sarcoma-related herpes-virus), most ganciclovir-resistant CMV, and most acyclovir-resistant HSV and VZV. Also active against HIV *in vitro* and *in vivo*. The frequency of CMV resistance *in vitro* is 20-30% after 6-12 months of foscarnet treatment (JID 1998;177:770). Studies of patients with CMV retinitis showed a mean decrease of 0.5 log HIV RNA/mL during foscarnet therapy (JID 1995;172:225). The major clinical experience is with CMV retinitis, which revealed that clinical effectiveness is equivalent to that of ganciclovir (NEJM 1992;326:213; Ophthalmology 1994;101:1250). In two trials foscarnet was associated with increased survival compared with ganciclovir (NEJM 1992;326:213; Am J Med 1993;94:175), but had more treatment-limiting side effects. Many question the relavance of these data in the era of HAART. *In vitro* activity versus HHV-8 is good, but results with foscarnet treatment of Kaposi sarcoma (KS) is variable; if KS is a true neoplasm, this treatment is of doubtful significance once transformance has occurred (Science 1998;282:1837).

Table 6-17: Dose Recommendations for Foscarnet

Indication	Dose regimen
CMV retinitis	Induction: 60 mg/kg IV q 8 h or 90 mg/kg IV q 12 h x 14 days Maintenance: 90-120 mg/kg IV qd[†]
CMV (other)	60 mg/kg IV q 8 h or 90 mg/kg IV q 12 h x 14-21 days, indications for maintenance treatment are unclear
Acyclovir-resistant HSV	40 mg/kg IV q 8 h or 60 mg/kg q 12 h x 3 weeks
Acyclovir-resistant VSV	40 mg/kg IV q 8 h or 60 mg/kg q 12 h x 3 weeks

[†] Survival and time to relapse may be significantly prolonged with maintenance dose of 120 mg/d vs 90 mg/d (JID 1993;168:444).

Pharmacology

Bioavailability: 58% absorption with oral administration, but poorly tolerated

T½: 3 hours

CSF levels: 15-70% plasma levels

Elimination: Renal exclusively

Administration: Controlled IV infusion using ≤24 mg/mL (undiluted) by central venous catheter or <12 mg/mL (diluted in 5% dextrose or saline) via a peripheral line. No other drug is to be given concurrently via the same catheter. Induction dose of 60 mg/kg is given over ≥1 hour via infusion pump with adequate hydration. Maintenance treatment with 90-120 mg/kg is given over ≥2 hours by infusion pump with adequate hydration. Many use 90 mg/kg/d for initial maintenance and 120 mg/kg/d for maintenance after re-induction for a relapse.

Table 6-18: Foscarnet Dose Adjustment In Renal Failure

CrCl (mL/min/kg)	60 mg/kg dose	90 mg/kg dose	120 mg/kg dose
>1.4	60	90	120
1.3	49	78	104
1.1	42	75	100
0.9	35	71	94
0.7	28	63	84
0.5	21	57	76

VI. Drugs

Side effects:

1. Dose-related renal impairment – 37% treated for CMV retinitis have serum creatinine increase to ≥2 mg/dL; most common in second week of induction and usually reversible with recovery of renal function within one week of discontinuation. Monitor creatinine 2-3x/week with induction and q 1-2 weeks during maintenance. Modify dose for creatinine clearance changes. Foscarnet should be stopped for creatinine clearance <0.4 mL/min/kg.

2. Changes in serum electrolytes including hypocalcemia (15%), hypophosphatemia (8%), hypomagnesemia (15%), and hypokalemia (16%). Patients should be warned to report symptoms of hypocalcemia: perioral paresthesias, extremity paresthesias, and numbness. Monitor serum Ca++, Mg++, K+, and PO4 and creatinine, usually ≥2x/week during induction and 1x/wk during maintenance. If paresthesias develop with normal electrolytes, measure ionized calcium at start and end of infusion.

3. Seizures (10%) related to renal failure and hypocalcemia.

4. Penile ulcers.

5. Miscellaneous: Nausea, vomiting, headache, rash, fever, hepatitis, marrow suppression

Pregnancy: Category C. No adequate studies in animals or humans.

Drug interactions: Concurrent administration with IV pentamidine may cause severe hypocalcemia. Avoid concurrent use of potentially nephrotoxic drugs such as amphotercin B, aminoglycosides, and pentamidine. Possible increase in seizures with imipenem.

FOSCAVIR – See Foscarnet (above)

FUNGIZONE – See Amphotericin B (p. 165)

GANCICLOVIR

Trade Name: Cytovene (Hoffman-LaRoche) and ganciclovir ocular implant: Vitrasert (Chiron Vision)

Forms and price: 500 mg vial @ $35.68, 250 mg caps @ $3.99/cap, 500 mg caps @ $7.99

Patient assistance program: (800) 285-4484. Patient must have CMV retinitis, no insurance coverage, and inability to pay plus outpatient treatment. Vitracert (ocular implant): (800) 843-1137.

Class: Synthetic purine nucleoside analog of guanine.

Active against herpes viruses including CMV, HSV-1, HSV-2, EBV, VZV, HHV-6 and HHV-8 (Kaposi sarcoma). About 10% of patients given ganciclovir ≥3 months for CMV will excrete resistant strains that are sensitive to foscarnet (JID 1991;163:716; JID 1991;163:1348). The frequency of ganciclovir resistance at 12 months is 26% (JID 1998;177:770). Ganciclovir is active *in vitro* against HHV-8, but the clinical experience with ganciclovir treatment of Kaposi sarcoma is variable; it may be necessary to treat HHV-8 seropositive patients prior to transformance if KS is a true neoplasm (Science 1998;282:1837).

Indications and dose regimen:

    CMV retinitis: 5 mg/kg IV q 12 h x 14-21 days, then maintenance with 5 mg/kg/day IV or 1.0 gm tid po. Comparative trials of ganciclovir vs foscarnet show these drugs are therapeutically equivalent for CMV retinitis with mean times to relapse of 40-60 days (NEJM 1992;326:213; Am J Med 1993;94:175). Patients with relapse were studied in ACTG 228, in which re-induction with the same agent (IV ganciclovir or IV foscarnet) was as effective as switching to the alternative. Combination treatment was superior in terms of time to progression, but was associated with a lower quality of life. In SOCA (Study of Ocular Complications of AIDS), ganciclovir was associated with a significant reduction in p24 antigen, suggesting inhibition of CMV limited HIV replication (JID 1995;172:613). With maintenance therapy the time to relapse is somewhat earlier with oral vs IV ganciclovir, but it avoids the inconvenience, cost, and complications of the indwelling IV catheter (NEJM 1995;333:615). Many authorities now prefer the sustained release ganciclovir implant (Vitrasert) for CMV retinitis, usually in combination with oral ganciclovir to prevent systemic CMV disease and contralateral retinitis (NEJM 1997;337:83;337:105).

    Other forms of disseminated CMV: Indications to treat are often not well established. The usual regimen is the induction dose used for retinitis; need for maintenance therapy is not clear except for CMV encephalitis and CMV radiculopathy. Oral ganciclovir has been FDA-approved only for maintenance therapy of CMV retinitis.

CMV prophylaxis: In one study oral ganciclovir (1 gm po tid) significantly reduced rates of CMV disease (primarily retinitis) in AIDS patients with a CD4 count <50/mm³. Disadvantages include cost (about $15,000/yr), the "pill burden" (12 tabs/day), side effects (neutropenia and possibly anemia), and possible promotion of ganciclovir resistance. In addition, another more recent study of oral ganciclovir (CPCRA 023) failed to show significant benefit. Routine use of oral ganciclovir for primary CMV prophylaxis is not currently recommended.

Pharmacology

Bioavailability: 3-5% in fasting state; 6-9% with meal. Administration of oral form with meals needs emphasis.

Serum level: Mean peak with IV induction doses is 11.5 µg/mL. (MIC50 of CMV is 0.1-2.75 µg/mL.) Mean peak with oral regimen is 1 µg/mL, which approximates the CMV median 50% inhibitory concentration. This is about 10% of the peak levels achieved with IV administration, but AUC is 18 µg/hr/mL for oral administration vs 26 µg/hr/mL with 5 mg/kg/day given IV (JID 1995;171:1431).

CSF concentrations: 24-70% of plasma levels; Intravitreal concentrations: 10-15% of plasma levels – 0.96 µg/mL (JID 1993;168:1506)

T½: 2.5-3.6 hours with IV administration; 3-7.3 with oral administration.

Elimination: IV form: 90-99% excreted unchanged in urine. Oral form: 86% in stool and 5% recovered in urine.

Table 6-19: Ganciclovir Dose Modification In Renal Failure

IV form	Capsule form
CrCl >80 mL/min ....5 mg/kg q 12 h	**CrCl** >70 mL/min ....1000 mg tid
50-79 mL/min ....2.5 mg/kg q 12 h	50-69 mL/min ....50 mg tid
25-49 mL/min ....2.5 mg/kg q 24 h	25-49 mL/min ....500 mg/day
<25 mL/min ....1.25 mg/kg q 24 h	<10 mL/min ....3x/wk post hemodialysis

Side effects: IV form: 1) Neutropenia with ANC <500/mm^3 (25-40%) requires discontinuation of drug in ≥20%; alternative is administration of G-CSF; discontinuation or reduced dose will result in increased ANC in 3-7 days. Monitor CBC 2-3x/wk and discontinue if ANC <500/mm^3 or platelet count <25,000/mm^3; 2) thrombocytopenia in 2-8%; 3) CNS toxicity in 10-15% with headaches, seizures, confusion, coma; 4) hepatotoxicity (2-3%); 5) GI intolerance (2%). Note: Neutropenia (ANC <500/dL) or thrombocytopenia (<25,000/dL) represents contraindications to initial use. Oral form: Neutropenia with ANC <500/dL in 18%, <750/dL in 35%; anemia with Hgb <8 gm% in 10%, <9.5% in 35%; serum creatinine >2.5 mg/dL in 4%, >1.5 mg/dL in 73%.

Pregnancy: Category C. Teratogenic in animals in concentrations comparable to those achieved in humans; should be avoided unless need justifies the risk.

Drug interaction: AZT increases the risk of neutropenia, and concomitant use is not recommended. Other marrow-toxic drugs include interferon, sulfadiazine, hydroxyurea, and TMP-SMX. Oral and IV ganciclovir increase AUC of ddI by 100% – monitor for adverse effect of ddI (MMWR 1999;48[RR-10]:48). Probenecid increases ganciclovir levels by 50%. Additive or synergistic activity with foscarnet *in vitro* against CMV and HSV. Use with caution with drugs that inhibit replication or rapidly dividing cells – dapsone, pentamidine, pyrimethamine, flucytosine, cytotoxic antineoplastic drugs (vincristine, vinblastine, doxorubicin), amphotericin B, trimethoprim-sulfamethoxazole, and nucleoside analogs.

G-CSF (FILGRASTIM)

Trade name: Neupogen (Amgen)

Forms and price: 300 µg in 1 mL vial and 480 µg in 1.6 mL vial; 300 µg $165.30

Patient instructions: Subcutaneous injections are usually self administered using abdomen or upper thighs; back of upper arms if injected by someone else. Injection sites should be rotated. The drug should be stored in a refrigerator at 36-46°F.

Note: 300 µg vial is the only form available. Pharmacists commonly instruct patients to discard unused portion; the cost-effective alternative is to retain the unused portion in refrigerated syringes for later use. For example, a 75 µg dose = 1 immediate dose and 3 syringes with subsequent doses.

Reimbursement assistance/appeal: (800) 272-9376. Patient must have lack of prescription drug insurance and financial need.

Product information: A 20-kilodalton glycoprotein produced by recombinant technique that stimulates granulocyte precursors

Indication: Neutropenia with ANC <500-750/mm^3 ascribed to 1) zidovudine (AZT) (Blood 1991;77:2109); 2) other drugs such as ganciclovir, TMP-SMX, hydroxyurea, and interferon; 3) cancer chemotherapy (lymphoma or Kaposi's sarcoma); or 4) HIV infection. Indications are arbitrary. Some authorities conclude that AIDS patients may tolerate low ANC levels better than cancer patients in terms of infectious complications (Arch Intern Med 1995;155:1965; Infect Control Hosp Epid 1991;12:429), and G-CSF is "not recommended for most patients" with neutropenia, according to the 1995 guidelines of USPHS/IDSA (MMWR 1995;44[RR-8]:1). Nevertheless, the incidence of bacterial infections appears to be increased 2-3 fold in patients with an ANC <500/mL (Lancet 1989;2:91; Arch Intern Med 1995;155:1965), and most HIV infected patients respond. A therapeutic trial in 258 HIV-infected patients with ANC of 750–1,000/mm³ showed G-CSF recipients had 31% fewer bacterial infections, 54% fewer severe bacterial infections and 45% fewer hospital days for these infections (AIDS 1998;12:65). USPHS/IDSA 1999 recommendations are that use of G-CSF or GM-CSF is "not routinely indicated" in neutropenic HIV-infected patients.

VI. Drugs

Dose: Initial dose is 5-10 µg/kg/day subcutaneously (lean body weight) usually about 5 µg/kg/day. For practical purposes the dose will be a convenient approximation of the calculated dose for a 1.0, 0.5 or 0.2 cc syringe. This may be increased by 1 µg/kg/day after 5-7 days up to 10 mcg/kg/day or decreased and given either daily or every other day. Monitor CBC 2x/wk and keep ANC >1,000-2,000/mL. If unresponsive after 7 days at 10 µg/kg/day, treatment should be discontinued.

Pharmacology

> **Absorption:** Not absorbed with oral administration. G-CSF must be given IV or SQ; SQ is usually preferred.

> **T½:** 3.5 hours (subcutaneous injection)

> **Elimination:** Renal

Side effects: Medullary bone pain is the only important side effect, noted in 10-20%, and usually controlled with acetaminophen.

Rare side effects: Mild dysuria, reversible abnormal liver function tests, increased uric acid, and increased LDH.

Pregnancy: Category C. Caused abortion and embryolethality in animals at 2-10x dose in humans; no studies in humans.

Drug interactions: Should not be given within 24 hours of cancer chemotherapy.

G-CSF: is also available from three suppliers as Leucoman (Sandoz), Leukine (Immunex), and Prokine (Hoechst-Roussel). This may also be used for neutropenia. There has been concern that stimulation of the monocyte/macrophage cells would enhance HIV replication, but this does not appear to be a problem with monitoring HIV RNA PCR (AIDS Res Hum Retroviruses 1996;12:1151). Dosing recommendations and indications are 250 µg/m² IV over 2 h qd.

GREPAFLOXACIN (Roxar) – See Fluoroquinolone Summary (page 207)

GROWTH HORMONE, HUMAN

Trade name: Serostim (Serona Labs)

Form and Price: Vials of 4 mg (about 12 IU), 5 mg (about 15 IU) and 6 mg (about 18 IU) @ $42/mg. The average cost is $252/day or $21,000 for a 12 week course.

Patient assistance program: (888) 628-6673

Class: Human growth hormone produced by recombinant DNA technology

Regimen: Administer SC at bedtime in the following doses:

>55 kg — 6 mg SC daily
45-55 kg — 5 mg SC daily
35-45 kg — 4 mg SC daily
<35 kg — 0.1 mg/kg SC daily
Assess at 2 weeks

Patient assistance program: (888) 628-6673 for compassionate use and for support above the cap of $36,000/calendar year for each qualified patient.

Indications (FDA labeling): Treatment of AIDS-associated wasting or cachexia

Clinical trials: In a therapeutic trial in 178 AIDS patients with wasting those receiving 12 weeks of somatropin treatment had a 1.6 kg increase in body weight and a 3.0 kg increase in lean body mass compared to placebo recipients. The somatropin recipients also had a 13% increase in median treadmill work output. There was no significant survival benefit (Ann Intern Med 1996;125:873). Another trial in 60 patients with wasting showed similar results (Ann Intern Med 1996;125:865). Drug cost at the doses used was over $1,000/week, raising questions about the cost-effectiveness (Ann Intern Med 1996;125:932). One option to reduce cost is to limit use to periods of OIs to reduce OI associate weight loss (AIDS 1999;13:1195). Preliminary experience suggests that Serostim is effective in reversing fat accumulation that complicates HAART (Ann Intern Med 1999;131:313). However, it is possible that it may exacerbate fat atrophy as a result of increased fat mobilization

Pharmacology:

Bioavailability with SC injection: 70-90%

T½: 3.9-4.3 hours

Elimination: Metabolized primarily in renal cells; also metabolized in the liver.

Dose in liver or renal failure: Decreased clearance but clinical significance and specific guidelines for dose modification are unknown.

Side effects: Growth hormone may cause dose-related fluid and sodium retention with edema, arthralgias and hypertension. The most common side effects are musculoskeletal discomfort (20-50%) and increased tissue turgor with swelling of hands and feet (25%); both usually subside with continued treatment. Other side effects include flu-like symptoms, rigors, back pain, malaise, carpal tunnel syndrome, chest pain, nausea and diarrhea. Side effects may be reduced by reduction in daily dose or by reduction in the number of doses/week.

Drug interactions: Not studied

Pregnancy: Category B

HALCION – See Triazolam (p. 274)

HUMATIN – See Paromomycin (p. 248)

HYDROXYUREA (HU)

Generic/Trade name: Hydrea (Bristol-Myers Squibb), Droxia (Bristol-Myers Squibb), and generic

Form and price: 500 mg caps (Hydrea); $1.42/500 mg cap (200, 300, 400 mg Droxia)

Dose: Optimum dose is not known. Usual dose is 500 mg bid or 1000 mg qd (with ddI ± additional agents)

Class: Hydroxyurea (HU) is used primarily for sickle cell disease and is not FDA approved for HIV. HU inhibits cellular ribonucleotide reductase, resulting in decreased intracellular deoxynucleoside triphosphates that are required for DNA synthesis (AIDS 1999;13:1433). This makes ddI a more potent inhibitor of HIV and *in vitro* studies show synergistic activity when HU is combined with didanosine (ddI) vs. HIV in resting lymphocytes (Proc Natl Acad Sci USA 1994;91:11017). Synergy was not demonstrated with concentrations that can be achieved clinically using hydroxyurea plus AZT (zidovudine) and ddC (zalcitabine). The cytostatic property causes blunting of the CD4 response. The combination with ddI may also magnify ddI toxicity as an inhibitor of mitochondrial replication.

Clinical trials: A trial of hydroxyurea (500 mg bid) + ddI (200 mg bid) in 12 patients with CD4 counts >250/mm³ demonstrated a mean decrease in viral load of 1.7 log and a median CD4 increase of 120/mm³. Six patients had decreases in viral load to <500 c/mL (JAIDS 1995;10:36). A subsequent study randomized 26 patients receiving monotherapy with ddI to the addition of hydroxyurea in doses of 500 mg/d vs. 1,000 mg/d. There was no significant decline in viral load with low doses; the high dose group had a median decline of 0.63 log (JID 1997;175:801). In ACTG 307 the mean decrease in VL with ddI monotherapy was 1.2 log compared to a decrease of 1.8 log with ddI/hydroxyurea. HU alone showed no antiviral activity (6ᵗʰ Retrovirus Conf, 1999, Chicago, Abstract 402). The combination of hydroxyurea/ddI/indinavir in 20 patients in early stage disease (mean CD4 of 448) showed all had HIV RNA levels <500/mL at 9 months (Lori et al, 5ᵗʰ Retroviral Conference, 1998, Abstract 655). The combination of HU, ddI and a PI for 10 patients with acute HIV infection resulted in a decrease in viral load to <50 c/mL in all 10 (6th Retrovirus Conf, 2/99, Chicago Abstract 401). The variable results in CD4 cell counts are ascribed to marrow suppression by hydroxyurea.

Many investigators use HU for intensification, primarily in regimens containing ddI. Most studies demonstrate a modest antiviral effect with no risk of resistance. The CD4 count response is usually blunted due to the cytotoxic effect of HU. Major uses of HU include primary HIV infection, intensification, salvage regimens and clinical settings in which high CNS levels are necessary. The drug should be given with ddI regimens containing due to demonstrable synergy. Conclusions about efficacy are limited by the lack of well controlled trials. The best results are with early stage therapy; the drug is poorly tolerated in salvage regimens.

Recent work has led to increasing concern that the synergy between HU and ddI is accompanied by a synergistic effect on ddI toxicity; with higher rates of peripheral neuropathy (AIDS 2000;14:273) and pancreatitis. ACTG 5025 was discontinued prematurely after 3 deaths ascribed to pancreatitis secondary to ddI + HU (7th CROI, Abstract 456).

Pharmacology

Bioavailability: Well absorbed.

T½: 2-3 hr

Penetration: Highly diffusable with good CNS penetrations (Science 1994;266:801)

Elimination: Half is degraded by the liver and excreted as respiratory CO_2 and in the urine as urea.

Side effects: Dose dependent bone marrow suppression with leukopenia, anemia and thrombocytopenia in 5-7% (AIDS 1999;13:1433). Leukopenia is most common and usually occurs first. Recovery from marrow depression is usually rapid with discontinuation of treatment. In sickle cell anemia patients receiving 2.5-35 mg/kg/day for painful crises, 10% had myelosuppression, and these patients had marrow recovery within two weeks following drug discontinuation. A CBC should be monitored during therapy at regular intervals.

Other side effects include GI intolerance which may be severe including stomatitis, nausea, vomiting, anorexia, diarrhea and constipation. Mild reversible dermatologic side effects are common and include a maculopapular rash, facial erythema, hyperpigmentation, oral ulceration, desquamation of the face and hands and partial alopecia (J Am Acad Derm 1997;36:178). Chronic leg ulcers may complicate therapy that exceeds 3 years (Ann Intern Med 1998;29:128).

Hydroxyurea potentiates the antiretroviral activity of ddI and appears to potentiate ddI toxicity, with increased rates of ddI-associated peripheral neuropathy (AIDS 2000;14:273) and possibly pancreatitis.

Rare side effects include dysuria, neurologic complications (drowsiness, disorientation, hallucinations, convulsions), hyperuricemia, renal failure, fever, chills, and alopecia.

Pregnancy: Category D

INDINAVIR (IDV)

Trade name: Crixivan (Merck)

Forms and price: 200, 333, and 400 mg capsules; $2.58/400 mg capsule; $105/wk.

Patient assistance program: (800) 850-3430

Product information: (800) 497-8383

Class: Protease inhibitor

Dose: 800 mg q8h in fasting state (1 hour before or 2 hrs after a meal), or with a light, non-fat meal, i.e., dry toast with jelly, juice, coffee (with skim milk & sugar) or corn flakes with skim milk. Patients should drink ≥48 oz fluids daily; 6-8 oz glasses of fluids/day, preferably water, to prevent indinavir renal calculi. Administration should be at 8 hour intervals; bid dosing is appropriate only when combined with ritonavir and possibly with nelfinavir.

Resistance: Mutations at codons 10, 20, 24, 32, 46, 54, 63, 71, 82, 84 and 90 correlate with reduced *in vitro* activity (AAC 1998;42:2775). Substitutions at positions 46 and/or 82 are major mutations that predict resistance. In general, at least 3 mutations are necessary to produce phenotype resistance. Overlap with ritonavir is extensive so that strains resistant to one are usually resistant to both. (The rationale for the RTV-IDV combination is for pharmacologic benefit in sustaining IDV levels.) The overlap with other PIs is less extensive but multiple mutations generally imply class resistance (Nature 1995;374:569).

Clinical trials: The mean decrease in viral load was 1-1.5 log in patients given indinavir alone and >2 log with indinavir plus ddI or indinavir plus AZT and 3TC (ACTG 320 and MSD trial 035). CD4 counts in these two trials increased an average of 80-150/mm³. In the indinavir plus AZT and 3TC trial (trial 035), viral load was <400 c/mL in 80% of the participants at two years (NEJM 1997;337:734).

Merck trial 035 has continued as an open label protocol; at 100 weeks approximately 78% had viral loads <50 c/mL by as-treated analysis (JAMA 1998;280:35). In ACTG 320 this same combination was significantly better than AZT/3TC in terms of survival, rate of HIV-related complications, CD4 response, reduction in viral load and quality of life among 1,156 participants with CD4 counts <200/mm³/prior AZT experience; the proportion who achieved viral load <500 c/mL at 24 weeks was 90% (NEJM 1997;337:725).

Merck 060/ICC 004 is a trial of IDV/AZT/3TC in 199 treatment naïve patients with CD4 counts >500/mm³. At 48 wks 79% had VL <50 c/mL by intent-to-treat analysis; the mean increase in CD4 count was 160/mm³. 8% had nephrolithiasis (7th CROI, Abstract 511).

Trials combining IDV with ritonavir (RTV) have demonstrated favorable pharmacokinetics with marked increases in IDV trough levels permitting bid dosing (6th Retroviral Conf., 1999, Chicago, Abstracts 362, 363, 364, 631, 677). The optimal dose regimen is not known. The regimen of 400 mg bid of both drugs is associated with trough IDV levels that are 3-4 fold higher and lower peak levels, which would be expected to reduce the risk of nephrohthiasis. However, the dose of 400 mg bid of RTV is often poorly tolerated. The alternative is to use IDV 800 mg bid plus RTV 100-200 mg bid; this is better tolerated but is associated with higher peak levels of IDV. Preliminary results from a trial involving RTV intensification in patients with detectable virus in IDV-containing regimens demonstrated increased IDV trough levels, and found that over half of patients achieved a viral load <50 c/mL (7th CROI, Abstract 534).

Indications: See Chapter 4.

Pharmacology

> **Bioavailability:** Absorption is 65% in fasting state or with only a light, non-fat meal. Full meal decreases IDV levels 77%; give 1 hr before or 2 hr after meal, with light meal or with ritonavir. Food has minimal effect on IDV when given with ritonavir.

> **T½:** 1.5-2 hours (serum); **Cmax:** peak >200 nM; 8 hrs post dose – 80 nM (95% inhibition *in vitro* at 25-100 nM). Penetraction into CSF is moderate (CSF: Serum = 0.16), but is superior to that of other PIs. The levels achieved are above the IC_{95} for most HIV isolates (AIDS 1999;13:1227). CSF trough levels of IDV are increased >5 fold when IDV is combined with RTV (7th CROI, Abstract 312).

> **Elimination:** Metabolized via hepatic glucoronidation and cytochrome P450(3A4)-dependent pathways. Urine shows 5-12% unchanged drug and metabolites.

> **Storage:** Room temperature

Indications (FDA): Indinavir is indicated for the treatment of HIV infection in adults when antiretroviral therapy is warranted.

Side effects: 1) Asymptomatic increase in indirect bilirubin to ≥2.5 mg/dL without an increase in transaminases noted in 10-15% of patients; 2) Mucocutaneous: Paronychia and ingrown toenails, dry skin, mouth, eyes – common; 3) Class adverse effect: Insulin-resistant hyperglycemia, fat redistribution, hyperlipidemia (increased triglyceride, cholesterol, LDL), osteoporosis; possible increased bleeding with hemophilia. 4) Nephrolithiasis ± hematuria in 5-15%. Patients should drink 48 oz of fluid daily to maintain urine output at ≥150 mL/hour during the 3 hours after ingestion;

stones are crystals of indinavir ± calcium (Ann Intern Med 1997;349:1294). Nephrolithiasis usually reflects elevated peak plasma levels of indinavir despite standard doses and most patients had virologic control with a reduced dose (600 mg tid) (AIDS 1999;13:473); 5) Nephrotoxicity with urine sediment changes and renal failure that is independent of nephrolithiasis; 6) Alopecia – all hair bearing areas (NEJM 1999;341:618); 7. GI intolerance with nausea; 8) Less common: increased transaminase levels, headache, nausea, vomiting, epigastric distress, diarrhea, metallic taste, fatigue, insomnia, blurred vision, dizziness, rash, and thrombocytopenia. Rare cases of fulminant hepatic failure and death. Fulminant hepatitis has been associated with steatosis and an eosinophilic infiltrate, suggesting a drug related injury (Lancet 1997;349:924). Gynecomastia reported (CID 1998;27:1539).

Drug interactions:

1. Concurrent use with antiretroviral agents

   Nucleosides: No effect; use standard doses

Table 6-20: Recommendations for Indinavir in Combination with Other PIs or with NNRTIs

Agent	AUC	Concurrent use regimen
Ritonavir*	IDV ↑ 5–8x	RTV 400 mg bid + IDV 400 mg bid or RTV 200 mg bid + IDV 800 mg bid or RTV 100 mg bid + IDV 800 mg bid
Saquinavir	SQV ↑ 4–7x IDV: No effect	No data (possible *in vitro* antagonism—JID 1997;176:265)
Nelfinavir	NFV ↑ 80% IDV ↑ 50%	IDV 1200 mg bid + NFV 1250 mg bid
Nevirapine	NVP: No effect IDV ↓ 28%	Standard doses
Delavirdine	DLV ? IDV ↑ 40%	DLV 400 mg tid + IDV 600 mg q 8 h
Efavirenz	EFV: No effect IDV ↓ 31%	EFV 600 mg qd + IDV 1,000 mg q 8 h
Amprenavir	APV ↑ 30–60% IDV: No effect	APV 800 mg tid + IDV 800 mg tid

* It is possible that IDV/RTV could be given once daily but data are limited (7th CROI, Abstract 512).

2. **Antimycobacterial agents:** Rifampin – concurrent use is contraindicated. Rifabutin – reduce RFB dose to 150 mg/day and increase IDV dose to 1000 mg tid

3. **Contraindicated for concurrent use:** Rifampin, astemizole, terfenadine, cisapride, midazolam, triazolam, ergotamines, simvastatin, lovastatin, St. John's wort.

4. **ddI:** Take ≥2 hours apart

5. **Other interactions:** Ketoconazole and itraconazole increase IDV levels 70%; decrease IDV dose to 600 mg q 8 h; **clarithromycin** levels increase 53% – no dose change; grapefruit juice reduces IDV levels 26%; norethindrone levels increase 26% and ethinylestradiol levels increase 24% – no dose change; anticonvulsants (phenobarbitol, phenytoin, carbamazepin) may decrease IDV levels substantially; monitor anticonvulsant level. Co-administration of IDV and sildenafil (Viagra) increases the AUC for sildenafil 4.4 fold (AIDS 1999;13:F10). The maximum recommended dose is 25 mg/48 hr. Methadone interactions have not been studied. St. John's wort reduces IDV AUC 57% (Lancet 2000;355:547).

Pregnancy: Category C. Negative rodent teratogenic assays; placental passage studies show high newborn : maternal drug levels in rats, low ratio in rabbits. Some authorities are concerned about the elevated indirect bilirubin and nephrolithiasis in the event that these complications may occur in the fetus.

INTERFERON

Trade name: Roferon (Hoffman-LaRoche), Intron (Schering), Infergen (Amgen)

Forms and price:

Interferon alfa-2a (Roferon): vials of 3, 9, 18, and 36 million units @ $34.97/3 mil units.

Interferon alfa-2a (Intron): vials of 3, 5, 10, 18, 25, and 50 million units; $34.93/3 million units.

Rebetron combination Therapy Pac consists of ribavirin for oral administration (200 mg caps) and Intron for parenteral administration in patients with hepatitis C infection (see ribavirin).

Patient assistance program (Roferon): (800) 443-6676; Cap program (983 million units ≤ yr.)

Patient assistance program (Intron): (800) 521-7157

Class: Interferon alfa is a family of highly homogeneous species-specific proteins of human origin (using donor cells, cultured human cell lines, or recombinant techniques with human genes) possessing complex antiviral, antineoplastic, and immunomodulating activities. The Alfa-2a and alfa-2b refer to similar subtypes prepared by recombinant techniques.

Activity: Broad spectrum antiviral agent with *in vitro* activity against HIV, HPV, HBV, HCV, HSV-1 & 2, CMV, VZV, etc.

Indications and regimen (Interferon alfa-2b)

Hepatitis C: 3 mil units IM or SC 3x/wk x 12-18 months (NEJM 1995;332:1457). Results are superior when interferon is given with ribavirin (Lancet 1998;351:83). See ribavirin for dosing instructions.

Hepatitis B: 5 mil units IM or SC daily or 10 mil units 3x/wk x 4 mos

Kaposi's sarcoma*: 30-36 mil units IM or SC (3-7x/wk) until KS lesions resolve, toxicity or rapid progression of KS (average 7 months) precludes further treatment.

* Best response rates (40-50%) in patients with CD4 counts >200/mm³ and no "B symptoms"; response is dose-related.

Pharmacology

Bioavailability: Protein with 165 amino acids and molecular weight of 18,000-20,000; absorption after oral administration is nil; bioavailability with SC or IM administration is 80%

T½: 2-5.1 hours

CSF level: None detected

Elimination: Metabolized by kidney

Side effects: All patients have side effects and especially with doses ≥18 mil units. Most side effects diminish in frequency and severity with continued administration:

1. Flu-like syndrome (50-98%); fever, chills, fatigue, headache, and arthralgias, usually within six hours of administration, lasting 2-12 hours. (Reduced with nonsteroidal anti-inflammatory agents)

2. GI intolerance (20-65%) with anorexia, nausea, vomiting, diarrhea, metallic taste, and abdominal pain

3. CNS toxicity with delirium or obtundation

4. Marrow suppression with neutropenia, anemia, or thrombocytopenia

5. Hepatotoxicity (10-50%) with increased transaminase levels

6. Dyspnea and cough

7. Rash ± alopecia (25%)

8. Proteinuria (15-20%)

Pregnancy: Category C. Abortifacient in animals with doses 20-500 x doses in humans. No data for humans. Use in pregnancy only when need justifies risk.

Drug interactions: AZT – increased hematologic toxicity; increased levels of theophylline, barbiturates.

INTRON – See Interferon (above)

INVIRASE – See Saquinavir (p. 262)

VI. Drugs

ISONIAZID (INH)

Trade names: Isotamine, Laniazide, Teebaconin, Rifamate, Nydrazid and generic

Forms: 50, 100, and 300 mg tabs; solution with 50 mg/5 mL for oral use; vial for injection with 1 gm/vial

Combinations: Caps with rifampin: 150 mg INH + 300 mg rifampin (Rifamate) and tabs with 50 mg INH + 120 mg Rifampin and 300 mg PZA (Rifater)

Price: INH – $0.02/300 mg tab; Rifater – $1.80/tab

Indications: Prophylaxis and treatment of tuberculosis

Table 6-21: Dose

	Daily	DOT	Pyridoxime (Vit B$_6$)
Prophylaxis x 9 mo	300 mg	900 mg 2x/wk	50 mg/d or 100 mg 2x/wk
Treatment	300 mg	900 mg 2-3x/wk	50 mg/d or 100 mg 2x/wk

Treatment with Rifamate: 2 caps/day

Treatment with Rifater:

<65 kg: 1 tab/10 kg/day

>65 kg: 6 tabs/day

Pharmacology

Bioavailability: 90%

T½: 1-4 hrs; 1 hr in rapid acetylators

Elimination: Metabolized and eliminated in urine. Rate of acetylation is generically determined. Slow inactivation reflects deficiency of hepatic enzyme N-acetyltransferase and is found in about 50% of whites and African-Americans. Rate of acetylation does not affect efficacy of standard daily or DOT regimens.

Dose modification in renal failure: Half dose with creatinine clearance <10 mL/min in slow acetylators.

Side effects: Hepatitis rates by age (Med Clin N Amer 1988;72:661)

Table 6-22: Correlation Between Age and Frequency of INH - associated Hepatotoxicity

	25 yrs	35 yrs	45 yrs	55 yrs	65 yrs
Definite	1.3%	5.9%	10.9%	17.5%	10.5%
Probable	6.3%	12.7%	20.4%	31.4%	25.5%

Patient should be warned of symptoms of hepatitis; some recommend LFTs at one and three months. Drug should be stopped if transaminase levels increase to >5 times upper limit of normal. Major risks are Etoh abuse and age (Ann Intern Med 1999;181:1014). These are the most frequently quoted data, but a recent review suggests the risk is greatly exaggerated. Using a strict definition of INH-associated hepatitis (transaminase levels >5x ULN + symptoms + resolution when INH was discontinued) in patients given preventive care showed a rate of only 0.1%.

Peripheral neuropathy due to increased excretion of pyridoxine which is dose-related and rare with usual doses; it is prevented by concurrent pyridoxine (10-50 mg/day) which is recommended for diabetics, alcoholics, pregnant patients, AIDS patients, and malnourished patients. Miscellaneous reactions: rash, fever, adenopathy, GI intolerance. Rare reactions: psychosis, arthralgias, optic neurpathy, marrow suppression.

Drug interactions:

Increased effects of coumadin, benzodiazepines, carbamazipine, cycloserine, ethionamide, phenytoin, theophylline

INH absorption decreased with Al++ containing antacids

Hepatitis: increased frequency with excessive alcohol

Ketoconazole: decrease ketoconazole level

Food: decreases absorption

Tyramine (cheese, wine, some fish): rare patients develop palpitations, sweating, urticaria, headache, and vomiting.

Pregnancy: Category C. Embryocidal in animals; not teratogenic. Large retrospective studies have shown no pattern of congenital abnormalities; small studies suggest possible CNS toxicity (CID 1995;21 suppl 1:S24). ATS recommendation is that pregnant women with positive PPD plus HIV infection should receive INH; begin after first trimester if possible.

ITRACONAZOLE

Trade name: Sporanox (Janssen)

Forms and price: 100 mg caps at $6.80/100 mg cap and 10 mg/mL oral solution in 150 mL bottles at $106.86 or $7.13/100 mg; intraconazole injection 10 mg/mL in 25 mL vials

Price for histoplasmosis (200 mg cap bid): $25.86/day

Price for thrush (100 mg solution/day): $7.13/day

Price comparison for thrush: nystatin (5cc 5x/d) = $1.40/day
ketoconazole (200 mg/d) = $3.07/day
fluconazole (100 mg/d) = $6.87/day

Comparison of oral formulations (caps vs oral solution): See next section on bioavailability.

Patient assistance program: (800) 544-2987. Patient must have no insurance and income/asset eligibility, which is individually reviewed. Drug is available for off-label indications.

Class: Triazole (like fluconazole) with three nitrogens in the azole ring; other imidazoles have two nitrogens.

Activity: *In vitro* activity against *H. capsulatum, B. dermatitidis, Aspergillus, Cryptococcus, Candida sp.* Strains of candida that are resistant to fluconazole are often sensitive to itraconazole (AAC 1994;38:1530).

Table 6-23: Itraconazole Indications and Dose Regimen

Histoplasmosis*:	200 mg po tid x 3 days, then 200 mg po bid indefinitely (induction with 1 gm amphotericin B preferred for moderately severe disseminated disease) (Ann Intern Med 1993;118:610).
Candida[†] Thrush: Vaginitis: Esophagitis:	200 mg po/day, maintenance: 100 mg/day 100-200 mg po bid x 1 day or 100-200 mg/day x 2-3 days 100-200 mg po tid
Aspergillus[†]:	200 mg po tid x 3 days, then 200 mg po bid (amphotericin B often preferred). Failure rate of itraconazole: CNS - 65%; sinusitis - 50%; pulmonary 15%.
Cryptococcosis[†]:	200 mg po tid x 3 days, then 200 mg po bid (efficacy is not established). ACTG trial showed fluconazole (200 mg/d) was superior to itraconazole (200 mg/day) for maintenance.
Coccidioidomycosis[†]:	400-800 mg/day, then 200 mg bid
Dermatophytic infections[†]:	Onchomycosis: Fingernails – 200 mg bid x 1 week x 2 separated by 3 weeks; Toenails – 200 mg bid x 1 week/month x 3-4 mo or 200 mg/d x 12 weeks; 100 mg po qd (other dermatophytic infections)
Parenteral Itraconazole	200 mg IV x 4 doses then 200 mg IV/d (systemic fungal infections)

*FDA-approved

[†]Alternative agents usually preferred

Pharmacology

Bioavailability: Requires gastric acid for absorption; average is 55% and improved when taken with food. May increase absorption in gastric achlorhydria with acidic drinks such as Coca-Cola, Pepsi Cola, and orange juice (AAC 1995;39:1671). Should follow serum levels to insure absorption. Usual therapeutic level anticipated with standard dose is >2 mcg/mL and <10 mcg/mL. The liquid formulation shows better absorption, and the supplier recommends a dose adjustment of one half that recommended for capsules. Some consider the liquid formulation to be preferred for all oral itraconazole therapy. Concerns are that nearly all studies were done with capsules, and bioavailability studies have shown substantial variation. Based on these concerns, some authorities prefer the liquid formulation only for thrush (topical effect), for patients with known achlorhydria, those with inadequate serum levels and when there is a need for H_2 blockers or proton pump inhibitors.

Reference lab for serum levels: 1) Dr. Michael Rinaldi, Dept. of Pathology, University of Texas Health Science Center, 7703 Floyd Curl Dr., San Antonio, Texas 78284-7750; telephone (210) 567-4131 or 2) The Histoplasmosis Reference Lab, 1001 West 10th St, OPW 441, Indianapolis, IN, 46202; telephone (317) 630-2515; Fax (317) 630-7522; CLIA # 15 D0647154; CPT #80299; Cost in both labs is $59. Specimen should be serum or plasma. Volume >0.5 mL (2-4 mL preferred) sent in frozen state. Specimen can be obtained about 2 hours post dosing, and should be done at ≥5 days of treatment to assure steady state has been reached. Goal is level of ≥1µg/mL.

T½: 64 hours

Elimination: Metabolized by liver by cytochrome P450 to metabolites including hydroxyitraconazole which is active *in vitro* against many fungi. Renal excretion is 0.03% of parent drug and 40% of administered dose as metabolites.

Dose modification with renal failure: None

Dose modification with liver disease: No data, manufacturer suggests monitoring serum levels

Side effects: Elevation of hepatic enzymes is seen in 4%, but clinically significant hepatitis is rare (Lancet 1992;340:251). Hepatic enzymes should be monitored in patients with prior hepatic disease, and patients should be warned to report symptoms of hepatitis. Most common side effects are GI intolerance (3-10%) and rash (1-9%, most common in immunosuppressed patients). Infrequent dose related toxicities include hypokalemia, hypertension, and edema. Ventricular fibrillation due to hypokalemia has been reported (J Infect 1993;26:348).

Pregnancy: Category C; teratogenic to rats, no studies in humans.

Drug Interactions: Impaired absorption with H2 blockers, omeprazole, antacids or sucralfate. Increases levels of indinavir (indinavir dose decreased to 600 mg tid) and saquinavir; no dose adjustment for invirase or nelfinavir. Should not be given concurrently with terfenadine (Seldane), cisapride, astemizole, triazolam (Halcion), lovastatin (Mevacor), simvastatin (Zocor), rifampin, rifabutin, phenytoin, or phenobarbital. Itraconazole increases levels of loratadine (Claritin) cyclosporine, oral hypoglycemics, calcium channel blockers and digoxin. Decreased itraconazole levels with administration of rifampin, rifabutin, phenobarbitol, carbamazepine, ddI, isoniazid, and phenytoin.

KETOCONAZOLE

Trade name: Nizoral (Janssen)

Forms and price: 200 mg tabs – $3.37; 2% cream in 15, 30, and 60 gm tubes; 30 gm – $28.21; shampoo 2% 120 mL – $20.74

Class: Azole antifungal agent

Patient assistance program: (800) 544-2987

Indications:

Thrush: 200 mg po 1-2x/day

Candida esophagitis: 200-400 mg po bid. Note: Fluconazole (200 mg/day) is superior, but initial treatment with ketoconazole may be cost-effective (Ann Intern Med 1992;117:655).

Candida vaginitis: 200-400 mg/day po x 7 days or 400 mg/day x 3 days

Pharmacology

Bioavailability: 75% with gastric acid; decreased bioavailability with hypochlorhydria (common in AIDS patients)

Administration with hypochlorhydria: Each 200 mg should be dissolved in 4 mL of 0.2 N hydrochloric acid. Use a straw to avoid contact with teeth. Alternatives are concurrent administration of 580 mg glutamic acid hydrochloride or 240 mL of the following acidic soft drinks: Coca-Cola©, Pepsi Cola©, Canada Dry© ginger ale, and Minute Maid© orange juice (AAC 1995;39:1671).

T½: 6-10 hours

Elimination: Metabolized by liver, but half-life is not prolonged with hepatic failure.

Dose modification in renal failure: None

Side effects: Gastrointestinal intolerance; temporary increase in transaminase levels (2-5%); dose-related decrease in steroid and testosterone synthesis with impotence, gynecomastia, oligospermia, reduced libido, menstrual abnormalities (usually with doses ≥600 mg/day for prolonged periods); headache, dizziness, asthenia; rash;

abrupt hepatitis with hepatic failure (1:15,000); rare cases of hepatic necrosis; marrow suppression (rare); hypothyroidism (genetically determined); hallucinations (rare).

Drug interactions:

Important interactions: Increase in gastric pH impairs ketoconazole absorption including antacids, H_2 blockers, proton pump inhibitors and ddI – take ≥2 hrs apart or use alternative antifungal agent (MMWR 1999;48[RR-10]:47); INH – decreases ketoconazole effect; Rifampin – decreased activity of both drugs; Generic – terfenadine (Seldane) and cisapride – ventricular arrhythmias (avoid concurrent use).

Protease inhibitors and NNRTIs: Indinavir levels increased 68% – reduce indinavir dose to 600 mg q 8 h; saquinavir levels increased 3 fold – no dose change; ritonavir increases ketoconazole levels >3 fold – use <200 mg ketoconazole/day. Amprenavir levels increased 31% and ketoconazole levels increased 44% - dose implications are unclear; nelfinavir – no dose changes. Nevirapine levels increased 15-30% and ketoconazole levels decreased 63% - combination is not recommended. Efavirenz and delavirdine - no data.

Other: Alcohol – possible disulfiram-like reaction; antacids, H2 blockers, ddI or omeprazole – decreased absorption of ketoconazole; oral anti-coagulants – increased hypoprothrombinemia; corticosteroids – increased levels of methylprednisolone; cyclosporine – increased cyclosporine activity; phenytoin – altered metabolism of both drugs; theophylline – increased theophylline levels.

Pregnancy: Category C. Embryotoxic and teratogenic in experimental animals with large doses; no studies in humans; use with caution.

LAMIVUDINE - (3TC)

Trade name: Epivir (Glaxo Wellcome)

Forms and price: 150 mg tablets at $4.32/tab or $60.48/week; Oral solution 10 mg/mL, bottles of 240 mL at $69.30/240 mL. Available in combination with zidovudine as Combivir (150 mg lamivudine + 300 mg zidovudine) for bid administration at $9.38/tab. For hepatitis B: 100 mg tabs @ $4.33 and oral solution 5 mg/mL at $4.33/100 mg.

Patient assistance: (800) 722-9294 (Mon-Fri 8:30 AM – 7:00 PM EST)

Class: Nucleoside analog

Indications: FDA approved "for use in combination with Retrovir (AZT) for the treatment of HIV infection when antiretroviral therapy is warranted based on clinical and/or immunologic evidence of disease progression." For chronic hepatitis B associated with evidence of HBV replication and active liver inflammation.

Regimen: 150 mg po bid; <50 kg – 2 mg/kg bid; take without regard to meals.
For hepatitis B: 100 mg/day x 52 wks

Resistance: Monotherapy with 3TC results in selection of strains with mutations in the RT gene at codon 184 that confer high grade resistance within weeks when 3TC is given alone or with AZT. This drug should never be given as monotherapy. The 184 mutation suppresses AZT resistance, but some polymorphisms can result in resistance to both agents. The 184 codon mutation confers partial resistance to ddI, ddC and abacavir. A preferable treatment strategy in the era of protease inhibitors is to prevent 3TC resistance by using a completely suppressive regimen. Recent studies have found that additional resistance mutations at codons 44 and 118 are associated with 3TC resistance, AZT resistance and multi-nucleoside resistance (7th CROI, Abstract 741).

Efficacy: Four comparative trials with 3TC plus AZT versus monotherapy revealed that the combination was superior based on surrogate marker endpoints. At 24 weeks the mean CD4 cell increase was 20-75/mm^3. Results with 3TC or AZT alone were inferior (NEJM 1995;333:1662). The presumed explanation for the superior results with AZT plus 3TC in AZT experienced patients is partially ascribed to reestablishment of susceptibility to AZT (Science 1995;269:696).

HIV Indications: See Chapter 4

Hepatitis B: Lamivudine is a potent inhibitor of HBV replication (NEJM 1995;333:1657). Treatment of HBV-HIV co-infected patients showed significant reductions in HBV DNA concentrations in 26 of 27 (Ann Intern Med 1996;125:705). For treatment of HBV, single daily doses of 100-300 mg for 3-6 months resulted in HBV DNA negativity in 80%; in patients with HBV and HIV, prolonged suppression was reported in 90% (Lancet 1995;345:396). A one year trial with 100 mg/day vs placebo showed that patients with chronic hepatitis B had reduced progression to fibrosis, elimination of HBV DNA and clearance of HBVe antigen (NEJM 1998;339:61). CAESAR was a large prospective study of nucleoside therapy for HIV. A subset analysis of 122 patients who received 3TC (150 mg bid) and had HBV co-infection with HBsAg at baseline found that 3TC recipients had a reduction in HBV DNA averaging 2.7 $\log_{10}$ at 52 weeks and reductions in ALT; 40% had loss of HBV DNA and 20% has loss of HBeAg (JID 1999;180:607). Resistance by similar point mutations for HBV and HIV have been reported (Lancet 1997;349:20).

Pharmacology

　　Bioavailability: 86%

　　T$\frac{1}{2}$: 3-6 hours; Intracellular T$\frac{1}{2}$: 12 hrs

　　CNS penetration: 13% (CSF: plasma ratio = 0.11). These levels exceed the IC$_{50}$ and have been shown to clear HIV RNA from CSF (Lancet 1998;351:1547).

　　Elimination: Renal excretion accounts for 71%

Dose modification in renal failure:

Table 6-24: Lamivudine Dose Adjustments With Renal Failure

Cr. Clearance	Dose HIV	Dose HBV
>50 mL/min	150 mg bid	100 mg/day
30-49 mL/min	150 mg qd	100 mg, then 50 mg/d
15-29 mL/min	150 mg, then 100 mg qd	100 mg, then 25 mg/d
5-14 mL/min	150 mg, then 50 mg qd	35 mg, then 15 mg/d
<5 mL/min	150 mg, then 25 mg qd	35 mg, then 10 mg/d
Hemodialysis	150 mg, then 25–50 mg qd	35 mg, then 10 mg/d

VI. Drugs

Side effects: Experience in >25,000 patients given 3TC through the Treatment IND showed minimal toxicity. Infrequent complications include headache, nausea, diarrhea, abdominal pain, and insomnia. Comparison of side effects in 251 patients given 3TC plus AZT and 230 patients given AZT alone in four trials (A3001, A3002, B3001, and B3002) indicated no clinical or laboratory complications uniquely associated with 3TC. Pancreatitis has been noted in 15% of pediatric patients given 3TC. The most common side effects in patients given 3TC plus AZT are headache (35%), nausea (18%), neuropathy (12%), neutropenia (7%), and anemia (3%). Most of these are ascribed to AZT. **Class side effect:** Lactic acidosis and steatosis

Hepatitis B: In HIV infected patients with HBV co-infection, discontinuation of 3TC may cause a recurrence of hepatitis. This is expressed with increases in HBV DNA levels and increases in ALT levels.

Pregnancy: Category C. Negative carcinogenicity and teratogenicity studies in rodents; placental passage studies in humans show newborn: maternal drug ratio of 1.0. Studies in pregnant women show that lamivudine is well tolerated and has pharmacokinetic properties similar to those of non-pregnant women (MMWR 1998;47[RR-2]:6).

Interactions: TMP-SMX (1 DS daily) increases levels of 3TC; however, no dose adjustment is necessary due to the safety profile of 3TC.

LAMPRENE – See Clofazimine (p. 184)

LEUKOVORIN (Folinic Acid)

Generic

Trade name: Wellcovorin (Burroughs Wellcome), generic

Forms and price:

Oral tabs: 5 mg, 10 mg, 15 mg, and 25 mg tabs

5 mg – $2.95; 25 mg – $21.00

Parenteral: 50, 100, and 350 mg; 3 mg/mL; 100 mg – $41.51

Class: Calcium salt or folinic acid

Indications: Antidote for folic acid antagonists

Note: Protozoa are unable to utilize leukovorin because they require p-aminobenzoic acid as a cofactor. It does not interfere with antimicrobial activity of trimethoprim. Usual use in HIV-infected patients is to prevent hematologic toxicity of pyrimethamine and trimetrexate. Therapy is usually oral, but should be parenteral if there is vomiting, NPO status, or the dose is >25 mg.

> Toxoplasmosis treatment: Pyrimethamine, 50-100 mg/day + leukovorin 10 mg/day x 6 weeks; maintenance leukovorin 5 mg/day

> Toxoplasmosis prophylaxis: Pyrimethamine/leucovorin, 25 mg/wk

> Trimetrexate: See this entry for dose regimen

Pharmacology

> Normal folate levels are 0.005-0.015 µg/mL, level <0.005 indicates folate deficiency and levels <0.002 cause megaloblastic anemia. Oral doses of 15 mg/day result in mean level of 0.268 µg/mL.

Side effects: Nontoxic in therapeutic doses. Rare hypersensitivity reactions.

LOPINAVIR/RITONAVIR (ABT-378/R)

Trade name: Kaletra

Form: Capsules containing ABT-378 – 400 mg plus ritonavir 100 mg.

Class: Protease inhibitor

Early Access Program: 1-888-711-7193. Criteria for inclusion: Investigator is unable to construct a viable regimen from available agents based on current treatment guidelines and the subject's previous antiretroviral use.

Dose: Three capsules (each containing ABT-378 133 mg/ritonavir 33 mg) bid

Activity: Lopinavir is approximately 10 times more potent than ritonavir vs wild type HIV. With ritonavir (400 mg lopinavir: 100 mg RTV) the mean C_{max} is 6-8 µg/mL and the IC_{50} value for wild type virus is 0.07 µg/mL. With bid dosing the trough levels of lopinavir exceed the EC_{50} by >50-fold throughout the dosing interval. For comparison, Cmin/EC_{50} values for single PI regimens range from 1-4.

Clinical trials: Trial M97-720 was a dose-finding phase II trial with ABT-378/r plus d4T and 3TC in 100 treatment naïve patients with VL >5,000 c/mL. At 72 weeks 80% had <50 c/mL by intent-to-treat analysis (87% of those with a baseline VL >100,000 c/mL) (7th CROI Abstract 515).

Trial M97-765 was a phase II study in 70 NNRTI-naïve patients with a viral load of 10^3-10^5 c/mL (median viral load 10,000 c/mL and median CD4 349/mm^3) on their PI regimen. Patients received ABT-378/r plus nevirapine and 2 NRTIs. At 48 weeks 60% had VL <50 c/mL by intent-to-treat analysis (7th CROI Abstract 532).

Pharmacology

Bioavailability: ABT-378 absorption ~ 80%, bioavailability improved with food. The addition of ritonavir remarkably increases concentrations, AUC and T$_{1/2}$ due to inhibition of the P450 CYP3A isoenzymes, which are the major excretory route for lopinavir. Lopinavir has minimal effect on RTV pharmacokinetics; the C$_{max}$ for RTV when given in the lopinavir/ritonavir formulation is approximately 0.6 µg/mL, compared to 11 µg/mL with standard doses of RTV (600 mg bid). The mean steady-state lopinavir plasma concentrations are 15- to 20-fold higher than those of ritonavir. Since ritonavir activity *in vitro* is 10-fold lower than lopinavir, RTV functions primarily as a pharmacologic enhancer and not as an antiretroviral agent, *per se*.

T$_{1/2}$: 5-6 hr.

Excretion: Metabolized primarily by P450 CYP3A isoenzymes. ABT-378/r inhibits CYP3A isoenzymes, but the effect is less than that of RTV, and similar to that of indivar.

Side effects: The drug is generally well tolerated, with <2% discontinuing ABT-378/r due to adverse drug reactions in phase II clinical trials through 48 weeks. The most common adverse reactions were gastrointestinal, with diarrhea of at least moderate severity in 10-20%. Laboratory abnormalities through 72 weeks included transminase increases (to >5x normal) in 8%, triglyceride increases (to >750 mg/dL) in 12%, and cholesterol increases (to >300 mg/dL) in 14% of treatment-naïve patients receiving ABT-378/r.

Drug interactions: The major effect is due to the inhibition of CYP3A isoenzymes to prolong the half-life of drugs metabolized by the route. The inhibition is less than that seen with therapeutic doses of ritonavir.

Drugs contraindicated for concurrent use: Astemizole, terfenadine, midazolam, triazolam, cisapride, pimozide, ergot derivatives, rifampin

Drugs that require a modified dose: Rifabutin – dose reduction necessary.

Dose recommendations with other antiretroviral agents: ABT-378/r 400 mg/100 mg bid plus one of the following: IDV 600 mg bid, SQV (Fortovase) 800 mg bid, APV 750 mg bid, NFV 750 mg bid, NVP 200 mg bid, EFV 600 mg hs. When dosed with EFV, ABT-378/r dose should be increased from 3 capsules (400 mg/100 mg) to 4 capsules (533 mg/133 mg) bid.

LORAZEPAM

Trade name: Ativan (Wyeth-Ayerst); generic

Forms: 0.5 mg, 1.0 mg and 2.0 mg tabs; 2 mg, 4 mg, 20 mg and 40 mg vials

Price: Generic: $0.02/.5 mg tab, $0.02/1.0 mg tab, $0.03/2 mg tab

Ativan: $0.68/5 mg tab; $0.89/1.0 mg tab; $1.29/2.0 mg tab

Class: Benzodiazepine, controlled substance category IV (see p. 176)

Indications and dose regimens:

Anxiety: 1-2 mg 2-3x/day; increase to usual dose of 2-6 mg/day in 2-3 divided doses

IV administration: 2 mg

Insomnia plus anxiety: 2-4 mg hs

Pharmacology

Bioavailability: >90%

T½: 10-25 hours

Elimination: Renal excretion of inactive glucuronide metabolite. Not recommended with severe hepatic and/or renal disease.

Side effects: See Benzodiazepines (p. 176). Additive CNS depression with other CNS depressants including alcohol. Warn patient of prolonged sedation and decreased recall for ≥8 hours. Injected lorazepam may reduce physical coordination 24-48 hours.

Pregnancy: Category D; fetal harm – contraindicated.

LOTRIMIN – See Clotrimazole (p. 184)

MARINOL – See Dronabinol (p. 194)

MEGACE – See Megestrol acetate (below)

MEGESTROL ACETATE

Trade name: Megace (Bristol-Myers Squibb)

Forms and price: 20 mg tab – $0.73; 40 mg tab – $1.29; oral suspension 40 mg/mL (8 oz) – $0.51/40 mg

Financial assistance program: (800) 272-4878 for patients without insurance coverage plus financial need.

Product information: (800) 426-7644

Class: Synthetic progestin related to progesterone

Indications: Appetite stimulant to promote weight gain in patients with HIV infection or neoplastic disease; a concern is that most weight gain is fat.

Usual regimen: Oral suspension: 400-800 mg (20 mL in one daily dose), up to 800 mg/day. Tablets: 80 mg po qid; up to 800 mg/day (suspension usually preferred).

Efficacy: Average weight gain in uncontrolled study – 0.5 kg/wk with average total weight gain of 4 kg (Ann Intern Med 1994;121:393; Ann Intern Med 1994;121:400). However, there was <5 lbs weight gain in 35% despite doses of 800 mg/day for 12 weeks and most of the gain is fat. Most authorities recommend use in combination with anabolic steroids, resistance exercises or both.

Pharmacology

Bioavailability: >90%

T½: 30 hrs

Elimination: 60-80% excreted in urine

Side effects: Most serious: Hypogonadism (which may exacerbate wasting), diabetes and adrenal insufficiency. Most common: Diarrhea, impotence, rash, flatulence, asthenia, hyperglycemia (5%), and pain. Less common or rare: carpal tunnel syndrome, thrombosis, nausea, vomiting, edema, vaginal bleeding, and alopecia; high dose (480-1,600 mg/day) – hyperpnea, chest pressure, mild increase in blood pressure, dyspnea, congestive heart failure. A review of FDA reports of adverse drug reactions with megestrol showed 5 cases of Cushing syndrome, 12 new onset diabetes and 17 cases of possible adrenal insufficiency (Arch Intern Med 1997;157:1651).

Drug interactions: No information

Pregnancy: Category D. Progestational drugs are associated with genital abnormalties in male and female fetuses exposed during first four months of pregnancy.

MEPRON – See Atovaquone (p. 172)

METHADONE

Generic; Trade name: Dolophine

Forms: 5 mg tab – $0.08
10 mg tab – $0.14
40 mg tab – $0.33
10 mg/5 mL (500 mL) – $0.11/10 mg
Usual yearly cost of medication for methadone maintenance averages $180

Class: Opiate schedule II. The FDA restricts physician prescribing of methadone for methadone maintenance to those licensed to provide this service and those attached to methadone maintenance programs. Licensed physicians can prescribe methadone for pain control.

Indications:

Detoxification for substantial opiate abstinence symptoms: Initial dose is based on opiate tolerance, usually 15-20 mg; additional doses may be necessary. Daily dose – 40 mg usually stabilizes patient; when stable 2-3 days, decrease dose 20%/day. Must complete detoxification in <180 days or considered maintenance.

Maintenance as oral substitute for heroin or other morphine-like drugs; initial dose 15-30 mg depending on extent of prior use, up to 40 mg/day. Subsequent doses depend on response. Usual maintenance dose is 40-100 mg/day, but higher doses are sometimes required. Most states limit the maximum daily dose to 80-120 mg/day.

Note: During first three months, and for all patients receiving >100 mg/day, observation is required six days/week; with good compliance and rehabilitation, clinic attendance may be reduced for observed ingestion 3 days/week with maximum two-day supply for home administration; after two years, clinic visits may be reduced to 2/wk with three-day drug supplies; after three years, visits may be reduced to weekly with a six-day supply.

Pain: 2.5-10 mg po, SC or IM q 3-4h or 5-20 mg po q 6-8h for severe chronic pain in terminally ill patients

Pharmacology

Bioavailability: >90% absorbed

T½: 25 hrs. Duration of action with repeated administration is 24-48 hours

Elimination: Metabolized by liver. Parent compound excreted in urine with increased rate in alkaline urine; metabolites excreted in urine and gut.

Side effects:

Acute toxicity: CNS depression – stupor or coma, respiratory depression, flaccid muscles, cold skin, bradycardia, hypotension.

Treatment: Respiratory support ± gastric lavage (even hours after ingestion due to pylorospasm) ± naloxone (but respiratory depression may last longer than naloxone, and naloxone may precipitate acute withdrawal syndrome).

Chronic toxicity: Tolerance/physical dependence with abstinence syndrome following withdrawal – onset at 3-4 days after last dose of weakness, anxiety, anorexia, insomnia, abdominal pain, headache, sweating, and hot-cold flashes.

Treatment: Detoxification.

Pregnancy: Category C. Avoid during first three months and use sparingly, in small doses, during last six months.

Drug interactions: Potentiates effects of other CNS depressants including alcohol and marijuana. Methadone levels are reduced with rifampin, rifabutin, nevirapine, efavirenz, ritonavir, and nelfinavir. Dose adjustment of methadone should be titrated. Opiate withdrawal is expected in a substantial number receiving methadone plus EFV or NVP (7th CROI, Abstract 88); it is uncommon with NFV (7th CROI, Abstract 87). There is no data for IDV, APV, DLV, or SQV. There is no evidence that methadone alters pharmacokinetics of PIs or NNRTIs. Methadone increases AZT levels (no dose adjustment necessary); it reduces AUC for d4T by 20% (no dose adjustment necessary) and reduces the AUC for ddI by 64% (dose adjustment probably necessary). These nucleosides have no important effect on methadone levels.

VI. Drugs

METRONIDAZOLE

Generic; Trade name: Flagyl (Searle); Femazol, Metizol, MetroGel, Metryl, Neo-Tric, Novonidazole, Protostat, Trikacids

Forms: 250 mg and 500 mg tabs, IV vials – 500 mg, vaginal gel 0.75%, 70 gm

Price: $0.08/250 mg tab, $0.16/500 mg tab; $33.83/500 mg IV, $35.16/70 gm vaginal gel

Class: Synthetic nitroimidazole derivative

Indications and dose regimens:

Gingivitis: 250 mg po tid or 500 mg po bid

Intra-abdominal sepsis: 1.5-2 gm/day po or IV in 2-4 doses

Amebiasis: 750 mg po tid x 5-10 days

Bacterial vaginosis: 2 gm x 1 or 500 mg po bid x 7 days

Trichomoniasis: 2 gm x 1 or 250 mg po tid x 7 days

C. difficile colitis: 500 mg po bid or 250 mg po tid x 10-14 days

Giardiasis: 250 mg po tid x 5-10 days

Pharmacology

Bioavailability: >90%

T½: 10.2 hours; serum level after 500 mg dose: 10-30 µg/mL

Elimination: Hepatic metabolism; metabolites excreted in urine

Dose adjustment in renal failure: None

Liver failure: Half-life prolonged; reduce daily dose in severe liver disease and monitor serum levels

Side effects: Most common – GI intolerance and unpleasant taste; Less common – glossitis, furry tongue, headache, ataxia, urticaria, dark urine; Rare -seizures; Prolonged use – reversible peripheral neuropathy; disulfiram (Antabuse)-type reaction with alcohol

Pregnancy: Category B. Fetotoxicity in animals. Contraindicated in first trimester – although 206 exposures during the first trimester showed no increase in birth defects; use during the last six months is not advised unless essential. For trichomoniasis CDC recommends 2 gm x 1 after first trimester. Alternative agents are available for most other conditions.

Drug interactions: Increases level of coumadin, lithium, and possibly astemizole, propulsid, and terfenadine (Seldane); the latter may cause ventricular arrhythmias and the combination should be avoided. Mild disulfiram-like reactions noted with alcohol (flushing, headache, nausea, vomiting, cramps, sweating). This is infrequent and unpredictable. Patients should be warned, and manufacturer recommends that alcohol be avoided. Concurrent use with disulfiram may cause psychoses or confusion; disulfiram should be stopped two weeks prior to use of metronidazole.

Note: Metronidazole is virtually completely absorbed with oral administration and should be given IV only if patient can take nothing by mouth.

MYAMBUTOL – See Ethambutol (p. 201)

MYCELEX – See Clotrimazole (p. 184)

MYCOBUTIN – See Rifabutin (p. 254)

MYCOSTATIN – See Nystatin (p. 245)

NEBUTEM – See Pentamidine (p. 249)

NELFINAVIR (NFV)

Trade name: Viracept (Agouron Pharmaceuticals)

Form and price: 250 mg tabs @ $2.15/250 mg tab or $135.15/week (750 mg tid) or $150.50/week (1250 mg bid); oral powder 50 mg/gm, 144 gm @ $2.10/250 mg

Class: Protease inhibitor

Dose: 1250 bid with meal or snack

Clinical trials:

1. Pre-registration trials showed the drug was well tolerated with 4% of 696 patients discontinuing treatment due to side effects. The major side effect was diarrhea in 10-30%; this was sufficiently severe to require discontinuation of nelfinavir in 1.6%. In more recent trials bid dosing with 1250 mg was as effective as the standard regimen of 750 mg tid.

2. Trial 511 included 297 treatment naive participants randomized to receive "triple therapy" (nelfinavir, 3TC and AZT) vs 3TC plus AZT. At 24 weeks viral load was <500 c/mL in 81% compared to 18% in the AZT/3TC arm; the average increase in CD4 cell count with "triple therapy" was 155/mm^3. At 52 weeks, the proportion with HIV RNA <500/mL was 75%, and the median increase in CD4 cells was 220/mm^3 (5th Retrovirus Conference, 1998, Abstract 372).

3. A retrospective analysis was conducted of 847 patients given PI containing regimens in London between 11/95 and 7/98 (6th Retrovirus Conf, 1999, Chicago, Abstract 171). The proportions who achieved viral loads <500 c/mL at 4 months were: IDV – 30%, RTV/SQV – 44%, RTV – 42% and NFV 64%. The proportions with VL <500 c/mL who subsequently relapsed were: IDV – 22%, RTV – 22%, RTV/SQV – 21% and NFV – 11%.

4. Dual-PI and PI/NNRTI regimens take advantage of pharmacokinetic interactions to reduce pill burden and/or dosing frequency. Combinations of NFV with RTV or IDV are poorly studied. The latter combination requires full doses of both drugs. The NFV/SQV combination has been more extensively studied, but requires a large number of pills. NFV has minimal drug interactions with NVP and EFV permitting standard doses in "triple target regimens" for salvage or for initial treatment of patients with a poor prognosis.

5. The COMBINE study compared NFV vs. NVP, each with AZT/3TC in 142 treatment naïve patients. Results at 24 weeks showed a superior virologic response in nevirapine recipients with 58% achieving VL <50 c/mL compared to 33% in the nelfinavir group (p=0.06) (7th CROI, Abstract 510). The high drop-out rate and surprisingly poor showing for NFV makes it hard to interpret this study

6. ACTG 364 evaluated 195 patients with extensive NRTI exposure given 1-2 new NRTIs plus NFV, EFV, or both. At 48 wks the proportions with VL <50 c/mL were: NFV – 22%, EFV – 44%, NFV/EFV – 67%.

Resistance: The primary mutation conferring NFV resistance is at codon 30 on the protease gene; this is virtually always seen with NFV phenotypic resistance (AAC 1998;42:2775). A condon 90 mutation is quite common and confers cross-resistance to other PIs. Other less important or secondary mutations are at codons 36, 46, 63, 71, 77, 84, 88 and 93 (7th CROI, Abstract 565). Some authorities feel cross resistance is less problematic with HFV, thus making salvage treatment with other PIs more likely to succeed.

VI. Drugs

Indications: See Chapter 4

Pharmacology

> **Bioavailability:** Absorption with meals is 20-80%. Food increases absorption 2-3 fold.
>
> **T½:** 3.5-5 hrs.
>
> **CNS penetration:** No detectable levels in CSF (JAIDS 1999;20:39)
>
> **Excretion:** Primarily by cytochrome P450 (3A4). Inhibits 3A4. Only 1-2% is found in urine; up to 90% is found in stool, primarily as oxidative metabolites.
>
> **Storage:** Room temperature
>
> **Dose modification in renal or hepatic failure:** None in renal failure; consider therapeutic drug monitoring with severe liver disease. It appears that autoinduction of NFV is blunted in severe liver disease, and there is also a reduction in the M8 active metabolite. Standard doses may give high or low levels.

Side effects: About 10-30% of 1,500 recipients have reported diarrhea or loose stools; most respond to Imodium and some respond to pancreatic enzymes. This is a secretory diarrhea, characterized by low osmolarity and high sodium, possibly due to chloride secretion (7th CROI, Abstract 62). Class adverse effects: fat redistribution, increased levels of triglycerides and/or cholesterol, hyperglycemia with insulin resistance and type 2 diabetes, osteoporosis and possible increased bleeding with hemophilia.

Drug interactions: The cytochrome P450 enzyme is inhibited by nelfinavir, primarily CYP3A.

NFV reduces levels of methadone 30-50% but in most cases no dose change is required (7th CROI, Abstract 87).

Drugs that require dose modifications: oral contraceptives, levels of ethinylestradiol decrease 47% - use alternative birth control method. Phenobarbital, phenytoin, and carbamazepine may decrease NFV levels substantially – monitor anticonvulsants levels. Sildenafil AUC increased 2-11 fold – do not exceed 25 mg/48 hrs. Rifabutin levels increased 2 fold and NFV levels decreased 32% – increase NFV dose to 1000 mg tid and decrease RFB dose to 150 mg/day.

Drugs that have no effect: ketoconazole; drugs with no data: clarithromycin

Table 6-25. Combinations with PIs and NNRTIs.

Drug	AUC	Regimen
IDV	IDV ↑ 50% NFV ↑ 80%	IDV 1200 mg bid NVP 1250 mg bid
RTV	RTV No change NFV ↑ 1.5x	RTV 400 mg bid NFV 500-750 mg bid
SQV	SQV ↑ 3-5x NVP ↑ 20%	SQV (Fortovase) 800 mg tid or 1200 bid NFV 1250 bid
APV	AMP ↑ 1.5x NVP ?	Inadequate data
NVP	NVP no change NFV ↑ 10%	Standard doses
EFV	NFV ↑ 20% EFV no change	Standard doses
DLV	DLV ↓ 50% NFV ↑ 2x	Inadequate data

VI. Drugs

NEUPOGEN – See G-CSF (p. 214)

NEVIRAPINE (NVP)

Trade name: Viramune (Roxane Labs, Inc. — distributor; Boehringer Ingelheim — manufacturer)

Forms and price: 200 mg tabs – \$4.24/200 mg tab or \$59.36/week; 50 mg/5 mL suspension

Patient assistant program: (800) 274-8651

Class: Non-nucleoside reverse transcriptase inhibitor

Clinical Trials: The largest clinical trial is the INCAS trial using nevirapine combined with AZT and ddI in treatment naïve patients. At 52 weeks 52% had undetectable virus (<400 c/mL).

The Atlantic Trial was a multicenter trial involving 235 patients who were randomized to receive ddI + d4T plus either NVP, IDV or 3TC. At 48 weeks 55-59% in all three groups had <400 c/mL by intent-to-treat analysis. The low viral load at entry (median of 15,000 c/mL) limits the conclusions that can be drawn from this study (39th ICAAC 9/99, Abstract LB-22).

The COMBINE study (7th CROI, Abstract 510) compares NVP and NFV, each in combination with AZT/3TC in 142 treatment naïve patients with a median baseline VL of 4.8 $\log_{10}$. Analysis at 24 weeks showed VL <20 c/mL in 58% of NVP recipients compared to 33% in the NFV group by intent-to-treat analysis (p=0.06). Concerns about this study are the high drop out rate and the atypically poor performance of NFV.

Switching therapy from a PI containing regimen to NVP due to lipodystrophy shows rapid improvement in blood lipid changes but minimal change in fat distribution (AIDS 1999;13:805).

Regimen: 200 mg po daily x 14 days ("lead-in" to reduce frequency of rash), then 200 mg twice daily. Patients experiencing a rash during the lead-in should not increase the dose until the rash has resolved. Patients with interrupted treatment >7 days should restart at 200 mg daily. Standard doses of each drug are recommended when NVP is combined with indinavir, ritonavir or nelfinavir; NVP should not be combined with saquinavir or with other NNRTIs (EFV or DLV). The pharmacokinetic properties of NVP support once daily dosing, e.g., 400 mg po bid.

Pregnancy: In a study carried out in Uganda, a single intrapartum dose of nevirapine (200 mg po at onset of labor) and a single dose given to the infant (2 mg/kg within 72 hours of birth) was superior to intrapartum AZT (600 mg at onset of labor, then 300 mg q 3h until delivery) plus AZT to the infant (4 mg/kg/d x 7 days). Perinatal transmission occurred in 13.1% of the NVP recipients vs. 21.5% of the AZT recipients (Lancet 1999;354:795).In the March 2000 DHHS guidelines NVP is now included as an option for prevention of perinatal transmission for HIV infected women who present at term with no prior therapy. A single oral dose of 200 mg is given at the onset of labor and a single dose (2 mg/kg) is given to the infant at 48-72 hrs (www.hivatis.org). Some authorities also feel that these findings justify more consideration of NVP for post-exposure prophylaxis.

Resistance: Monotherapy is associated with rapid and high level resistance with RT mutations at codons 101, 103, 106, 108, 135, 181, 188 and/or 190; the most important are codons 103 and 181, which increase the IC_{90} by >100 fold (JAIDS 1995;8:141). There is cross resistance with delavirdine; cross resistance with efavirenz is more variable; it requires the presence of the K103N mutation, which causes cross-resistance to all currently available NNRTIs. There is evidence that administration of NVP with AZT may predispose to emergence of the K103N mutation. There is no cross resistance with nucleoside analogs or protease inhibitors. With nevirapine alone or nevirapine combined with AZT there is >100-fold reduction in sensitivity to nevirapine within 8 weeks. Thus, nevirapine *must* be used in combination with two nucleoside analogs and/or at least one protease inhibitor, and optimal results are anticipated when it is used in nucleoside analog-naïve patients (Ann Intern Med 1996;124:1019). Although the 103 mutation confers resistance to all NNRTIs, many patients who fail NVP will retain sensitivity to EFV.

Indications: See Chapter 4

Pharmacology

Bioavailability: 93% and not altered by food, fasting, ddI or antacids

T½: 25-30 hours

CNS penetration: CSF levels are ,45% peak serum levels
(CSF: plasma ratio=0.45)

Serum half life: 25-30 hours

Metabolism: Metabolized by cytochrome P450 (3A4) to hydroxylated metabolites that are excreted primarily in the urine which accounts for 90% of the oral dose. Nevirapine autoinduces hepatic cytochrome P450 enzymes of the CYP3A type reducing its own plasma half-life over 2-4 weeks from 45 hours to 25 hours.

Dose-modification with renal or hepatic failure: NVP is extensively metabolized by the liver, and nevirapine metabolites are largely eliminated by the kidney so either organ may alter pharmacokinetics; experience in liver or renal disease is limited, so use standard doses with caution.

VI. Drugs

Side effects: The major toxicities are life threatening cutaneous and hepatic reactions during the initial 8 weeks. Patients should be warned to promptly report symptoms of a hypersensitivity reaction – fever, rash, arthralgias or myalgias. Some authorities advocate monitoring ALT and AST during the first 8 weeks with the following responses based on recommendations of the European Medicines Evaluation Agency (statement 4/12/00 – www.eudra.org/emea.html).

AST/ALT	Hypersensitivity*	Recommendation
AST or ALT >2x ULN	No Yes	Continue NVP and monitor D/C NVP and do not rechallenge
AST or ALT >5x ULN	No	D/C NVP: may rechallenge when LFTs normal 200 mg qd x 14 d, then 400 mg qd
Unknown	Yes	Perform LFTs

* Fever, rash arthralgias, myalgias, eosinophilia and/or renal failure.

The most common toxicity is rash, which is seen in about 17%; the usual rash is maculopapular and erythematous with or without pruritis located on the trunk, face and extremities. Many patients with rashes required hospitalization and 7% of all patients required discontinuation of the drug compared to 4.3% given delavirdine and 1.7% given efavirenz. NNRTIs should be discontinued for severe rash, or rash accompanied by fever, blisters, mucous membrane involvement, conjunctivitis, edema, arthralgias, or malaise. Steven-Johnson Syndrome has been reported, and three deaths ascribed to rash have been reported with nevirapine (Lancet 1998;351:567).

Drug interactions: Nevirapine, like rifampin, induces CYP3A families of the cytochrome P450 mechanism. Maximum induction takes place 2-4 weeks after initiating therapy. Major concern is enhanced metabolism by this mechanism. Methadone: NVP may substantially lower opiate levels and may cause opiate withdrawal; patients receiving methadone may require increases in methadone doses to >150 mg/day (6th Retrovirus Conf, 1999, Chicago, Abstract 372).

Drugs that are contraindicated or not recommended for concurrent use:
Rifampin and ketoconazole

Table 6-26: Dose Recommendations for Nevirapine Plus Protease Inhibitor Combinations

PI	PI level	NVP level	Regimen recommended
Indinavir	↓ 28%	No change	IDV 1000 mg q 8 h NVP standard
Ritonavir	↓ 11%	No change	Standard doses
Saquinavir	↓ 25%	No change	Not recommended
Nelfinavir	↑ 10%	No change	Standard doses
Amprenavir	?	?	No data

Drugs that required dose modification with concurrent use: Nevirapine decreases AUC for ethinyl estradiol by about 50%; alternative methods of birth control should be used. Nevirapine reduces clarithromycin AUC by 30% but the increase in levels of the 14-OH metabolite, which has antibacterial activity that compensates, means that no dose adjustment is necessary. Rifabutin levels decreased 16% – no data for RBT dose. No data for phenobarbital, phenytoin, carbamazepine, simvastatin and lovastatin. NFV decreases methadone levels, but also decreases protein-binding of methadone – no dose change was required (7th CROI, Abstract 87).

Pregnancy: Class C. Negative rodent teratogenicity assays; placental passage in humans shows a newborn : maternal ratio of 1.0. Pharmacokinetic studies show the elimination half life of nevirapine is longer in pregnant women, with a mean of 66 hours compared to 45 hours in non-pregnant women.

NIZORAL – See Ketoconazole (p. 228)

NORTRIPTYLINE

Generic; Trade names: Aventyl (Lilly) and Pamelor (Sandoz)

Forms and price: 10 mg caps – $0.12; 25 mg caps – $0.16; 50 mg caps – $0.19; 75 mg caps – $0.24; oral suspension 10 mg/5 mL (480 mL) – $0.47/10 mg

Class: Tricyclic antidepressant

Indications and dose regimens:

> **Depression:** 25 mg hs initially; increase by 25 mg every 3 days until 75 mg, then wait 5 days, and obtain level with expectation of level of 100-150 ng/dL.

> **Peripheral neuropathy:** 10-25 mg hs; increase dose over 2-3 weeks to maximum of 75 mg hs

Pharmacology

Bioavailability: >90%

T½: 13-79 hours, mean – 31 hours

Elimination: Metabolized and renally excreted

Side effects: Anticholinergic effects (dry mouth, dizzy, blurred vision; constipation, urinary hesitancy), orthostatic hypotension (less compared to other tricyclics), sedation, sexual dysfunction (decreased libido), and weight gain.

Pregnancy: Category D. Animal studies are inconclusive and experience in pregnant women is inadequate. Avoid during first trimester, and when possible limit use in the last two trimesters.

Drug interactions: The following drugs should not be given concurrently – adrenergic neuronal blocking agents, clonidine, other alpha-2 agonists, excessive alcohol, fenfluramine, cimetidine, and MAO inhibitors. Drugs that increase nortriptyline levels – cimetidine, quinidine, fluconazole.

NORVIR – See Ritonavir (p. 258)

NYSTATIN

Generic; Trade names: Mycostatin (Apothecon, Bristol-Myers Squibb)

Forms and price:

Lozenges – 200,000 units – $ 1.01/Mycostatin lozenge

Cream – 100,000 u/gm, 15 gm – $1.46; 30 gm – $2.18 (generic); 15 gm $14.48 (Mycostatin)

Ointment – 100,000 u/gm, 15 gm – $1.46; 30 gm – $3.60 (generic); 15 gm – $14.48 (Mycostatin)

Suspension – 100,000 u/mL, 60 mL – $4.39; 480 mL – $20.64 (generic); 60 mL – $21.84 (Mycostatin)

Oral tabs – 500,000 units – $.12/tab (generic); $.55/tab (Mycostatin)

Vaginal tabs – 100,000 units – $0.11/tab (generic); $.73 tab (Mycostatin)

Patient assistance program (Bristol-Myers Squibb): (800) 272-4878

Class: Polyene macrolide similar to amphotericin B

Activity: Active against *Candida albicans* at 3 µg/mL and other *Candida* species at higher concentrations

Indications and dose regimens:

Thrush – 5 mL suspension to be gargled 5x/day x 14 days

Vaginitis – 100,000 unit tab intravaginally 1-2x/day x 14 days

Note: some studies suggest topical treatment with imidazoles (eg, clotrimazole, miconazole) may be superior

Pharmacology

Bioavailability: Poorly absorbed and undetectable in blood following oral administration

Therapeutic levels persist in saliva for two hours after oral dissolution of two lozenges.

Side effects: Infrequent, dose-related GI intolerance (transient nausea, vomiting, diarrhea)

OCTREOTIDE (Somatostatin)

Trade name: Sandostatin (Sandoz)

Forms and price: Concentrations of 50, 100, 200, 500, and 1000 µg/mL in 20 and 50 mL vials; 1 mg vial – $121.41

Patient assistance program: (888) 455-6655

Class: Synthetic polypeptide related to somatostatin

Indications: Occasional AIDS patient with uncontrolled chronic secretory diarrhea, usually due to cryptosporidiosis or microsporidiosis. A controlled trial showed minimal benefit, but the drug was more effective at higher doses when used for a more prolonged period of time (Gastroenterology 1995;108;1753).

Dose: Standard initial dose is 50-100 µg SC 1-3x daily, usually 100 µg tid initially and then increased to 500 µg tid x ≥8 weeks. Maximum doses of 1,500-3,000 µg/day in 2 or 3 daily doses have been given.

Side effects: Cholelithiasis or biliary sludge in 15-20%; baseline ultrasound of gall bladder is sometimes recommended. GI: nausea, vomiting, cramping, and diarrhea in 5-15%; these side effects usually resolve and rarely require discontinuation of the drug; CNS: headache, dizziness, lightheadedness, asthenia in 1-2%. Endocrine: Hyperglycemia in 1-2%

OFLOXACIN – See Fluoroquinolone Summary (page 207)

Class: Antimalarial

Indications and dose:

> *P. carinii* pneumonia: Primaquine 15 mg (base)/day + clindamycin 600-900 mg
> q 6-8 h IV or 300-450 mg qid po

Pharmacology

> **Bioavailability:** Well absorbed

> **T½:** 4-10 hours

> **Elimination:** Metabolized by liver

Side effects: Hemolytic anemia in patients with G-6-PD deficiency; its severity depends
on drug dose and genetics of G-6-PD deficiency: In African-Americans the reaction is
usually mild, self-limited and asymptomatic; in patients of Mediterranean or certain
Asian extractions, hemolysis may be severe. Hemolytic anemia may also occur with
other forms of hemoglobinopathy. Warn patient of dark urine as sign and/or measure
G-6-PD level prior to use in susceptible individuals. Other hematologic side effects:
methemoglobinemia, leukopenia. GI: nausea, vomiting, epigastric pain (reduced by
administration with meals). Miscellaneous: headache, disturbed visual accommoda-
tion, pruritis, hypertension, arrhythmias.

PROCRIT – See Erythropoietin (p. 199)

PYRAZINAMIDE (PZA)

Generic

Forms and price: 500 mg tabs $1.12 (usually 2 gm/day at $4.48/day)

Class: Derivative of niacinamide

Indication and regimen: Tuberculosis

> Daily regimen: 20-35 mg/kg in 3-4 daily doses up to 2 gm/day; up to 60 mg/day
> for drug-resistant TB

> Twice weekly regimen: 50-70 mg/kg up to 4 gm/day

> Thrice weekly regimen: 50-70 mg/kg up to 3 gm/day

Treatment with Rifater (tabs with 50 mg INH, 120 mg rifampin and 300 mg PZA):

> <65 kg: 1 tab/10 kg/day

> >65 kg: 6 tabs/day

Pharmacology

> **Bioavailability:** Well absorbed; absorption is reduced about 25% in patients
> with advanced HIV infection (Ann Intern Med 1997;127:289).

T½: 9-10 hours

CSF levels: Equal to plasma levels

Elimination: Hydrolyzed in liver; 4-14% of parent compound and 70% of metabolite excreted in urine

Renal failure: Usual dose unless creatinine clearance <10 mL/min – 12-20 mg/kg/day

Hepatic failure: Contraindicated

Side effects: Hepatotoxicity in up to 15% received >3 gm/day – transient hepatitis with increase in transaminases, jaundice, and a syndrome of fever, anorexia, and hepatomegaly; rarely, acute yellow atrophy. Monitor LFTs. Hyperuricemia is common, but gout is rare. Nongouty polyarthralgia in up to 40%; hyperuricemia usually responds to uricosuric agents. Use with caution in patients with history of gout. Rare – rash, fever, acne, dysuria, skin discoloration, urticaria, pruritis, GI intolerance, thrombocytopenia, sideroblastic anemia.

Pregnancy: Category C. Not tested in animals or in humans. Conclusion is that risk of teratogenicity is unknown, so INH, rifampin, and ethambutol are preferred. PZA is advocated for pregnant women if resistant *M. tuberculosis* is suspected or established.

PYRIMETHAMINE

Generic

Trade name: Daraprim (Glaxo Wellcome)

Forms and price: 25 mg tabs; $0.41/tab

Patient assistance program: (800) 722-9294

Class: Aminopyrimidine-derivative antimalarial agent that is structurally related to trimethoprim.

Indications and dose regimens:

> **Toxoplasmosis: Treatment** – Pyrimethamine 50-100 mg/day po plus sulfonamide (sulfadiazine, sulfamethoxazole, or trisulfapyrimidine) 4-8 gm po/d x ≥6 weeks plus leukovorin 10 mg/day po or pyrimethamine 50-100 mg/d po plus clindamycin 600 mg q 6-8 h IV or 300-450 mg q 6 h po plus leukovorin 10 mg/day po

> **Toxoplasmosis: Prophylaxis** – Pyrimethamine 25 mg po 2x/wk plus dapsone 50 mg po 2x/wk plus leukovorin 25 mg/wk

Pharmacology

Bioavailability: Well absorbed

T½: 54-148 hours (average – 111 hours)

Elimination: Parent compound and metabolites excreted in urine

Dose modification in renal failure: None

Side effects: Reversible marrow suppression due to depletion of folic acid stores with dose-related megaloblastic anemia, leukopenia, thrombocytopenia, and agranulocytosis; prevented or treated with folinic acid (leukovorin)

GI intolerance: Improved by reducing dose or giving drug with meals

Neurologic: Dose-related ataxia, tremors, or seizures

Hypersensitivity: Most common with pyrimethamine plus sulfadoxine (Fansidar)

Pregnancy: Category C. teratogenic in animals

Drug interactions: Lorazepam – hepatotoxicity

REBETOL – See Ribavirin (below)

RETROVIR – See Zidovudine (AZT, ZDV) (p. 283)

RIBAVIRIN

Trade name: Rebetol (Schering Corp.)

Form: 200 mg capsule
Ribavirin is provided as a Therapy Pak (Rebetron) in combination with interferon (Intron).

Indication (FDA labeling): Ribavirin in combination with interferon is recommended for treatment of chronic hepatitis C in patients with compensated liver disease who have not previously been treated and those who have relapsed after interferon monotherapy.

Clinical trials: The major study was a multicenter trial comparing interferon alfa vs. ribavirin/interferon for hepatitis C patients with compensated liver disease, detectable HCV RNA and relapse following interferon therapy alone (NEJM 1998;339:1485). Among 345 patients, a virologic response (<100 c/mL HCV by RT-PCR) was noted in 46% in the ribavirin arm compared to 5% in the group receiving interferon only. The frequency of post-treatment biopsies showing histologic improvement was 51% vs. 30% favoring ribavirin. Two other trials showed similar results with superior outcomes in patients treated with ribavirin plus interferon vs. interferon alone [Lancet 1998;351:1426; NEJM 1998;339:1493]. The number with a sustained virologic response among recipients of combination therapy in these trials was 30-50%; for those with non-genotype 1 it was 60-70%.

Regimen:

Table 6-27: Ribavirin Regimen

Dose Weight	Ribavirin	Interferon
<75 kg	2 x 200 mg caps AM 3 x 200 mg caps PM	3 million units 3x/wk
>75 kg	3 x 200 mg caps bid	3 million units 3x/wk

Pharmacokinetics

   Oral Bioavailability: 64%, absorption increased with high fat meal

   T½: 30 hrs.

   Elimination: Metabolized by phosphorylation and deribosylation; there are few or no P450 enzyme-based drug interactions. Metabolites are excreted in the urine. The drug should not be used with severe renal failure.

Side effects: About 6% of patients receiving ribavirin/interferon discontinue therapy due to side effects. The main side effect of ribavirin is hemolytic anemia which is noted in the first 1-2 weeks of treatment and usually stabilizes by week 4. In clinical trials the mean decrease in hemoglobin was 3 gm/dL and 10% of patients had a hemoglobin <10 gm/dL. Patients with a hemoglobin level <10 gm/dL or decrease in hemoglobin ≥2 gm/dL *and* a history of cardiovascular disease should receive a modified regimen: ribavirin 600 mg/day + interferon 1.5 million units 3x/wk. The drugs should be discontinued if the hemoglobulin decreases to ≤8.5 gm/dL or if the hemoglobulin persists at <12 gm/dL in patients with a cardiovascular disease. Other side effects ascribed to ribavirin include leukopenia, hyperbilirubinemia, increased uric acid and dyspnea.

Note: See Interferon (p. 222) for side effects ascribed to that agent.

Drug interaction: Ribavirin probably interacts with thymidine-phosphorylated nucleoside analogues such as AZT and d4T (Science 1987;235:1376); the significance of this interaction is unknown.

Pregnancy: Category X

RIFABUTIN

Trade name: Mycobutin (Pharmacia & Upjohn)

Forms and price: 150 mg caps – $4.41

Patient assistance program: (800) 242-7014

Class: Semisynthetic derivative of rifampin B that is derived from *Streptomyces mediterranei*.

Activity: Active against most strains of *M. avium* and rifampin-sensitive *M. tuberculosis*; cross resistance between rifampin and rifabutin is common with *M. tuberculosis* and *M. avium*.

Indications and dose:

M. avium prophylaxis: 300 mg po qd. Efficacy established (NEJM 1993;329:828); azithromycin or clarithromycin usually preferred

Tuberculosis: Preferred rifamycin for use in combination with protease inhibitors or NNRTIs (MMWR 1998;47:[RR-20]). Usual dose for TB treatment and prophylaxis: 300 mg/day
Nucleosides: No dose adjustment
PIs and NNRTIs: See Table 6-28

Pharmacology

Bioavailability: 12-20%

T½: 30-60 hours

Elimination: Primarily renal and biliary excretion of metabolites

Dose modification in renal failure: None

Side effects: Common – brown-orange discoloration of secretions; urine (30%), tears, saliva, sweat, stool, and skin. Infrequent – rash (4%), GI intolerance (3%), neutropenia (2%). Rare side effects – flu-like illness, hepatitis, hemolysis, headache, thrombocytopenia, myositis. Major concern is uveitis which presents as red and painful eye, blurred vision, photophobia, or floaters. This is dose-related, usually with doses >450 mg/day, or with standard dose (300 mg/day) plus concurrent use of drugs that increase rifabutin levels: clarithromycin and fluconazole (NEJM 1994;330:868). Treatment is with topical corticosteroids and mydriatics. These patients should be seen by an ophthalmologist.

Pregnancy: Category C. High doses in rabbits caused skeletal abnormalities; no data in humans.

Drug interactions: Rifabutin induces hepatic microsomal enzymes (cytochrome P450), although the effect is less pronounced than for rifampin. Concurrent treatment with rifabutin reduces the activity of amprenavir (80% decrease), coumadin, barbiturates, benzodiazepines, ß-adrenergic blockers, chloramphenicol, clofibrate, oral contraceptives, corticosteroids, cyclosporine, diazepam, dapsone, digitalis, doxycycline, haloperidol, oral hypoglycemics, ketoconazole, methadone, phenytoin, quinidine, theophylline, trimethoprim, and verapamil. Drugs that inhibit cytochrome P450 and prolong the half life of rifabutin: erythromycin, clarithromycin, (4-fold increase), ciprofloxacin, and azoles (fluconazole, itraconazole and ketoconazole). With concurrent rifabutin and fluconazole, the levels of rifabutin are significantly increased, leading to possible rifabutin toxicity (uveitis, nausea, neutropenia) or increased efficacy (CID 1996;23;685).

Table 6-28: Rifabutin Interactions and Dose Adjustments With Antiretroviral Drugs (MMWR 1998;47[RR-20]:14)

Agent	AUC for		Comment
	ART agent	RBT	
Nucleosides	NC	NC	Use standard doses
Amprenavir	↓14%	↑193%	AMP–standard; RBT–150 mg/d
Delavirdine	↓80%	↑100%	(Contraindicated)
Efavirenz	NC	↓35%	EFV–standard; RBT–450 mg/d
Indinavir	↓34%	↑173%	IDV–1000 mg q 8h; RBT–150 mg/d
Nevirapine	↓16%	↓	No data
Nelfinavir	↓32%	↑200%	NFV–1,000 mg tid; RBT–150 mg/d
Ritonavir	NC	↑293%	RBT– 150 mg qod; RTV – standard
Saquinavir (Fortovase)	↓40%	?	Not recommended

NC = No change

Preliminary data suggest that RBT may be given with RTV/SQV (400 mg/400 mg bid) with no dose adjustment for PIs and RBT given at 150 mg q 3 d or 300 mg q 7 d (7th CROI, Abstract 91).

Comments:

1. There is an as yet unsubstantiated concern that widespread use of rifabutin will promote rifampin resistance to *M. tuberculosis*.

2. Rifampin and rifabutin are related drugs, but *in vitro* activity and clinical trials show that rifabutin is preferred for *M. avium* and rifampin is preferred for *M. tuberculosis*.

3. Clarithromycin plus ethambutol is the preferred regimen for treatment of disseminated *M. avium* infection.

4. Drug interactions are similar for rifabutin and rifampin although rifabutin is a less potent inducing agent of hepatic microsomal enzymes.

5. Uveitis requires immediate discontinuation of drug and ophthalmology consult.

RIFAMATE – See Isoniazid (p. 224) or Rifampin (below)
(Ann Intern Med 1995;122:951)

RIFAMPIN

Generic; Trade name: Rifadin (Hoechst Marion Roussel) and Rimactane (Ciga-Geigy); Combination with INH: Rifamate and Rifater

Forms: 150 and 300 mg caps; caps with 150 mg INH plus 300 mg rifampin (Rifamate); tabs with 50 mg INH + 120 mg rifampin + 300 mg pyrazinamide (Rifater); 600 mg vials for IV use

Price: $1.61/300 mg cap; $79.38/600 mg vial; Rifater – $1.80/tab

Active against: *M. tuberculosis, M. kansasii, S. aureus, H. influenzae, S. pneumoniae, Legionella,* and many anaerobes.

Indication: Tuberculosis (with INH, PZA, and SM or ETH)

> **Dose:** 600 mg/day
>
> **DOT:** 600 mg 2-3x/wk
>
> **Prophylaxis (alone or in combination with PZA or ETH):** 600 mg/day

Protease inhibitors + active TB: The U.S. Public Health Service suggest (MMWR 1996;45:922):

> **Protease inhibitor not started:** Give standard four drug TB regimen and then give protease inhibitor.
>
> **Rifampin + antiretroviral agents:** The use of rifampin to treat tuberculosis in patients receiving protease inhibitors (ritonavir, indinavir, saquinavir, nelfinavir or amprenavir) or NNRTIs (nevirapine, delavirdine or efavirenz) is always contraindicated (MMWR 1998;47[RR-20]:12).

Rifamate treatment: 2 caps/day

Rifater treatment:

> <65 kg – 1 tab/10 kg
>
> >65 kg – 6 tabs/day
>
> **Other infections:** *S. aureus* (with vancomycin, fluoroquinolones, or penicillinase-resistant penicillin): 300 mg po bid

Pharmacology

> **Bioavailability:** 90-95%, less with food. Absorption is reduced 30% in patients with advanced HIV infection; significance is unknown (Ann Intern Med 1997;127:289).
>
> **T½:** 1.5-5 hours, average – 2 hrs
>
> **Elimination:** Excreted in urine (33%) and metabolized
>
> **Dose modification in renal failure:** None

Side effects: Common – orange-brown discoloration of urine, stool, tears (contact lens), sweat, skin. Infrequent – GI intolerance; hepatitis, usually cholestatic changes in first month of treatment (no increase in risk when given with INH); jaundice (usually reversible with dose reduction or continued use); hypersensitivity, especially

VI. Drugs

pruritis ± rash (3%); flu-like illness with intermittent use – dyspnea, wheezing, purpura, leukopenia. Rare side effects – thrombocytopenia, leukopenia, hemolytic anemia, increased uric acid, and BUN. Frequency of side effects that require discontinuation of drug: 3%.

Pregnancy: Category C. Dose-dependent congenital malformations in animals. Isolated cases of fetal abnormalities noted in patients, but frequency is unknown. Large retrospective studies have shown no risk of congenital abnormalities; case reports of neural tube defects and limb reduction (CID 1995;21 suppl 1:S24). May cause postnatal hemorrhage in mother and infant if given in last few weeks of pregnancy. Must use with caution.

Drug interactions: Rifampin induces hepatic P450 enzymes resulting in reduced levels of amprenavir, atovaquone, coumadin, barbiturates, benzodiazepines, beta-adrenergic blockers, chloramphenicol, clarithromycin, clofibrate, oral contraceptives, corticosteroids, cyclosporine, diazepam, dapsone, delavirdine, digitalis, doxycycline, efavirenz, erythromycin, haloperidol, indinavir, oral hypoglycemics, ketoconazole, methadone, nelfinavir, nevirapine, phenytoin, quinidine, saquinavir, theophylline, trimethoprim, and verapamil. The following drugs inhibit cytochrome P450 enzymes and prolong the half life of rifampin: indinavir, ritonavir, clarithromycin, crythromycin, ciprofloxacin, and azoles (fluconazole, itraconazole, and ketaconazole). Efavirenz has no significant effect on rifampin levels, but rifampin reduces efavirenz levels by 20-26%. Concurrent use with protease inhibitors or NNRTIs (with the possible exception of ritonavir and efavirenz) are contraindicated (see Rifabutin for treatment guidelines using antiretroviral agents with TB treatment).

RIFATER – See INH (p. 224) or Rifampin (above)
(Ann Intern Med 1995;122:951)

RITONAVIR (RTV)

Trade name: Norvir (Abbott Laboratories)

Forms and price: 100 mg soft gel capsules @ $1.86/100 mg cap; liquid formulation – 600 mg/7.5 mL @ $31.71/240 mL

Patient assistance program: (800) 659-9050

Class: Protease inhibitor

Trials: The activity of ritonavir has been extensively studied, initially alone and later in combination with NRTIs. More recent studies have examined RTV in combination with other PIs, because RTV as a single agent is poorly tolerated and because it dramatically increases the levels and half life of most other PIs by inhibition of the P450 metabolic pathway.

1. Study 247 was a multinational, randomized, double-blind, placebo-controlled trial in 1,090 HIV-infected patients who had been receiving nucleoside analog

therapy for at least nine months and had CD4 cell counts ≤100 cells/µL. Ritonavir 600 mg bid was added to each patient's baseline regimen, which could have consisted of up to two approved nucleoside analogs. There was a 44% reduction in the risk of death (4.8% for ritonavir vs 8.4% for placebo; p=0.02), and a 47% reduction in the risk of the combined endpoint of disease progression of death (15.7% for ritonavir and 33.1% for placebo; <0.001) (Lancet 1998;351:543). Note: The addition of a protease inhibitor to a failing regimen is no longer recommended.

2. Ritonivar/saquinavir: There is great interest in combining RTV with other PIs due to both the poor GI tolerance of RTV at full therapeutic doses and its potent inhibition of cytochrome P450 metabolic pathways. In combination with RTV, the AUCs and trough levels for saquinavir, indinavir, amprenavir and nelfinavir are increased. The greatest experience is with RTV/SQV (Invirase or Fortovase), which has been used extensively for initial and for salvage therapy. The IRIS Study demonstrated that RTV/SQV/d4T was as effective as indinavir plus 2 NRTIs in the treatment of PI naïve patients (6th Retrovirus Conf., 1999, Chicago, Abstract 630). In M96-462 120 of 141 patients (85%) treated with RTV/SQV had VL <200 c/mL at 144 weeks, although 11% required intensification with NRTIs (7th CROI, Abstract 533). The Prometheus trial compared RTV/SQV (alone) with RTV/SQV/d4T as initial therapy in 208 patients with intensification using d4T at 12 weeks if the VL was >500 c/mL. At 48 weeks 63% and 68% had VL <500 c/mL without intensification, respectively (7th CROI, Abstract 526). The use of RTV/SQV is more challenging in salvage therapy: A trial of RTV + SQV + 2 NRTI was used in patients who failed nelfinavir (6th Retrovirus Conf, 1999, Chicago, Abstract 392). At 60 weeks 58% of participants had a viral load <500 c/mL. Not surprisingly, a relatively low viral load at the time of the switch predicted success.

3. RTV/IDV: Recent trials have studied the combination of RTV with IDV. Pharmacokinetic studies demonstrate a highly favorable impact on IDV levels with high trough levels of IDV, which presumably decrease subtherapeutic levels and permit bid dosing. Peak levels were also reduced compared to IDV given alone q 8 h, and this would be expected to lead to a reduced risk of nephrolithiasis. Several regimens have been tested: RTV 100-200 mg bid plus IDV 800 mg bid or RTV 400 mg bid + IDV 400 mg bid. The 400/400 mg bid regimen shows a good pharmacokinetic profile with lower IDV peak levels (which may reduce rates of nephrolithiasis) and high trough levels, but the 400 mg dose of RTV is often poorly tolerated. The 100-200/800 mg bid regimen is better tolerated, but gives higher peak levels of IDV. An alternative strategy is to intensify with RTV in patients with virologic failure on IDV-containing regimens (7th CROI, Abstract 534).

4. RTV/NFV: RTV has also been combined with NFV using regimens of RTV 400 mg bid plus NFV 500–750 mg bid. Results of a small pilot trial demonstrate good antiviral activity, but high rates of diarrhea (6th Retroviral Conf, 1999, Chicago, Abstract 393).

5. RTV/APV: Ritonavir increases AMP AUC 2.5 fold and increases AMP trough levels 10 fold (7th CROI, Abstracts 77 and 78). Dosing recommendations are APV 600 mg bid + RTV 100 mg bid *or* APV 1200 mg qd + RTV 200 mg qd. If EFV is added: RTV 200 mg bid + AMP 1200 mg bid + EFV 600 mg hs.

6. ABT 378/r: See page 232.

Resistance: Phenotypic resistance correlates with mutations on the protease gene at codons 46, 63, 71, 82 and 84 (J Virol 1995;69:701). Patients failing monotherapy have multiple mutations at 9 codons: 20, 33, 36, 46, 62, 71, 82, 84 and 90 (Nat Medicine 1996;2:760; 7th CROI, Abstract 565). The initial mutation was at codon 82, which was consistently seen and appeared necessary for phenotypic resistance (AAC 1998;42:2775). This was followed by mutations at codons 54, 71 and 36; codon 84 and 90 mutations occurred late and less frequently.

Dose: 600 mg bid when used as a single PI or 100-400 mg bid when used with another PI. Administration with food improves tolerability but is not required. Separate dosing with ddI by ≥2 hours.

Recommended dose escalation regimen to improve GI tolerance: Day 1 & 2: 300 mg bid; Day 3-5: 400 mg bid; Day 6-13: 500 mg bid; Day 14 and thereafter: 600 mg bid

Dose regimen for ritonavir/saquinavir (hard gel or soft gel capsule)

Patients already taking ritonavir: Add saquinavir 400 mg bid

Patients already taking saquinavir: Reduce saquinavir to 400 mg bid and add ritonavir at 300 mg bid x 2 days, then 400 mg bid

Patients naïve to both: Start saquinavir 400 mg bid and ritonavir 300 mg bid. Dose escalate ritonavir to 400 mg bid on day 3.

Pharmacology

Bioavailability: 60-80% (not well determined). Levels increased 15% when taken with meals. CNS penetration: No detectable levels in CSF.

T½: 3–5 hours

Elimination: Metabolized by cytochrome P450 3A4>2D6. RTV is a potent inhibitor of P450 3A4.

Dose modification in renal or hepatic failure: Use standard doses for renal failure; consider empiric dose reduction in severe hepatic disease.

Side effects: The most frequently reported adverse events are GI intolerance (nausea, diarrhea, vomiting, anorexia, abdominal pain, taste perversion), circumoral and peripheral paresthesias and asthenia. GI intolerance is often severe and improved by the graduated dose regimen and with continued administration for ≥1 month. Side effects are less severe in the reduced doses used in the dual PI combinations. Hepatotoxicity with elevated transaminase levels are more frequent and more severe with RTV than with other PIs; there does appear to be a modest increased risk with hepatitis B or C co-infection (JAMA 2000;238:74). This risk may be reduced with lower RTV doses used in PI combinations. Laboratory changes include elevated triglycerides, cholestrol, transaminases, CPK and uric acid. **Class adverse reactions:** Insulin resistant hyperglycemia, fat redistribution, elevated triglycerides and cholesterol, osteoporosis, and possible increased bleeding with hemophilia.

Drug interactions: Ritonavir is a potent inhibitor of cytochrome P450 enzymes, including 3A41 and 2D6 and can produce large increases in the plasma concentrations of drugs that are metabolized by that mechanism.

Use with the following agents is contraindicated: amiodarone, astemizole, bepridil, bupropion, cisapride, clorazepate, flecainide, lovastatin, meperidine, midazolam, ergot alkaloids, quinidine, pimozide, propoxyphene, simvastatin, terfenadine, triazolam, and zolpidem.

Drugs that require dose modification: Clarithromycin AUC increased 77%, but the clinical consequences are unknown (CID 1996;23:685). Methadone levels are decreased 36%; consider dose increase. Desipramine levels are increased 145% decrease desipramine dose. Didanosine reduces absorption of ritonavir and should be taken ≥2 hours apart. Ketoconazole levels increased 3x – do not exceed 200 mg ketoconazole/day. Rifampin reduces RTV levels 35% – no data on combination use and concern for hepatotoxicity. Rifabutin levels increased 4x – RBT dose of 150 mg qod or 150 mg 3 day/wk. Ethinylestradiol levels decreased 40% – use alternative method of birth control. Theophylline levels decreased 47% – monitor theophylline levels. Phenobarbital, phenytoin and carbamazepine interaction ill-defined – monitor anticonvulsant levels. Sildenafil AUC increased 2-11 fold – do not use >25 mg/48 hr. A potentially fatal reaction has been reported with RTV and MDMA ("Ecstasy") (Arch Intern Med 1999;159:2221).

VI. Drugs

Table 6-29: Ritonavir Interactions with Antiretroviral Drugs

Drug	Effect	Recommendation
Saquinavir	SQV – ↑2x RTV – No change	Saquinavir 400 mg bid + Ritonavir 400 mg bid
Nevirapine	RTV – ↑70% NVP – No change	Standard dose
Nelfinavir	NFV – 1.5x RTV – No change	Ritonavir 400 mg bid + Nelfinavir 500-750 mg bid
Delavirdine	DLV – No change RTV – ↑70%	No data (Standard dose)
Indinavir	IDV – ↑ 2-5x RTV – no change	Indinavir 400 mg bid + Ritonavir 400 mg bid *or* Indinavir 800 mg + Ritonavir 100-200 mg bid
Efavirenz	EFV – ↑21% RTV – ↑18%	Ritonavir 600 mg bid (500 mg for intolerance) + Efavirenz 600 mg/day
Amprenavir	APV – ↑2.5x RTV – no change	APV 1200 mg qd + RTV 200 mg qd *or* APV 600 mg bid + RTV 100 mg qd. With EFV/APV/RTV use: RTV 200 mg bid, APV 1200 mg bid + EFV 600 mg hs

Pregnancy: Category B. Negative rodent teratogenic assays; placental passage studies in rodents show newborn : maternal drug ratio of 1.15 at midterm and 0.15 – 0.64 at late term.

ROFERON – See Interferon (p. 222

SANDOSTATIN – See Octreotide (p. 246)

SAQUINAVIR (SQV)

Trade name: Invirase (hard gel capsule); Fortovase (soft gel capsule) (Hoffman-LaRoche)

Form and price: 200 mg cap (hard gel, Invirase) @ $2.16/200 mg and 200 mg cap (soft gel, Fortovase) @ $1.08/200 mg. Cost/week (Fortovase) is $136.

Reimbursement hotline and Patient Assistance Program: 9 AM – 8 PM EST; (800) 282-7780

Preparations and dosing: The soft gel capsule of saquinavir was introduced in November 1997 as the preferred formulation due to improved bioavailability. The only role for Invirase is for use in combination with ritonavir when Fortovase is not tolerated. The cost/gm is twice the cost for Fortovase.

Standard dose (Fortovase): 1200 mg po tid or 400 mg po bid with ritonavir 400 mg po bid. Note: The twice daily regimen of SQV 1600 mg bid as a single PI has been tested, but the results were considered inadequate for FDA approval as of April, 2000. **(Invirase):** 400 mg po bid with ritonavir 400 mg po bid

Class: Protease inhibitor

Trials: Most trials have evaluated the Invirase formulation of saquinavir either alone or in combination with ritonavir. Trials with Fortovase show better bioavailability and better efficacy.

1. Combination treatment of ritonavir plus saquinavir showed a 2-3 log decrease in plasma HIV RNA levels that was sustained ≥52 wks

2. An open label study (NV 15355) compared Invirase and Fortovase, each in combination with two nucleosides in treatment naïve patients with an average CD4 count of 429/mm³. By intent-to-treat analysis 57% of Fortovase recipients and 38% of Invirase recipients had undedectable virus (<400 c/mL). At 48 weeks 51% of Fortovase recipients had <50 c/mL at 48 weeks. These results were sustained at 72 wks. As expected, VL <500 c/mL at 12 weeks or <50 at 24 wks predicted a durable viologic response (6th Retroviral Conf, 1999, Chicago, Abstract 165).

3. Combinations of saquinavir with ritonavir or nelfinavir (plus NRTIs) in treatment-naïve patients with CD4 counts >200 are highly potent with plasma HIV RNA levels <500 c/mL in 80-85%; these combinations are also favored in patients with failed PI containing regimens (5th Conference on Retroviruses & Opportunistic Infections, 1998, Abstracts 388, 394b, 396, 422, 423, 427, 510).

4. The CHEESE Study compared Fortovase vs indinavir, each in combination with AZT/3TC in treatment naïve patients (or AZT <12 mo) with VL >10,000 c/mL and CD4 count <500. By intent-to-treat analysis 80% in each group had <400 c/mL and 71-74% had <50 c/mL at 24 weeks. There was an unexplained statistically significantly greater increase in the CD4 count among SQV recipients (mean increase 162 vs. 85/mm³) (AIDS 1999;13:F53). The 48 wk data continued to show comparable results for viral load and CD4 response.

5. The SPICE Study randomized 157 PI naïve patients to Fortovase + 2 NRTIs, nelfinavir (NFV) + 2 NRTIs, Fortovase + NFV + 2 NRTIs or Fortovase + NFV. At 48 weeks 45-66% had <400 c/mL and 35-51% had <50 c/mL by intent-to-treat analysis. Results were inferior in the regimen lacking NRTIs; the quadruple treatment regimen was well tolerated and possibly superior in patients with prior NRTI treatment or high baseline viral load. The dose used in the combination PI regimen was Fortovase 800 mg + NFV 750 mg tid. There is also evidence supporting twice-daily dosing of this combination (1200/1250 bid) (JAIDS 2000;23:128).

6. ACTG 359 compared SQV/RTV (400/400 mg bid) with SQV/NFV (800 mg tid/750 mg tid) in 277 patients who failed IDV. The responses were comparable but unimpressive, suggesting that NNRTI containing regimens are superior for salvage (7th CROI, Abstract 235).

Resistance: Genotypic resistance is greatest with mutations at L90M (most common; three-fold decrease in sensitivity) and G48V (less common; 30-fold decrease in sensitivity). Minor mutations conferring resistance are at codons 10, 20, 24, 30, 36, 54, 63, 71, 82, and 84. There is now evidence that patients with clinical resistance to saquinavir frequently have mutations associated with resistance to ritonavir and saquinavir, and clinical resistance to nelfinavir has been demonstrated following saquinavir failure, despite the lack of the characteristic mutation at D30N.

Pharmacology

Bioavailability: Absorption of hard gel capsule is 4% with high fat meal; absorption of the soft gel capsule (Fortovase) is superior to Invirase but % absorption is not established. Food increases SQV levels with Fortovase 6-fold. Fortovase should be taken within two hours of a large meal to increase absorption. Invirase absorption is not influenced by food when taken with RTV. CNS penetration is nil (CSF: serum ratio is 0.02).

T½: 1-2 hours

Elimination: Hepatic metabolism by cytochrome P450 isoenzyme CYP_3A_4; 96% biliary excretion; 1% urinary excretion

Storage: Room temperature

Dose modification in renal or hepatic failure: Use standard dose for renal failure; consider empiric dose reduction for hepatic failure.

Side effects: Gastrointestinal intolerance with nausea, abdominal pain, diarrhea in 5-15% (Invirase), 20-30% (Fortovase); headache and hepatic toxicity; hypoglycemia in patients with type 2 diabetes (Ann Intern Med 1999;131:980). Class adverse effects: fat redistribution, increased levels of triglycerides and/or cholesterol, hyperglycemia with insulin resistance and type 2 diabetes, osteoporosis and possible increased bleeding with hemophilia.

Drug interactions:

Drugs that require dose modification with concurrent use: Sildenafil AUC↑ 2-11x – use ≤25 mg/48 hr.

Drug interactions of uncertain significance: Dexamethasome decreases SQV levels. Phenobarbital, phenytoin, and carbamazepine may decrease SQV levels substantially - monitor anticonvulsant levels. Ketoconazole increases SQV levels 3x – standard dose. Clarithromycin increases SQV levels 177% and SQV increases clarithromycin levels 45% – standard dose. Oral contraceptives – no data.

80%, rifabutin reduces saquinavir levels by 40%. Clarithromycin or azithromycin should be used for MAC prophylaxis rather than rifabutin. For treatment of TB consider INH, ethambutol, PZA ± ciprofloxacin or use a different protease inhibitor with rifabutin in place of rifampin. Other drugs that induce CYP_3A_4 (phenobarbital, phenytoin, nevirapine, dexamethasone, and carbamazepine) may decrease saquinavir levels; these combinations should be avoided if possible.

Drugs that are contraindicated for concurrent use: terfenadine, astemizole, cisapride, triazolam, midazolam, rifampin, rifabutin and ergot alkaloids simvastatin, lovastatin. Pregnancy: Category B. Studies in rats showed no teratogenicity or embryotoxicity.

Table 6-30: Combination Therapy with Fortovase Plus 2nd PI or an NNRTI

Drug	AUC*	Regimen*
RTV	SQV ↑ 20x RTV no change	SQV 400 mg bid RTV 400 mg bid
IDV	IDV no change SQV ↑ 4-7x	Avoid (possible antagonism)
APV	APV ↓ 32% SQV ↓ 19%	Insufficient data
EFV	EFV ↓ 62% SQV ↓ 12%	Not recommended
NVP	NVP no change SQV ↓ 25%	Insufficient data
DLV	DLV no change SQV ↑ 5x	SQV 800 mg tid DLV standard
NFV	NFV ↑ 20% SQV ↑ 3-5x	SQV 800 mg tid NFV standard

* All data and recommended regimens are for the Fortovase formulation of SQV. The exception is SQV/RTV, which may be Fortovase (preferred) or Invirase.

Pregnancy: Category B. Studies in rats showed no teratogenicity or embryotoxicity.

SEPTRA – See Trimethoprim-Sulfamethoxazole (p. 276)

SEROSTIM (Somatropin; Human Growth Hormone)
– See Growth Hormone (p. 216)

SPORANOX – See Itraconazole (p. 225)

STAVUDINE (d4T)

Trade Name: Zerit (Bristol-Myers Squibb)

Forms and price: 15 mg cap – $3.86; 20 mg cap – $4.02; 30 mg cap – $4.18; and 40 mg cap – $4.33 or $60.62/week for 40 mg bid; solution 1 mg/mL, 200 mL

Financial assistance: (800) 272-4878. For patients without insurance coverage plus financial need.

Indications: d4T is relatively easy to administer (bid dosing) and generally well tolerated except for patients with peripheral neuropathy. AZT should not be combined with d4T due to pharmacologic antagonism (JID 1996;173:355). The mechanism of pharmacologic antagonism is disputed.

D4T has become a favored regimen for initial therapy due to tolerability. In DuPont 043 d4T/3TC/EFV was highly effective, and had efficacy superior to that seen in the DuPont 006 trial with AZT/3TG/EFV. The difference may have been due to improved adherence with the d4T containing regimen. In contrast, START 1 compared d4T/3TC vs. AZT/3TC, each in combination with indinavir, and found no difference in virologic outcome at 48 weeks; nevertheless, the CD4 count increased significantly more in the d4T recipients. In START 2 (IDSA 11/99, Abstract 14), a comparison of d4T/ddI/IDV vs. AZT/3TC/IDV d4T recipients had a superior virologic response that was marginally significant (61% vs. 45% for VL <500 c/mL) and a superior CD4 response that was statistically significant (150/mm^3 vs. 106/mm^3). A trial in Thailand comparing AZT/3TC/SQV vs. ddI/d4T/SQV also showed that d4T recipients had a significantly better CD4 response (7th CROI, Abstract 524).

An area of controversy with respect to d4T is its role in potentiating ddI peripheral neuropathy or pancreatitis and its role relative to other NRTIs in causing mitochondrial toxicity and lipodystrophy (7th CROI, Abstracts 52, 55, 302, 756).

Dose: >60 kg – 40 mg po bid; <60 kg – 30 mg po bid; Dose reduction for peripheral neuropathy: 20 mg po bid

Resistance: Mutation at codon 75 of the RT gene produces *in vitro* resistance that is not seen *in vivo*. Phenotypic resistance testing of patients in ACTG 306 who had received d4T >6 months showed no phenotypic resistance despite virologic failure (7th CROI, Abstract 733). The multi-nucleoside resistance mutations (Q151M complex and the T69-insertion mutation) result in resistance to d4T. It has now been observed that multi-nucleoside resistance can occur in d4T-treated patients, as can mutations traditionally thought of as "AZT-resistance mutations."

Pharmacology:

Bioavailability: 86% and not influenced by food or fasting

T½: (serum) 1 hour; **Intracellular T½:** 3.5 hours

CNS penetration: 30-40% (JAIDS 1998;17:235)
(CSF: plasma ratio = 0.16-0.97)

Elimination: Renal – 50%

Dose modification in severe liver disease: No guidelines; use standard dose with caution

Table 6-31: Dose modification in renal failure

Creatinine Clearance	Body >60 kg	Weight <60 kg
>50 mL/min	40 mg bid	30 mg bid
26-50 mL/min	40 mg qd	30 mg qd
10-25 mL/min	20 mg qd	15 mg qd
Hemodialysis	20 mg qd post dialysis	15 mg qd post dialysis

Side effects:

1 . Peripheral neuropathy: Frequency is 5-15% but up to 24% in some trials. Risk appears to be substantially increased when d4T is combined with ddI or ddI and hydroxyurea (AIDS 2000;14:273). Onset is usually noted at 2-6 months after treatment is started and usually resolves if d4T is promptly stopped. Peripheral neuropathy due to HIV infection or alternative nucleoside analog treatment (ddI, ddC) represents a relative contraindication to d4T. Dose adjustment after resolution of peripheral neuropathy if d4T is needed: ≥60 kg – 20 mg bid, <60 kg – 15 mg bid.

2. Subjective complaints are infrequent and include headache, GI intolerance with diarrhea or esophageal ulcers.

3. Elevated transaminase levels are common (8%), but generally do not interfere with continued therapy

Drug interactions:

ddI and ddC: Overlapping toxicity with peripheral neuropathy, although implications for therapy are unclear.

Drugs that cause peripheral neuropathy should be used with caution or avoided: ddC, ethionamide, ethambutol, INH, phenytoin, vincristine, glutethimide, gold, hydralazine, and long-term metronidazole. Concurrent use with ddI has been shown to be safe and effective.

Methadone reduces levels of d4T, but this is not thought to be sufficiently severe to require d4T dose adjustment; d4T has no effect on methadone levels.

Pregnancy: Category C. Rodent teratogenicity assay is negative; placental passage in rhesus monkeys showed a newborn : maternal drug ratio of 0.76. No studies in humans.

STREPTOMYCIN

Generic: Available from Pfizer at no charge. Order information – (800) 254-4445; FAX order request – (800) 251-4445. Initial request – 2 month supply (six 10-packs of 1 gm or 2.5 mL ampules). Comparative wholesale price for aminoglycosides (usual daily dose, 70 kg patient); streptomycin – free; gentamicin – $5.20 (400 mg); capreomycin – $20.86 (1 gm); tobramycin $37.40 (400 mg); amikacin – $1,200 (1 gm).

Form: Ampules with 1 gm/2.5 mL

Class: Aminoglycoside

Indication: Tuberculosis

Dose: Daily regimen – 15 mg/kg IM* up to 1 gm/day

DOT regimen – 25-30 mg/kg IM* up to 1.5 gm for twice weekly treatment and up to 1.0 gm for thrice weekly treatment

* Injections should be made in the upper outer quadrant of the buttock or mid-lateral thigh; deltoid muscle may be used if well developed. Injection sites should be alternated.

Pharmacology

Bioavailability: Not absorbed with po administration

T½: 5-6 hours

Peak levels: (1 gm dose) – 25-30 mcg/mL. **CNS levels:** Low

Elimination: Renal (30-80% recovered in urine)

Dose modification in renal failure: CrCl >50 mL/min – 15 mg/kg/day; 10-50 mL/min – 15 mg/kg q 24-72 h; <10 mL/min – 15 mg/kg q 72-96 h

Side effects: Ototoxicity, especially nausea, vomiting, and vertigo – dose- and duration-related; hearing loss is less common and may be irreversible. Patients should be warned that tinnitus, roaring noises, or sense of fullness in ears indicates the drug should be discontinued. Caloric stimulation tests and audiometric tests are advised with long courses, with selected high-risk patients (elderly, renal failure), and with complaints suggesting ototoxicity. Vestibular dysfunction is usually reversible within 2-3 months if the drug is promptly discontinued. Other less common forms of neurotoxicity include peripheral neuritis, arachnoiditis, encephalopathy, and respiratory paralysis. Renal failure is uncommon except with age >65 years, prior renal failure, and/or concurrent nephrotoxic drugs. Paresthesias – perioral and hands in 15% (not important). Streptomycin contains a sulfite that may cause allergic-type reactions including anaphylaxis, rash, urticaria, and eosinophilia. Serious reactions are rare and are more common in asthmatic patients.

Drug interactions: Increased nephrotoxicity and ototoxicity with other drugs that have these side effects, especially other aminoglycosides. Ototoxicity is potentiated by co-administration of ethacrynic acid, furosemide, mannitol, and possibly other diuretics.

Pregnancy: Category D. This and other aminoglycosides have been implicated in irreversible congenital deafness. Streptomycin is the only major antituberculosis drug with established toxicity to the fetus.

SULFADIAZINE

Generic: Eon Labs (718) 276-8600 and Goldline

Forms: 500 mg tabs – $0.55/500 mg tab

Class: Synthetic derivatives of sulfanilamide which inhibit folic acid synthesis

Indications and doses:

> **Toxoplasmosis:** Initial treatment 1-2 gm po qid x ≥6 weeks; maintenance, 500 mg-1 gm po qid indefinitely

> **Nocardia:** 1 gm po qid x ≥6 months

> **UTIs:** 500 mg-1 gm po qid x 3-14 days

Pharmacology

> **Bioavailability:** >70%

> **T½:** 17 hours

> **Elimination:** Hepatic acetylation and renal excretion of parent compound and metabolites

> **CNS penetration:** 40-80% of serum levels

> **Serum levels for systemic infections:** 100-150 µg/mL

> **Dose modifications in renal failure:** CrCl >50 mL/min – 0.5-1.5 gm q 4-6 h; 10-50 mL/min – 0.15-1.5 gm q 8-12 h (half dose); <10 mL/min – 0.5-1.5 gm q 12-24 h (one-third dose)

Side effects: Hypersensitivity with rash, drug fever, serum-sickness, urticaria; crystalluria reduced with adequate urine volume (≥1,500 mL/day) and alkaline urine – use with care in renal failure; marrow suppression – anemia, thrombocytopenia, leukopenia, hemolytic anemia due to G-6-PD deficiency.

Drug interactions: Decreased effect of cyclosporine, digoxin; increased effect of coumadin, oral hypoglycemics, methotrexate (?), and phenytoin.

Pregnancy: Category C. Competes with bilirubin for albumin to cause kernicterus – avoid near term or in nursing mothers.

SUSTIVA – See Efavirenz (p. 195)

3TC – See Lamivudine (p. 229)

TESTOSTERONE

Source: Testosterone cypionate (Keene, Forest, Hyrex, Upjohn, Hauck) and Testosterone ethanthate (Hyrex, Forest, Rugby, Gynex, Hauck)

Testosterone scrotal patch (Testoderm patch, Alza Pharmaceuticals)

Testosterone non-scrotal patch (Androderm, SmithKline Beecham and Testoderm TTS patch, Alza Pharmaceuticals)

Form and price: Vials of 100 and 200 mg/mL @ $12.71–$20.65/10 mL vial or about $2/week.

Testoderm scrotal patch @ $2.51/4 mg/24 hr patch $3.36/5 mg/24 hr TTS patch and $2.62/6 mg/24 hr patch or $17-$23/week.

Androderm non-scrotal patch @$3.50/5 mg/24 hr patch or about $24.50/week.

Indications: (For men only)

1. Hypogonadism: Normal testosterone levels in adult men are 300-1,000 ng/dl at 8 am, representing peak levels with circadian rhythm. Prior studies show subnormal testosterone levels in 45% of patients with AIDS and 27% of HIV-infected patients without AIDS (Am J Med 1988;84:611; AIDS 1994;7:46; J Clin Endocrinol 1996;81:4108). Testing should be done in the morning and should measure free (unbound) levels. Replacement therapy is recommended for men with low or low-normal levels. Restoration of normal testosterone levels can be achieved with testosterone enanthate 200 mg IM q 2 weeks, a 5 mg Androderm patch applied nightly or a 5 mg Testoderm TTS patch applied each morning.

2. Wasting: Testosterone is an anabolic steroid that may restore nitrogen balance and lean body mass in patients with wasting (JAIDS 1996;11:510; JAIDS 1997;16:254; Ann Intern Med 1998;129:18).

Regimen: 200-400 mg IM q 2 weeks. The dose and dosing interval may need adjustment; many use 100-200 mg IM q week given by self administration to avoid low levels in the second week; many initiate therapy of wasting with 300-400 mg q 2 wks with taper to 200 mg when weight is restored or combine with other anabolic steroids.

Transdermal systems: Advantages are rapid absorption, controlled rate of delivery, avoidance of first pass hepatic metabolism, avoidance of IM injections and possibly less testicular shrinkage. Two delivery systems are available: trans-scrotal and non-trans-scrotal. Trans-scrotal patches (Testoderm) are available in 10 and 15 mg sizes to deliver 4 and 6 mg testosterone, non-scrotal. The patch is placed on the scrotum in the morning, adherence is achieved with a hair dryer, and the patch is worn for 22-24 hours. Serum testosterone levels peak at 3-8 hours. After one month, a morning testosterone level should be obtained. Testoderm TTS is a non-scrotal patch with 5 mg testosterone. Another non-scrotal patch (Androderm) consists of a liquid reservoir containing 12.2 g testosterone that delivers 2.5 mg of testosterone/day or a liquid reservoir containing 24.3 mg that delivers 5 mg testosterone daily. The usual dose is a system that delivers 5 mg/day.

Controlled substance: Schedule C-III

Pharmacology:

> **Bioavailability:** Poor absorption and rapid metabolism with oral administration. The cypionate and enathate esters are absorbed slowly from IM injection sites

> **Elimination:** Hepatic metabolism to 17 ketosteroids that are excreted in urine

Side effects: Androgenic effects — acne, flushing, gynecomastia, increased libido, priapism and edema. Other side effects include aggravation of sleep apnea, salt retention, increased hematocrit, possible promotion of Kaposi's sarcoma and promotion of breast or prostate cancer. In women there may be virilization with voice change, hirsutism and clitoral enlargement. Androgens may cause cholestatic hepatitis. Patches are associated with local reactions, especially pruritus and occasionally blistering, erythema and pain. Local reactions are more common with Androderm patches than Testoderm or Testoderm TTS patches.

Drug interactions: May potentiate action of oral anticoagulants

THALIDOMIDE

Trade Name: Thalomid (Celgene Corp; (888) 423-5436)

Form and price: 50 mg capsule @ $7.50/50 mg or $30.00-$60.00/day for daily doses of 200-400 mg/day

Availability: Thalidomide is FDA approved for marketing through a restricted distribution program called "System for Thalidomide Education and Prescribing Safety" (STEPS). Only physicians registered with the program may prescribe thalodamide and only pharmacists registered with the program may dispense the drug. To register call (888) 423-5436. **Requirements for female patients:** 1) Women of childbearing potential must have a negative pregnancy test within 24 hours of initiating treatment and this must be verified in writing; 2) There must be weekly pregnancy tests during the first month of treatment and monthly thereafter; 3) Must use two reliable forms of contraception simultaneously unless continuously sexually inactive, post-hysterectomy or post-menapausal >24 mo.; and 4) There must be a signed agreement to these conditions. **Requirements for male patients:** 1) Acceptance of a condom for contraception even with vasectomy unless the female partner is post-hysterectomy or post-menopausal >24 mo., and 2) There must be a signed agreement to these conditions.

Patient assistance: (888) 423-5436

FDA labeling: Moderate to severe erythema nodosum leprosum

Regimen: 200 mg po qd or bid

Mechanism: Presumed mechanism for HIV-associated wasting is the reduction in TNF-alpha production (J Exp Med 1991;173:699). Thalidomide also has numerous other anti-inflammatory and immunomodulatory properties (Internat J Dermat 1974;13:20; PNAS 1993;90:5974).

Clinical Trials:

Aphthous ulcers: In a placebo-controlled trial using thalidomide (200 mg/day) in patients with oral aphthous ulcers, 16/29 (53%) in the thalidomide arm responded compared to 2/28 (7%) in the placebo group (NEJM 1997;336:1489). ACTG 251 was a placebo-controlled trial involving 45 patients given thalidomide (200 mg/day x 4 weeks followed by 100 mg/d for responders and 400 mg/day for non-responders for oral or esophageal ulcers). Among 23 recipients of thalidomide, 14 (61%) had a complete remission in 4 weeks and, 21 (91%) had a complete remission or partial response. In another ACTG trial for patients with aphthous ulcers of the esophagus, thalidomide (200 mg/d) was associated with a complete response at 4 weeks in 8 of 11 (73%) (JID 1999;180:61).

Wasting: Two placebo-controlled trials and three open label studies demonstrated that thalidomide (daily doses of 50-300 mg/day) for 2-12 weeks was associated with a mean weight gains of 2.4%-6.5%. Suggested initial dose is 100 mg po qd with increases up to 200 mg/day (AIDS 1996;10:1501). The higher dose is often poorly tolerated due to sedation.

Other possible uses in HIV-infected patients include prurigo nodularis (200-400 mg/day), post-herpetic neuralgia (100-300 mg/day), and AIDS-associated proctitis (300 mg/day) (J Am Acad Derm 1996;35:969).

Pharmacology (AAC 1997;41:2797)

Bioavailability: Well absorbed

T½: 6-8 hrs. Peak levels with 200 mg dose are 1.7 µg/mL; levels >4 µg/mL are required to inhibit TNF-alpha (PNAS 1993;90:5974; J Exp Med 1993;177:1675; J Am Acad Derm 1996;35:969). It is not known if thalidomide is in semen.

Elimination: Non-renal mechanisms, primarily non-enzymatic hydrolysis in plasma to multiple metabolites. There are no recommendations for dose changes in renal or hepatic failure.

Side effects: Major concern is in pregnant women due to high potential for birth defects, including absent or abnormal limbs; cleft lip; absent ears; heart, renal or genital abnormalities, and other severe defects (Nat Med 1997;3:8). Maximum vulnerability is 35 to 50 days after the last menstrual period when a single dose is sufficient to cause severe limb abnormalities in most patients (J Am Acad Derm 1996;35:969). It is *critical* that any woman of child bearing potential not receive thalidomide unless great precautions are taken to prevent pregnancy (pills and barrier protection). Since thalidomide may be in semen, condom use is recommended for men. Through 7/99 the FDA noted that 3000 patients had been treated and there were no documented exposures during pregnancy.

Drowsiness: Most common side effect is the sedation for which the drug was once marketed. Administer at bedtime to minimize this side effect.

Fever and rashes: These were the most frequent drug limiting toxicities noted in 36% of thalidomide treated HIV-infected patients in one study (CID 1997;24:1223).

Neuropathy: Dose-related paresthesias and/or pain of extremities, especially with high doses or prolonged use. This complication may or may not be reversible; it is not known if the risk is increased by diabetes, alcoholism or use of neurotoxic drugs including ddI, d4T or ddC. Symptoms may start after the drug is discontinued. Neuropathy is a contraindication to the drug.

HIV: Thalidomide may cause modest increase in plasma levels of HIV RNA (0.4 log10/mL).

Neutropenia: Discontinue thalidomide if ANC is <750/mm^3 without an alternative cause.

Less common side effects include dizziness, mood changes, bradycardia, tachycardia, bitter taste, headache, nausea, pruritus or hypotension.

Drug interactions: The greatest concern is in women of childbearing potential who take concurrent medications that interfere with the effectiveness of contraceptives. Concurrent use of drugs that cause sedation or peripheral neuropathy may increase the frequency and severity of these side effects.

Pregnancy: Category X

3TC – See Lamivudine (p. 229)

TRAZODONE

Trade name: Desyrel (Mead Johnson) and generic

Forms: 50 mg, 100 mg, 150 mg and 300 mg tabs

Price: Generic – $0.07/50 mg, $0.12/100 mg and $0.58/150 mg tab
Desyrel – $1.47/50 mg, $2.57/100 mg, $2.21/150 mg and $3.94/300 mg tab

Class: Non-tricyclic antidepressent (see Table 7-1, p. 281)

Indications and dose regimens:

Depression, especially when associated with anxiety or insomnia; 150 mg/day in two doses; if insomnia or daytime sedation, give as single dose at hs. Increase dose 50 mg every 3-4 days up to maximum dose of 400 mg/day for outpatients and 600 mg/day for hospitalized patients.

Insomnia (25-100 mg q hs)

Pharmacology

Bioavailability: >90%, improved if taken with meals

T½: 6 hours

Elimination: Hepatic metabolism, then renal excretion

Side effects: Adverse effects are dose- and duration-related, are usually seen with doses >300 mg/day, and may decrease with continued use, dose reduction, or schedule change.

Major side effects – sedation in 15-20%; orthostatic hypotension (5%); nervousness; fatigue; dizziness; nausea and vomiting. Rare – anticholinergic effects (dry mouth, blurred vision, constipation, urinary retention); priapism (1/6,000); agitation; cardiovascular and anticholinergic side effects are less frequent and less severe compared to tricyclics.

Pregnancy: Category B

Drug interactions: Increased levels of phenytoin and digoxin; alcohol and other CNS depressants potentiate sedative side effects; increased trazodone levels with fluoxetine; may potentiate effects of anti-hypertensive agents.

TRIAZOLAM

Trade name: Halcion (Upjohn)

Forms and price: 0.125 mg tab – $0.71; 0.25 mg tab – $0.78

Class: Benzodiazepine, controlled substance category IV

Indications and dose regimens:

Insomnia: 0.125-0.5 mg (usually 0.25 mg) hs for 7-10 days

Note: Current FDA guidelines state that triazolam should be prescribed for short-term use (7-10 days), the prescribed dose should not exceed a one-month supply, and use for more than 2-3 weeks requires re-evaluation of patient.

Pharmacology

Bioavailability: >90%

T½: 1.5-5 hours

Elimination: Metabolized by liver to inactive metabolites that are renally excreted.

Side effects: See Benzodiazepines p. 169. Most common are drowsiness, incoordination, dizziness, and amnesia. Anecdotal reports of delirium, confusion, paranoia, and hallucinations.

Interactions: Contraindicated for concurrent use with all protease inhibitors and delavirdine; "caution" with nevirapine.

Pregnancy: Category X

TRICYCLIC ANTIDEPRESSANTS

Tricyclic antidepressants elevate mood, increase physical activity, improve appetite, improve sleep patterns, and reduce morbid preoccupations in most patients with major depression. The following principles apply:

Indications:

1. **Psychiatric indications:** Major depression – response rates are 60-70%. Low doses are commonly used for adjustment disorders including depression and anxiety.

2. **Peripheral neuropathy:** Controlled trials have not shown benefit in AIDS-associated peripheral neuropathy, but clinical experience is extensive and results in diabetic neuropathy are good. If used, choice of agents depends on time of symptoms (JC Shlay, JAMA 280:1590,1998). Night pain: amitriptyline (sedating) 25 mg hs increasing to up to 75 mg/day. Day pain: nortriptyline (less sedating and less anticholinergic effect) 30 mg hs increasing to 90 mg hs.

Pharmacology: Well absorbed, extensively metabolized, long half-life, variable use of serum levels (see below).

Serum levels: Efficacy correlates with serum levels so that therapeutic monitoring includes drug levels to titrate dose.

Dose: Initial treatment of depression is 4-8 wks which is required for therapeutic response. Much or all of the initial dose is given at hs, especially if insomnia is prominent or if sedation is a side effect. Common mistakes are use of an initial dose that is too high resulting in excessive anticholinergic side effects or oversedation. The dose is increased q 3-4 days depending on tolerance and response. Treatment of major depression usually requires continuation for 4-5 months after response. Multiple recurrences may require long-term treatment.

Side effects: Anticholinergic effects (dry mouth, dizziness, blurred vision, constipation, tachycardia, urinary hesitancy, sedation) sexual dysfunction, orthostatic hypotension, weight gain.

Relative contraindications: Cardiac conduction block, prostatism, and narrow angle glaucoma. Less common side effects – mania, hypomania, allergic skin reactions, marrow suppression, seizures, tardive dyskinesia, tremor, speech blockage, anxiety, insomnia, Parkinsonism, hyponatremia; cardiac conduction disturbances, and arrhythmias (most common serious side effect with overdosage).

TRIMETHOPRIM

Generic

Forms and price: 100 mg tab – $0.17; 200 mg tab – $0.25
(See trimethoprim-sulfamethoxazole, next page)

Indications and dose regimen:

> PCP (with sulfamethoxazole as TMP-SMX or with dapsone): 5 mg/kg po tid or qid (usually 300 mg tid or qid) x 21 days

> UTIs: 100 mg po bid or 200 mg x 1/day x 3-14 days

Pharmacology

> **Bioavailability:** >90%

> **T½:** 9-11 hrs.

> **Excretion:** Renal

> **Dose modification with renal failure:** CrCl >50 mL/min – full dose; 10-50 mL/min – half dose

Side effects: Usually well tolerated; most common – pruritis and skin rash; GI intolerance; marrow suppression – anemia, neutropenia, thrombocytopenia; antifolate effects – prevent with leukovorin; reversible hyperkalemia in 20-50% of AIDS patients given high doses (Ann Intern Med 1993;119:291,296; NEJM 1993;238:703).

Drug interactions: Increased activity of phenytoin (monitor levels) and procainamide; levels of both dapsone and trimethoprim are increased when given concurrently.

Pregnancy: Category C. Teratogenic in rats with high doses; limited experience in patients shows no association with congenital abnormalities.

TRIMETHOPRIM-SULFAMETHOXAZOLE (TMP-SMX, COTRIMOXAZOLE)

Generic; Trade name: Septra (Glaxo Wellcome), Bactrim (Roche)

Table 6-32: Forms and Price

	Single strength 80/400 mg*	Double strength 160/800 mg	IV preparation 16 mg/mL 80 mg/mL
Generic	$0.07	$0.07	10 mL $ 3.53
Bactrim	$0.78	$1.28	10 mL $16.00
Septra	$0.98	$1.54	10 mL $15.60

* 80 mg trimethoprim plus 400 mg sulfamethoxazole.

Activity: TMP-SMX is effective in treatment or prophylaxis of infections involving *P. carinii*, methicillin-sensitive *S. aureus*, Legionella, *Listeria*, and common urinary tract pathogens. Recent studies show increasing rates of mutations in the dihydropteroate synthase gene of *P. carinii* which are associated with increased resistance to sulfonamides and dapsone; the clinical significance is unclear (JID 1999;180:1969). *S. pneumoniae* is becoming more resistant to TMP-SMX (CID 1998;27:764).

Indications and dose regimen:

PCP prophylaxis: 1 DS/day; alternatives are 3 DS/wk, or 1 SS/day

Graduated initiation to reduce adverse effects (ACTG 268): Oral preparation (40 mg trimethoprim and 200 mg sulfamethoxazole/5mL) – 1 mL/day x 3 days, then 2 mL/day x 3 days, then 5 mL/day x 3 days, then 10 mL/day x 3 days, then 20 mL x 3 days, then 1 TMP-SMX DS tab/day

Desensitization: See next page.

PCP treatment: 5 mg/kg (trimethoprim component) po or IV q 8 h x 21 days, usually 5-6 DS/day

Toxoplasmosis prophylaxis: 1 DS/day

Isospora: 5 mg/kg (trimethoprim) po bid, usually 2 DS po bid or 1 DS tid x 2-4 weeks; may need maintenance with 1-2 DS/d

Salmonellosis: 5-10 mg/kg (trimethoprim) po/day (usually 1 DS bid) x 2-4 weeks

Nocardia: 4-6 DS/day x ≥6 mos

Urinary tract infections: 1-2 DS/day x 3-14 days

Prophylaxis for cystitis: 1/2 SS tab daily

Pharmacology

Bioavailability: >90% absorbed with oral administration (both drugs)

T½: Trimethoprim, 8-15 hrs; sulfamethoxazole 7-12 hrs

Elimination: Renal; T½ in renal failure increases to 24 hrs for trimethoprim and 22-50 hrs for sulfamethoxazole

Renal failure: CrCl >50 mL/min – usual dose; 10-50 mL/min – half dose; <10 mL/min – avoid (some suggest further reduction in dose may be used)

Side effects: Noted in 10% of patients without HIV infection and about 50% of patients with HIV. Most common: nausea, vomiting, pruritis, rash, fever neutropenia, and increased transaminases. Many HIV-infected patients may be treated through side effects (GI intolerance and rash) if symptoms are not disabling; alternative with PCP prophylaxis is dose reduction usually after drug holiday (1-2 weeks) and/or "desensitization" (see below). Mechanism of most sulfonamide reactions is unclear and cause of increased susceptibility with HIV is also unclear. Rash: Most common is erythematous, maculopapular, morbilliform, and/or pruritic rash, usually 7-14 days after treatment is started. Less common are erythema multiforme, epidermal necrolysis, exfoliative dermatitis, Stevens-Johnson syndrome, urticaria, and Schonlein-Henoch purpura.

VI. Drugs

GI intolerance is common with nausea, vomiting, anorexia, and abdominal pain; rare side effects include *C. difficile* diarrhea/colitis and pancreatitis. **Hematologic side effects** include leukopenia, neutropenia, anemia, and/or thrombocytopenia. Rate is increased in patients with HIV infection and with folate depletion. Some respond to leukovorin (5-15 mg/day), but this is not routinely recommended. **Neurologic** toxicity may include tremor, ataxia, apathy, and ankle clonus that responds promptly to drug discontinuation. **Hepatitis** with cholestatic jaundice and hepatic necrosis has been described. **Hyperkalemia** in 20-50% of patients given trimethoprim in doses >15 mg/kg/d (NEJM 1993;328:703). **Meningitis** (Am J Med Sci 1996;312:27).

Protocol for oral "desensitization" or "detoxification":

1. Rapid desensitization (CID 1995;20:849)
   Serial 10-fold dilutions of oral suspension (40 mg TMP, 200 mg SMX/5 mL) given hourly over four hours.

Table 6-33: Rapid TMP-SMX Desensitization Schedule

Time (hr)	Dose (TMP/SMX)	Dilution
0	0.004/0.02 mg	1:100,000 (5 mL)
1	0.04/0.2 mg	1:1,000 (5 mL)
2	0.4/2.0 mg	1:100 (5 mL)
3	4/20 mg	1:10 (5 mL)
4	40/200 mg	(5 mL)
5	160/800 mg	tablet

2. Eight-day protocol
   Serial dilutions prepared by pharmacists using oral suspension (40 mg TMP, 200 mg SMX/5 mL). Medication is given four times daily for seven days in doses of 1cc, 2cc, 4cc, and 8cc using following dilutions.

Table 6-34: Eight Day TMP-SMX Desensitization Schedule

Day	Dilution	Day	Dilution
1	1:1,000,000	5	1:100
2	1:100,000	6	1:10
3	1:10,000	7	1:1
4	1:1,000	8	Standard suspension - 1 mL
		≥9	1 DS tab/day

Pregnancy: Category C. Teratogenic in animals. No congenital abnormalities noted in 35 children born to women who received TMP-SMX in first trimester. Use with caution due to possible kernicterus, although no cases of kernicterus have been reported (CID 1995;21 suppl 1:S24).

Drug interactions: Increased levels of oral anticoagulants, phenytoin, and procainamide. Risk of megaloblastic anemia with methotrexate.

VALACYCLOVIR – See p. 160

VANCOMYCIN

Generic

Trade name: Vancocin (Lilly)

Forms and price:

> **Parenteral:** 0.5 gm vial @ $12.61/500 mg
>
> **Oral:** Parvules 125 mg – $5.35; $20.40/day
> 500 mg vial for 4 oral doses – $7.80 ($7.80/day)

Class: Tricyclic glycopeptide antibiotic

Activity: Nearly all gram-positive bacteria including all *S. aureas*, 5-20% of hospital strains of *Enterococcus faecium* are resistant

Indications and regimens:

> Deep infections involving MRSA and *S. epidermidis*, infections involving other gram-positive bacteria in penicillin-allergic patients: 1 gm IV q 12 h infused ≥1 hr (± rifampin or gentamicin). *C. difficile* colitis: 125 mg po qid x 10-14 days

Pharmacology

> **Bioavailability:** Not absorbed with po administration, but may accumulate in serum with inflamed gut plus renal failure
>
> **T½:** 4-6 hrs
>
> **Elimination:** Renal
>
> **Dose modification in renal failure:** CrCl >50 mL/min – 15 mg/kg IV q 12 h, clearance 10-50 mL/min – 15 mg/kg q 3-10 days; clearance <10 mL/min – 15 mg/kg q 10 days.

Side effects:

> 1. **Red man syndrome** – hypotension and flushing ± dyspnea, urticaria, pruritis, and/or wheezing ascribed to histamine release from mast cells which is

VI. Drugs

directly related to rate of infusion. This usually begins shortly after infusion starts and may require antihistamines, corticosteroids, or IV fluids; most patients benefit from dose reduction, prolongation of infusion, and/or pretreatment with antihistamine.

2. **Ototoxicity and nephrotoxicity.** Infrequent and most likely with renal failure, high doses, long courses, and concurrent use of nephrotoxic or ototoxic drugs. Many authorities feel that current supplies of vancomycin are not nephrotoxic if used alone, but vancomycin appears to promote nephrotoxicity of other nephrotoxic drugs such as aminoglycosides. Relationship to serum levels is unclear and value of serum levels to monitor toxicity is unclear.

3. Thrombophlebitis and pain at infusion site.

4. Hypersensitivity reactions are rare; most reactions are the result of histamine release due to rapid infusion.

VIBRAMYCIN – See Doxycycline (p. 193)

VIDEX – See Didanosine (p. 191)

VIRACEPT – See Nelfinavir (p. 238)

VIRAMUNE – See Nevirapine (p. 241)

VITRASERT – See Ganciclovir (p. 212)

VITRAVENE – See Fomivirsen (p. 209)

WIN RHO [Rho (D) immune globulin]:

Trade name: Win Rho (Univax, North American Bio, Inc.; Cangene Corp.)

Form and price: Vials of 600 IU @ $103.00 and 1500 IU @ $235.00. Usual dose: 50 µg/kg or 3500 IU (70 kg). With hemoglobin levels <10g/dL, give 25-50 mg/kg to reduce the severity of anemia. Cost of IVIG (1000 mg/kg): $3,570-$4,569 (Med Letter 1996;38:8). Cost of Win Rho (AWP) is $1,081.50 for 5000 units.

Indication: Idiopathic thrombocytopenic purpura (ITP) in patient who is Rh positive. Advantages over IVIG: Short infusion time, modest cost reduction and, in some cases, availability.

Mechanism: This product was developed to provide anti-D globulin to prevent Rh isoimmunization in Rh negative pregnant women with an Rh positive fetus. Injection of anti-D into Rh positive patients with ITP coats the patient's D+ RBCs with antibodies and this spares splenic clearance of antibody-coated platelets (Trans Med Rev 1992;6:17).

Clinical trials: The average increase in platelets including patients with HIV-associated ITP is 50,000/mm[3] (Am J Hematol 1986;22:241; Blood 1991;77:1884). The response is somewhat delayed compared to IVIG. The effect lasts an average of 3 weeks. Note: Patients must have intact spleen and be Rho (D) positive for a biologic effect with treatment for ITP.

Regimen: Initial dose-50 µg/kg IV over 3-5 minutes. May repeat at 3-4 days and may increase dose up to 80 µg/kg. Most patients require maintenance doses of 25-60 µg/kg

Side effects: Hemolysis with decreases in hemoglobin of ≥2 gm/dL in 5-10%. Monitor CBC. Fever and chills 1-2 hours after infusion (presumably due to hemolysis) in 10%; this can be avoided or reduced in severity with acetaminophen, benedryl, prednisone or increasing infusion time to 15-20 minutes. Vial should not be shaken due to possible damage of protein or formation of aggregates.

Pregnancy: Category C

Note: Patients must have intact spleen and be Rho(D) positive for a biologic effect with treatment for ITP

XANAX – See Alprazolam (p. 164)

ZALCITABINE (ddC)

Trade name: Hivid (Hoffman-LaRoche)

Forms and price: 0.375 mg – $1.83; 0.75 mg tab – $2.30; cost/week – $48.09

Class: Nucleoside analog

Financial assistance: (800) 285-4484. Patients must not be able to obtain drug from any other source – insurance, Medicaid, or state-sponsored program; no income or asset criteria.

Indications: In ACTG 155 the addition of ddC after ≥6 months treatment with AZT provided no clear benefit based on clinical parameters -delayed progression and prolonged survival (Ann Intern Med 1994;122:24). ACTG 175 confirmed this finding, but also demonstrated that ddC plus AZT was superior to AZT monotherapy in AZT-naïve patients with CD4 counts of 200-500/mm[3] (NEJM 1996;335:1081). Studies of three drug regimens that include ddC show "triple therapy" with a PI is superior to 2 NRTIs alone, but did not address the relative merits of ddC compared to other NRTIs (NEJM 1996;334:1011).

Resistance: Codon mutations on the RT gene that confer resistance are at positions 65, 69, 74 and 184. The codon 74 mutation suppresses AZT resistance. Resistance to ddC appears to be uncommon during combination treatment (JAIDS 1994;7:135; JID 1996;173:1354). In Delta 1 there were no detectable mutations conferring ddC resistance after 112 weeks of treatment (Lancet 1996;348:283).

Regimen: 0.75 mg po tid

Pharmacology

> **Bioavailability:** 70-88%

> **T½:** 1.2-2 hours

> **Intracellular T½:** 3 hours; CSF levels: 20% serum levels
> (CSF: plasma ratio = 0.09–0.37)

> **Elimination:** Renal excretion – 70%

> **Dose adjustment in renal failure:** CrCl >50 mL/min – 0.75 mg po tid; 10-50 mL/min – 0.75 mg po bid; <10 mL/min – 0.75 mg po qd

Side effects:

1. The major clinical toxicity is peripheral neuropathy, noted in 17-31% of patients in initial trials. It is more frequent than with ddI or d4T (NEJM 1996;335:1099). Patients should be warned. Features are bilateral sensori-motor neuropathy with numbness and burning in distal extremities usually after 2-6 months of therapy followed by shooting or continuous pain. Symptoms usually resolve slowly if the drug is promptly discontinued; with continued use it may be irreversible and require narcotics. Frequency depends on dose and duration of ddC treatment. Pain requiring narcotics or progressive pain for ≥1 week represents a contraindication to future use; patients with less severe pain that resolves to mild intensity may be rechallenged with half dose.

2. **Stomatitis and aphthous esophageal ulcers** are seen in 2-4% (Ann Intern Med 1992;117:133) and usually resolve with continued ddC treatment.

3. **Pancreatitis** is noted in <1% of patients, but more frequently in those with a history of prior pancreatitis or elevated amylase levels at time treatment was started.

4. **Rash** is common after 10-14 days of treatment, it is a red maculopapular rash over the trunk and extremities and it usually resolves spontaneously.

5. **Class adverse reactions:** NRTIs may cause lactic acidosis and steatosis.

Interactions: Drugs that cause peripheral neuropathy should be used with caution or avoided: ddI, d4T, ethambutol, cisplatin, disulfiram, ethionamide, INH, phenytoin, vincristine, glutethimide, gold, hydralazine, and long-term metronidazole.

Pregnancy: Category C. Teratogenic and embryolethal in doses >1000 x those used in patients; carcinogenicity studies – thymic lymphomas in rodents; placental passage in rhesus monkeys show newborn : maternal drug ratio of 0.3-0.5; no studies in humans.

ZERIT – See Stavudine (p. 266)

ZIAGEN – See Abacavir (p. 158)

ZIDOVUDINE (AZT, ZDV)

Trade name: Retrovir (Glaxo Wellcome); Combivir (3TC/AZT)

Forms and price: 100 mg tabs and 300 mg tabs; $1.68/100 mg tab and $4.43/300 mg tab; $7.96/day; $2,905/year;
IV vials – 10 mg/mL, 20 mL (200 mg) -$16.74;
Combivir (3TC, 150 mg plus AZT 300 mg) @ $8.62/tab.

Patient assistance program: (800) 722-9294. Eligibility based on lack of third party drug coverage, monthly income criteria using Medicaid guidelines, and asset information; forms are reviewed on an individual basis.

Class: Nucleoside analog

Table 6-35: Indications and Regimen

Condition	Regimen (Always use in combination)
HIV infection	300 mg bid or 200 mg po tid (daily dose 600 mg)*
Pregnancy (ACTG 076 protocol)	300 mg bid or 200 mg tid during 2nd and 3rd trimesters*; IV during delivery - 2 mg/kg for 1 hr, then 1 mg/kg/hr until delivery; infant receives 2 mg/kg q6h x 6 wks (MMWR 1998;47:[RR-3]:38)
HIV-associated ITP	200-400 mg po 2-3x/day (daily dose 600-1,200 mg) (Response may be dose-related; see AIDS 1993;7:209). HAART may supplant need for high dose AZT.
HIV-associated dementia	200-400 mg po 2-5x/day (daily dose 600-1,200 mg). HAART may supplant need for high dose AZT
HIV exposure (healthcare workers)	200 mg po tid or 300 mg po bid x 28 days*
Renal failure or severe liver disease	Creatinine cl <20 mL/min 300-400 mg/day. Hemodialysis – 300 mg/day Severe hepatic failure – 100 mg tid
IV formulation	1 mg/kg q 4 h
IV Intrapartum	2 mg/kg IV x 1 hr, then 1 mg/kg/hr until delivery

* Twice daily dosing appears to be as effective as tid or q 4 h dosing (JAIDS 1997;15:283). GI tolerance may be better with lower doses at more frequent intervals and when taken with meals.

Resistance: The first codon mutation to appear that confers AZT resistance is at position 70; this is followed by resistant mutations at 215, 41, 67 and 219. A total of 3-6 mutations result in a 100 fold decrease in sensitivity. About 5-10% of recipients of AZT plus ddI develop a 151 codon mutation and a larger number have the T 69 SSS insertion; both mutations confer high level resistance to AZT, ddI, ddC, d4T, 3TC and abacavir. The M184V mutation that confers high level 3TC resistance delays or restores susceptibility to AZT unless there are multiple AZT resistance mutations. It has been postulated that prolonged AZT exposure may reduce response to d4T due to impaired d4T phosphorylation but supporting data are inconsistent. Analysis of patients with early HIV infection indicates that 5-10% have genotypic mutations associated with reduced susceptibility to AZT.

Pharmacology

Bioavailability: 60%; high fat meals may decrease absorption
CSF levels: 60% serum levels (CSF: plasma ratio = 0.3–1.35)
(Lancet 1998;351:1547)

T½: 1.1 hours; Renal failure: 1.4 hrs.

Intracellular T½: 3 hours

Elimination: Metabolized by liver to glucuronide (G-ZVD) that is renally excreted

Dose modification in renal failure or hepatic failure: In severe renal failure (CrCl <18 mL/min) half life is increased from 1.1 to 1.4 hrs and GZVD half life increased from 0.9 to 8.0 hours. Recommendation is to use 300-400 mg/day with creatinine clearance <20 mL/min and 300 mg/day with hemodialysis. With severe liver disease, some authorities advocate 100 mg tid.

Side effects

1. **Subjective:** GI intolerance, altered taste (dysguesia), insomnia, myalgias, asthenia, malaise, and/or headaches are common and are dose related (Ann Intern Med 1993;118:913). Most patients can be managed with symptomatic treatment.

2. **Marrow suppression** which is related to marrow reserve, dose and duration of treatment and stage of disease. Anemia may occur within 4-6 wks and neutropenia is usually seen after 12-24 wks. Marrow exams in patients with AZT-induced anemia may be normal or show reduced RBC precursors. Severe anemia should be managed by discontinuing AZT or giving erythropoietin concurrently. With neutropenia, an ANC <750/mm^3 should be managed by discontinuing AZT or giving G-CSF concurrently.

3. **Myopathy:** Rare dose related complication possibly due to mitochondrial toxicity. Clinical features are leg and gluteal muscle weakness, elevated LDH and CPK, muscle biopsy showing ragged red fibers and abnormal mitochondrial

(NEJM 1990;322:1098) and response to discontinuation of AZT within 2-4 weeks.

4. **Macrocytosis:** Noted within four weeks of starting AZT in virtually all patients and serves as an indicator of adherence.

5. **Hepatitis** with reversible increases in transaminase levels, sometimes within 2-3 weeks of starting treatment.

6. **Lactic acidosis and severe hepatomegaly with steatosis** are rare complications ascribed to all nucleoside analogs. This complication should be considered in patients with tachypnea, dyspnea and reduced serum bicarbonate. At risk are obese women and patients with hepatitis or other liver disease.

7. **Fingernail discoloration** with dark bluish discoloration at base of nail noted at 2-6 weeks.

8. **Carcinogenicity:** Long-term treatment with high doses in mice caused vaginal neoplasms; relevance to humans is not known. (See below.)

Drug interactions: Additive or synergistic against HIV with ddI, ddC, alpha interferon, and foscarnet; acyclovir is neutral; antagonism with ribavirin, ganciclovir and d4T. AZT and d4T should not be given concurrently due to in vitro and *in vivo* evidence of antagonism. Methadone increases levels of AZT 30-40%; AZT has no effect on methadone levels (JAIDS 1998;18:435). Marrow suppression usually precludes concurrent use with ganciclovir. Other marrow-suppressing drugs should be used with caution: TMP-SMX, dapsone, pyrimethamine, flucytosine, interferon, adriamycin, vinblastine, sulfadiazine, vincristine, amphotericin B, and hydroxyurea. Early studies suggested acetaminophen increased risk of AZT-induced granulocytopenia, possibly by competitive inhibition of glucuronidation, but most clinicians feel intermittent use of acetaminophen is safe. Probenecid increases levels of AZT.

Pregnancy: Advocated for pregnant women beyond first trimester to prevent vertical transmission.

Positive in rodent teratogen assay at near lethal doses. Studies in humans show newborn : maternal ratio of 0.85. Prolonged high doses to pregnant rodents were complicated by the development of squamous epithelial vaginal tumors in 3-12% of female offspring (Fundam Appl Toxicol 1996;32:148). The relevance of these studies to humans is questioned because the dose used in rodents was 10-12x higher and AZT in humans is largely metabolized, whereas unmetabolized AZT is excreted in urine of mice. Most importantly, long term data concerning the safety of *in utero* AZT exposure in humans is available from participants in ACTG 076 which shows no difference between AZT recipients and the placebo group in infants followed up to 6 years in terms of immunologic abnormalities, neurologic complications, abnormal growth and tumors (AIDS 1998;12:1805; JAMA 1999;281:151). An expert NIH Panel reviewed these data in January 1997 and concluded that the risk of perinatal transmission exceeded the hypothetical concerns of transplacental carcinogensis. Nevertheless, they advised that pregnant women be warned of this risk.

VI. Drugs

ZITHROMAX – See Azithromycin (p. 173)

ZOVIRAX – See Acyclovir (p. 160)

VII. SYSTEMS REVIEW

PSYCHIATRIC DISORDERS

Glenn Treisman, M.D. and Joseph Schwartz, M.D.

I. INTRODUCTION

Patients present with symptoms. It is the clinician's job to determine a diagnosis to explain the symptoms. Treatment then extends logically from the diagnosis. Symptomatic treatments are the exception and are usually confined to those situations where the diagnosis is unknown or there are no acceptable treatments for a given diagnosis. In order to diagnose a psychiatric problem it is important to keep in mind a structure for psychiatric problems.

An approach that the authors have found useful is based on the four perspectives of psychiatry outlined by McHugh and Slavney. Looking at symptoms through these four lenses minimizes the likelihood that some important aspect of a case will be neglected. They are the perspectives of diseases, dimensions, behaviors, and life stories.

The application of these perspectives assumes that a thorough history and examination has been obtained and that, as new clinical information becomes available including progress in treatment or lack thereof, the diagnosis and treatment plan will be open to revision. This chapter is organized around specific psychiatric problems (symptoms), their differential diagnoses, and the appropriate treatments.

II. SPECIFIC PSYCHIATRIC PROBLEMS

A. Sadness

1. *Major depression*

Up to twenty percent of HIV infected patients suffer from major depression at the time of their initial presentation for treatment. Depression is known to interfere with adherence with medical treatments. HIV, a neurotropic virus, may join a list that currently includes stroke and Parkinson's disease as causes of major depression. Whether idiopathic and predating seroconversion (and potentially contributing to transmission behaviors) or developing after seroconversion as a result of neurologic damage caused by HIV itself, the diagnostic features and treatment are the same.

The core features of the diagnosis are low mood, decreased energy, and a diminished opinion of self worth. Frequently associated symptoms are disturbed sleep, loss of appetite, loss of pleasure from activities, poor concentration, and thoughts of suicide. Early morning awakening is particularly indicative of a major depressive disorder. There can be psychomotor slowing or agitation.

Treatment is pharmacologic usually with adjunctive, supportive psychotherapy. A treatment algorithm is on page 289. Drug selection should be individualized. Patients at risk for suicide, for example, are more safely treated with SSRIs. Tricyclic antidepressants, on the other hand, are useful for patients with insomnia or peripheral neuropathy. A table of commonly used antidepressants is presented on page 281. Low doses should be used initially, and dose increases should be gradual to reduce unwanted side effects. With some agents (particularly the tricyclic antidepressants) blood levels may be useful.

2. *Bipolar illness*

Although the topic of bipolar illness is covered later in the mania section, it is important to consider this diagnosis in the differential diagnosis of depression since bipolar patients often present in the depressed phase. Identification of a history of mania or hypomania is important since use of antidepressants without concomitant mood stabilizers can precipitate a manic episode. Often mood stabilizers (such as lithium or valproate) are started first and antidepressants are added once the patient has a therapeutic blood level.

3. *Demoralization, grief, and adjustment disorder*

These three terms can be considered together and are often used interchangeably. They are understandable psychological reactions to difficult life circumstances. Often the circumstances are peripheral to HIV, such as poverty, homelessness, fragmented families, loss of loved ones, etc. The diagnosis of HIV itself can be a demoralizing life event, as can the progression of disease, with the associated symptom burden, loss of function, and risk of death.

Patients may react psychologically to these life circumstances with sadness, anxiety, insomnia (especially difficulty falling asleep as opposed to the early morning awakening characteristic of major depression), and feeling overwhelmed. Self attitude is typically not appreciably changed. Symptoms often wax and wane and may come in paroxysms especially following the loss of a loved one. An identifiable life stressor is required for the diagnosis. The reaction is usually transient, resolving with time as coping skills develop or when life circumstances improve.

Some patients, because of their temperaments, are particularly vulnerable to stressful or demoralizing life events. Depending on the personality classification scheme adhered to, these individuals are often labeled borderline or histrionic. A more useful understanding of their vulnerabilities involves recognition that such patients are extreme on the dimensions of both extroversion (focused on the present and seek rewards rather than avoiding consequences) and instability (relatively small events provoke strong emotions that come on quickly and resolve quickly). In these patients strong emotions often lead to problematic behaviors.

The treatment is psychological rather than pharmacological. Psychotherapy should be supportive and encouraging rather than exploratory and probing. The focus should be on the here and now and on problem solving. Group therapy and encouragement of social and family interactions are often important components of treatment. Severe insomnia can be treated with adjunctive pharmacologic agents as described below.

It is very important to remember the danger of being too ready with psychological explanations and thereby miss treatable diseases such as major depression. Thorough assessment and reassessments are necessary. Failure to improve with psychotherapy after several weeks may warrant the tentative reformulation of the diagnosis as major depression with a trial of an antidepressant medication.

4. *Substance induced depression*

Depression can occur in association with intoxication with a variety of substances (including alcohol, opiates, and benzodiazepines) or as part of a withdrawal syndrome (especially amphetamines and cocaine). The diagnosis is based on the assumption of a causal connection between the drug use and the mood symptoms and is confirmed when symptoms resolve with abstinence. Treatment initially is targeted at detoxification and treatment of withdrawal symptoms, and then quickly focuses on stopping the behavior of drug use. Comorbid idiopathic mood disorders are common. Lack of symptom resolution with abstinence or a history of depression or mania preceding and perhaps triggering relapses of drug or alcohol use should prompt the treatment of the underlying mood disorder. Substance abuse is considered in more depth below.

5. *Depression due to other medical problems*

This list of general medical problems and pharmacologic agents associated with depression is too extensive to be addressed within the scope of this book. Almost any central nervous system disorder can cause depression. Stroke has been previously mentioned. In the HIV population, CNS infections such as toxoplasmosis and chronic meningitis are important to consider. Endocrine disorders also should not be overlooked, especially hypothyroidism. Treatment is targeted at the underlying disorder. If depressive symptoms remain, then antidepressants should be used.

Table 7-1. Selected Antidepressants

DRUG	START DOSE	USUAL THERAPEUTIC DOSE	SERUM LEVEL	ADVANTAGES	MOST COMMON SIDE EFFECTS
nortriptyline (Pamelor)	10-25 mg q hs	50-150 mg q hs, titrate to level	70-125 ng/dl	Promotes sleep Blood levels useful	Anticholinergic alpha blocking*
desipramine (Norpramin)	10-25 mg q hs	50-200 mg q hs, titrate to level	>125 ng/dl	May promote sleep Blood levels useful	Anticholergic alpha blocking*
fluoxetine (Prozac)	10 mg qd	20 mg qd	unclear	Little sedation, few side effects	Insomnia, agitation, nausea, anorexia
Sertraline (Zoloft)	25-50 mg	50-150 mg qd	unclear	Little sedation, few side effects	Insomnia, agitation, nausea, anorexia
trazodone (Desyrel)	50-100 mg qd	50-150 mg for sleep 200-600 mg for depression	unclear	Helps with SSRI-induced insomnia	Sedation Rare priapism
imipramine (Tofranil)	10-25 mg q hs	100-300 mg q hs	200-250 ng/dl	Promotes sleep	Anticholinergic alpha blocking*
amitriptyline (Elavil)	10-25 mg q hs	100-300 mg q hs	200-250 ng/dl	Promotes sleep	Anticholinergic alpha blocking*
paroxetine (Paxil)	10 mg qd	20-30 mg/d	unclear	Little sedation, few side effects	Insomnia, agitation, nausea
venlafaxine (Effexor)	37.5 mg bid	75 mg bid or tid	unclear	Little sedation, few side effects	Insomnia, agitation, nausea
nefazodone (Serzone)	50 mg bid	300-400 mg/d in divided doses	unclear	Less insomnia, orthostatis, dizziness, and restlessness than to SSRI agents	Not well known - new class

*Anticholinergic alpha blocking: sedation and orthostasis.　　SSRI = Selective Serotonin Reuptake Inhibitor

B. Euphoria

1. *Bipolar illness*

If in clear consciousness (absence of delirium) and not in the context of drug intoxication (absence of substance-induced mania), persistent pathological euphoria is almost always due to bipolar illness. Symptoms of mania include elevated mood, increased energy, and an increased sense of self worth and well being. Patients often have psychomotor agitation, rapid speech, thought disorder, and a decreased need for sleep. Odd mixtures of depressed and manic states or rapid alternations occur less frequently. Manic patients rarely come in for treatment themselves unless they have experienced prior episodes and have gained insight through treatment. More commonly those close to the patient bring them in because their behavior has become disruptive. The incidence of mania is substantially increased in AIDS (possibly 9%), and it frequently presents concurrently with dementia.

The treatment of mania in patients with HIV infection is more complicated than in the general population because of a higher incidence of medication side effects at lower blood levels, higher blood levels at lower doses, and the potential for drug-drug interactions. Lithium and valproate are useful treatments. Dosing should start low and be increased slowly with close monitoring of blood levels. Advancing HIV disease has been associated with erratic swings in previously stable lithium levels, even on fixed doses with good compliance. Renal function with lithium and liver function with valproate require close monitoring. Often neuroleptics can be useful at low doses, such as haloperidol 1-2 mg qhs or bid. Their use is not limited to the acute stage; they can also be useful for ongoing prophylactic therapy and even as monotherapy. This is particularly true when other mood stabilizers are not tolerated, as is common in patients with HIV dementia. Carbamazepine is an alternative that may cause significant side effects in advanced HIV, and only the most preliminary data are available to support the use of the newer anticonvulsants such as gabapentin, lamotrigine, and topiramate.

2. *Delirium*

Delirium can present with any mood state (or in fact any psychiatric symptom at all). It is distinguished by a fluctuating level of consciousness. Treatment focuses on identifying the cause and removing it. Low dose neuroleptics may help with agitation but may also contribute to the delirium.

3. *Drug intoxication*

This should always be considered in euphoric patients. The diagnosis is made by taking a thorough history, often with the help of collateral informants, and supplemented by toxicology assays.

C. Delusions, hallucinations, and acute agitation

Delusions (fixed, false, idiosyncratic beliefs) and hallucinations (perceptions in the absence of stimuli) are often called "psychotic symptoms." Because of the imprecision associated with the use of this latter term, it is best avoided. Delusions, hallucinations, and acute agitation are signs associated with a variety of disorders but are pathognomonic of none. Treatment usually consists of adjunctive and often short term use of traditional neuroleptics or the newer atypical antipsychotics, in low doses. Patients with HIV infection, especially those in the later stages of the illness, are particularly sensitive to the extrapyramidal and delirium producing side effects of antipsychotic agents. The newer agents (such as risperidone, olanzapine, and quetiapine) have a decreased risk of producing these side effects.

1. *Delirium*

Delusions or hallucinations, especially visual hallucinations, should prompt the clinician to consider delirium by looking for the fluctuating level of consciousness that is its core feature.

2. *Dementia*

Severe dementia can be associated with delusions and/or hallucinations. Treatment is symptomatic.

3. *Affective disorders*

Both major depression and bipolar illness can have associated delusions and/or hallucinations. They are usually mood congruent; when they are not this should prompt the search for an alternative or additional diagnosis such as delirium.

4. *Schizophrenia*

HIV infection is not a risk factor for schizophrenia, but for many patients with schizophrenia, the associated chaos and impairment of sound judgment puts them at risk for contracting HIV. Schizophrenia is believed to be a disease, although information regarding pathology is preliminary and etiology is unknown. Although delusions and hallucinations are common, they are neither necessary nor sufficient for the diagnosis. Other possible symptoms, none of which are pathognomonic, include thought disorder, disorganized behavior, and affective flattening. The diagnosis is a complicated one and is best left to those with specialty training.

D. Anxiety

Several authors have suggested that anxiety disorders are more common in persons with HIV. Anxiety is a common complaint, but it is necessary to evaluate each patient thoroughly and make a diagnosis before initiating treatment. The common practice of treating the symptom of anxiety with benzodiazepines often leads to problems with toxicity or dependence that far outweigh the benefit.

1. *Panic disorder*

This condition may mimic a variety of non-psychiatric disorders. Patients frequently present with a bewildering array of symptoms including cardiovascular, respiratory, and neurologic. A careful general medical evaluation is necessary to rule out other diagnoses, such as hyperthyroidism, arrhythmia, asthma, pneumonia, cocaine intoxication and alcohol withdrawal, prior to the initiation of psychiatric treatment. Symptoms respond well to benzodiazepines, but for long term treatment tricyclic antidepressant and SSRIs are preferred. Panic disorder frequently responds at lower doses than those needed to treat major depression. Because of a heightened awareness of even mild side effects, extremely slow titrations are often required and supportive psychotherapy can help ensure continued compliance with treatment. Cognitive-behavioral psychotherapy is particularly helpful with anticipatory anxiety and learned avoidance.

2. *Generalized anxiety disorder*

Controversial and poorly understood, this diagnosis may not reflect a single diagnosis but rather the combination of a variety of anxiety-causing factors, including diseases (both psychiatric and non-psychiatric), learned behaviors, temperament, and stress. The diagnosis is made when patients suffer from prominent and persistent anxiety and other more specific diagnoses cannot be made. There may or may not be clear environmental provocations, and functioning is impaired. Major depression with associated anxiety should always be ruled out whenever the diagnosis of generalized anxiety disorder is considered.

For patients who are temporarily disposed to anxiety, non-pharmacologic treatments (such as cognitive-behavioral psychotherapy, deconditioning, relaxation training, and biofeedback) are often most helpful. Buspirone may help in some chronic anxiety conditions and is generally well tolerated. Tricyclic antidepressants have also been used. Beta blockers can control the peripheral symptoms of anxiety (such as palpitations and tremor) but may cause dizziness and syncope. Though commonly prescribed, benzodiazepines may cause more problems than benefits because of dose escalation, dependence, withdrawal, and intoxication.

3. *Obsessive compulsive disorder*

Although probably not increased in frequency in HIV, it is common enough in the general population (lifetime prevalence of about 2%) to warrant special mention. Patients have recurrent intrusive thoughts (obsessions) and/or behaviors (compulsions). In HIV infected patients with obsessive compulsive disorder the SSRIs are generally effective. Anafranil tends to be poorly tolerated. The preferred agents are fluoxetine, sertraline, and fluvoxamine. Often far higher doses are required than are typically used for major depression.

4. *Other causes*

The differential diagnosis of anxiety includes major depression, demoralization, endocrine abnormalities such as hyperthyroidism and pheochromocytoma, CNS lesions, obsessional personality, and drug intoxication and withdrawal.

E. Substance abuse

This is a disorder of motivated behavior. It is best understood as a condition in which a hunger or drive accelerates out of control and causes an increase in behaviors that satisfy the drive. Though there are a variety of initiating factors, exposure to the substance itself is the most important. It is the ability of the substance to reinforce its self-administration that ultimately provokes addiction. Treatment of drug and alcohol disorders can best be considered in three steps. Although oversimplified here, this approach will benefit many patients. The availability of a consultant for treatment of substance abuse is very valuable.

1. *Detoxification*

Intoxicated patients are not able to respond to therapy or to understand the cognitive steps necessary for effective treatment. At this stage patients often need persuasion, confrontation, and enthusiastic support to get them to cooperate with the detoxification. Detoxification can occur both in the inpatient and outpatient settings and may be accomplished by using the following guidelines. Drugs in the sedative-hypnotic class (alcohol, benzodiazepines, and barbiturates) are best detoxified by using long-acting benzodiazepines titrated to relieve abnormal vital signs and subjective "shakes." Because these agents have significant street value, careful and frequent follow-up is required for patients receiving an outpatient detoxification using benzodiazepines. Only small quantities should be prescribed at a time. Tricyclic antidepressants such as desipramine may be useful in people with intense cocaine cravings. In fact, low mood is one of the classic symptoms during cocaine detoxification, and the syndrome can be indistinguishable from major depression. These drugs should be prescribed with caution, since overdoses can be life-threatening. Detoxification from opiates can be accomplished with clonidine to control autonomic symptoms, short term opiate replacement with buprenorphine or methadone, or a combination of the two. Opiate detoxification is often extremely difficult to achieve as an outpatient.

2. *Treatment of Co-Morbid Conditions*

Although detoxification is the first step in the treatment of substance abuse, treatment of co-morbid disorders such as major depression, bipolar disorder, schizophrenia, personality disorders, and chronic pain should be initiated as soon as the problems are recognized. If these underlying issues are not addressed, they may drive continued drug use. Treatment of co-morbid conditions may be unavailable in detoxification centers which provide referred treatment for substance abuse disorders. Co-morbid conditions should be carefully looked for in patients who chronically fail treatment.

3. Maintenance Treatment and Relapse Prevention

Patients need ongoing and long term treatment to maintain their sobriety. This phase of treatment may often be best accomplished by using a twelve step program such as AA or NA. It may also be accomplished through individual therapy or group therapy. This phase of treatment is aimed at identifying triggers to substance abuse, decreasing exposure to substances, and putting in place a plan for the treatment of relapse. Because relapse is the rule rather than the exception, a careful plan for early intervention is critical to successful treatment. Monitoring with periodic urine toxicologies and breath alcohol measurements can provide a surprisingly useful incentive for patients to avoid temptation and can help identify relapses early.

F. Insomnia

Idiopathic insomnia requiring symptomatic treatment is much less common than secondary insomnia which requires treatment of the underlying diagnosis. Most of the disorders discussed here are covered in more depth earlier in the chapter.

1. Major depression

This is the most important diagnosis to avoid missing in a patient reporting insomnia. Often insomnia is the chief complaint in a patient with major depression. A thorough evaluation is required of any patient reporting insomnia, especially early morning awakening (a hallmark of major depression). It is often helpful to take advantage of the sedating properties of tricyclic antidepressants if insomnia is a significant feature. Trazodone, either as monotherapy or as an adjunctive agent, is also often useful.

2. Demoralization, grief, and adjustment disorder

These diagnoses are often characterized by initial insomnia (difficulty falling asleep). Patients with a clear temporary cause for insomnia, such as hospitalization, travel, or anxiety about a procedure, can usually be safely and effectively treated with almost any sedative. Chloral hydrate, 500 mg with the option of one repeat, is safe and effective for the short-term treatment of insomnia. Low dose trazodone is often helpful when the need for pharmacologic assistance will extend for days to weeks. Consultation is indicated for patients who require long-term treatment.

3. Primary insomnia

This diagnosis is restricted to those situations when, after a thorough evaluation, no cause for insomnia can be found. This is generally a disorder of elderly patients, but has also been described in many chronic medical conditions including HIV. Treatment recommendations in general have included the sedative/hypnotic drugs and the sedating antihistamines, although a variety of other medications have been used. In patients with substance abuse, benzodiazepines and other medications that can lead to dependence should be used with great caution.

4. *Other causes*

Other causes of insomnia which are beyond the scope of this chapter include diabetes mellitus causing nocturnal polyuria, congestive heart failure causing orthopnea, tuberculosis causing night sweats, and sleep apnea.

Figure 7-1: Depression

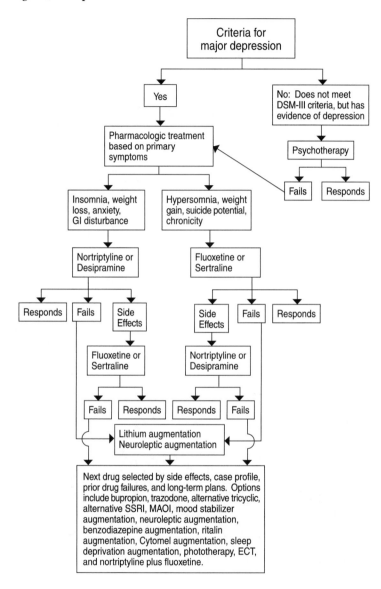

Table 7-2: Pulmonary Infection: Differential Diagnosis

Agent	Course*	Frequency, Setting	Typical Findings	Diagnosis	Treatment
BACTERIA					
S. pneumoniae	Acute; purulent sputum ± pleurisy	Common, all stages HIV infection; incidence is 150-fold higher than in healthy controls; recurrence rate at 6 mos is 6-24%	Lobar or bronchopneumonia ± pleural effusion	Blood cultures often positive Sputum GS, Quellung, culture (sensitivity of culture is 50%; prior antibiotics usually preclude growth)	Oral: Amoxicillin, cefurox, cefprozil, cefpodoxime, fluoroquinolone IV: Cefotaxime, ceftriaxone, fluoroquinolone
H. influenzae	Acute; purulent sputum	Incidence is 100-fold higher than in healthy controls; most infections are caused by unencapsulated strains	Bronchopneumonia	Sputum GS and culture (sensitivity of culture is 50%; prior antibiotics usually preclude growth)	Oral: Amox-CA, Azithro, TMP-SMX, fluoroquinolone, cephalosporin IV: Cefotaxime, ceftriaxone
Gram-neg bacilli	Acute; purulent sputum	Uncommon, except with nosocomial infection or neutropenia, *P. aeruginosa* is relatively common in late-stage disease, cavitary disease, or chronic antibiotic exposure (median CD4-50)	Lobar or bronchopneumonia	Sputum GS and culture (sensitivity is >80%, but specificity is poor)	Need *in vitro* susceptibility tests
Staph. aureus	Acute; sub-acute, or chronic; purulent sputum	Uncommon except with IDU and tricuspid valve endocarditis with septic emboli	Bronchopneumonia, cavitary disease, septic emboli with cavities ± effusion	Blood and sputum GS and culture (sputum culture is sensitive but specificity is poor). Blood cultures are nearly always positive with endocarditis.	MSSA: Naf/oxacillin, cefuroxime, TMP-SMX, clindamycin MRSA: Vancomycin
Legionella	Acute; mucopurulent sputum	Uncommon, but 40-fold higher than rate in persons without HIV	Bronchopneumonia; sometimes multiple infiltrates in non-contiguous segments	Sputum DFA stain (*L. pneumophila* only); sputum culture; urinary antigen (*L. pneumophila* serogroup 1 only, but this accounts for 70% of cases)	Fluoroquinolone, macrolide

Agent	Course*	Frequency, Setting	Typical Findings	Diagnosis	Treatment
Nocardia	Chronic or asymptomatic; sputum production (−50)	Uncommon; frequency higher with chronic corticosteroid use (median CD4 −50)	Nodule or cavity	Sputum or FOB; GS, modified AFB stain and culture; should alert lab	Sulfonamide/TMP-SMX
FUNGI					
Cryptococcus	Chronic, subacute, or symptomatic	Up to 8-10% in AIDS patients; late-stage HIV infection (median CD4 − 50); 80% have cryptococcal meningitis	Nodule, cavity, diffuse or nodular infiltrates	Sputum, induced sputum, or FOB stain and culture; serum cryptococcal antigen usually positive; CSF analysis indicated if antigen or organism found at any site	Fluconazole Amphotericin B
Pneumocystis carinii	Acute or subacute; nonproductive cough; dyspnea	Very common in late stages of HIV infection (CD4 <200) (median CD4 without prophylaxis − 100; with prophylaxis − 20; >95% have <200); infrequent in patients compliant with TMP-SMX prophylaxis; main predictor of prophylaxis failure is late-stage disease with very low CD4 count (JAMA 1995;273:1197)	Interstitial infiltrates with characteristic ground glass appearance; negative x-ray in early stages about 15-20%; atypical findings in 20%; atypical findings: upper lobe infiltrates, focal infiltrates, nodules, cavitary disease or mediastinal lymphadenopathy	Cytopathy of induced sputum (mean yield of 60% in proven cases) and FOB with BAL (mean yield of 95%); yield is lower in patients receiving aerosolized pentamidine; technical expertise is highly variable	TMP-SMX or Pentamadine Dapsone/Trimethoprim Clindamycin/Primaquine Atovaquone Trimetrexate pO_2 <70 or A-a gradient >35 mm: Prednisone
Histoplasma capsulatum‡	Chronic or subacute	Up to 15% of AIDS patients in endemic area; usually advanced HIV infection with disseminated histoplasmosis (median CD4 − 50); common features: fever, weight loss, hepatosplenomegaly, lymphadenopathy	Diffuse nodular infiltrates, nodule, focal infiltrate, cavity, hilar adenopathy (NEJM 1986;314:83; Medicine 1990;69:361)	Sputum, induced sputum, or FOB stain and culture; serum and urine polysaccharide antigen assay is best non-cultural technique with yield of 85% (blood) and 97% (urine) – available only through	Itraconazole or Amphotericin B

Table 7-2: Pulmonary Infection: Differential Diagnosis (Continued)

Agent	Course*	Frequency, Setting	Typical Findings	Diagnosis	Treatment
				J. Wheat, Indianapolis (800)HISTO-DG @ $70/assay, serology + in 50-70%; yield with culture of sputum – 80%, marrow – 80%; blood cultures positive in 60-85%	
MYCOBACTERIA					
Tuberculosis (MTB)[‡]	Chronic, subacute, or asymptomatic; usually has productive cough ± hemoptysis	Frequency is 5% (170-fold increase) in all AIDS pts, higher in some cities: NYC, Newark, Miami; with IDU, and in African American patients (median CD4 – 200 to 300)	Variable: focal infiltrates, reticulonodular, cavitary disease, hilar adenopathy, lower and middle lobe involvement common, pleural effusion; early-stage HIV infection-upper lobe cavitary; late-stage HIV-pneumonitis mid or lower lobes or miliary pattern with minimal granuloma formation. Extrapulmonary TB is common – esp meningitis, adenopathy	Sputum AFB stain and culture, if no sputum production-induced sputum or FOB; requires 1-4 weeks for growth in Bactec system with rapid ID by Gen Probe; requires 3-8 weeks for growth on conventional media; sensitivity of sputum AFB smear – 50% Drug sensitivity tests should be done on all isolates; requires reporting	See pp. 292-295
M. avium complex	Chronic or asymptomatic	Moderate for disseminated disease, but uncommon for pulmonary disease; late stage HIV (median CD4 – 20)	Variable	Sputum, FOB or induced sputum AFB stain and culture; must distinguish from MTB (DNA probe or radiometric culture technique); MA may colonize airways without	Clarithromycin + ethambutol ± rifabutin

Agent	Course*	Frequency, Setting	Typical Findings	Diagnosis	Treatment
				causing pulmonary disease; requires 1-2 weeks for growth in Bactec system	
M. kansasii	Chronic or asymptomatic	Uncommon: Late-stage HIV (median CD4 – 50)	Cavitary disease, nodule, cyst, infiltrate, or normal chest x-ray	Sputum, induced sputum, or FOB, AFB stain and culture	INH, ethambutol + rifampin ± clarithromycin or ciprofloxacin
Coccidioides immitis⁵	Chronic or sub-acute	Up to 10% of AIDS patients in endemic area; usually advanced HIV infection (median CD4 – 50); disseminated disease in 20-40%	Diffuse nodular infiltrates, focal infiltrate, cavity; hilar adenopathy (CID 1996;23:563)	Sputum, induced sputum, or FOB stain and culture; KOH of expectorated sputum is rarely positive; PAP stain or silver stain of BAL positive in 40%; culture of BAL usually positive; serology (CF) positive in 70%; skin test positive in <10% Blood cultures positive in 10%	Fluconazole, itraconazole or Amphotericin B
Candida	Chronic or sub-acute	Common isolate, rare cause of pulmonary disease (median CD4 count – 50)	Bronchitis; rare cause of pulmonary infiltrate	Recovery in sputum or FOB specimen is meaningless (up to 30% of all expectorated sputum and FOB cultures in unselected patients yield *Candida* sp.); must have histologic evidence of invasion on biopsy	Fluconazole or Amphotericin B
Aspergillus	Acute or sub-acute	Up to 4% of AIDS patients; usually advanced HIV infection (median CD4 – 30); about 50% have severe neutropenia (ANC <500/mm³) ± chronic steroids; disseminated disease is uncommon	Focal infiltrate, cavity – often pleural-based, diffuse infiltrates or reticulonodular infiltrates	Sputum stain and culture; false positive and false negative cultures common; most reliable tests are positive stain of respiratory secretions in typical setting or biopsy	Amphotericin B or Itraconazole

Table 7-2: Pulmonary Infection: Differential Diagnosis (Continued)

Agent	Course*	Frequency, Setting	Typical Findings	Diagnosis	Treatment
				evidence of tissue invasion; yield with BAL is high; most are *A. fumagitus*	
VIRUSES					
CMV	Subacute or chronic	Common isolate, rare cause of pulmonary disease; advanced HIV infection (median CD4 count – 20)	Interstitial infiltrates	Yield with FOB is 20-50%, culture requires more than 1 week; shell culture 1-2 days; diagnosis of CMV pneumonitis (disease) requires CMV seen on cytopath or biopsy, progressive disease, **and** no alternative pathogen	Ganciclovir, Foscarnet or Cidofovir
Influenza	Acute, purulent sputum	Influenza is common; influenza pneumonia is rare; any stage of HIV infection; frequency and course minimally different than in patients without HIV infection	Bronchopneumonia, interstitial infiltrates	Culture of throat washing and serology; most rely on epidemiology in community and typical symptoms. Bacterial super infection is common with *S. pneumoniae*, *S. aureus* and *H. influenza*	Amantadine/Ramantadine Neuramidase inhibitors
HSV, VZV, RSV, Parainfluenza	Acute	Rare causes of pneumonia	Diffuse or nodular pneumonia, bronchopneumonia	Culture or sputum or FOB commonly yields HSV as a contaminant from upper airways; RSV is rare in adults, but increased frequency in immuno-suppressed host, easily detected with DFA stain of respiratory secretions and possibly treatable with aerosolized ribavirin	HSV, VZV: Acyclovir RSV: Ribivarin (?)

Agent	Course*	Frequency, Setting	Typical Findings	Diagnosis	Treatment
Miscellaneous					
Kaposi's sarcoma	Asymptomatic or chronic progressive couple and dyspnea	Moderately common in patients with cutaneous KS and advanced HIV disease	Interstitial, alveolar, or nodular infiltrates, hilar adenopathy, (25%) scan usually negative pleural effusions (40%); gallium	FOB often shows discolored endobronchial nodule(s); yield with histopath of biopsy from FOB or transthoracic needle biopsy is only 20-30%. Pulmonary infiltrate on x-ray with negative gallium scan is highly suggestive	Taxol Liposomal daunorubacin or doxorubicin Adriamycin, bleomycin/ vincristin or vinblastin
				Suspect with enigmatic pulmonary infiltrates, chronic course, cutaneous lesions, and/or bloody pleural effusion	
Lymphoma	Chronic or asymptomatic	Uncommon, but may be presenting site	Interstitial, alveolar, or nodular infiltrates, cavity, hilar adenopathy, pleural effusions	Requires tissue for histopath; yield with FOB biopsy is poor – open lung biopsy often required	CHOP BACOD + G-CSF
Lymphocytic interstitial pneumonia (LIP)	Chronic or subacute	Uncommon in adults (median CD4 count – 200 to 400)	Diffuse reticulonodular infiltrates, on chest x-ray – resembles PCP; CD4 count is higher and LDA is lower; course is subacute and resembles PCP	Requires tissue for histopath; yield with FOB biopsy is 30-50% – open lung biopsy often required	Prednisone (?)

Table 7-2: Pulmonary Infection: Differential Diagnosis (Continued)

Agent	Course*	Frequency, Setting	Typical Findings	Diagnosis	Treatment
Aspiration	Acute or sub-acute	Accounts for 5-10% of pneumonia cases	Infiltrates in dependent pulmonary segment + cough and fever ± cavitation/empyema	It is not possible to verify anaerobic bacterial pneumonia; putrid drainage is diagnostic	Clindamycin Betalactam – Betalactamase inhibitor
Enigmatic	Acute or sub-acute	Accounts for most acute pneumonias	Most are presumably due to *S. pneumoniae* or *P. carinii* – distinguish based on CD4 count, tempo and x-ray changes	Antibiotic treatment precludes recovery of *S. pneumoniae* or *H. flu;* it does not reduce yield of *P. carinii*	TMP-SMX/cephalosporin or fluoroquinolone

* Course: Acute – symptoms evolve over days; subacute – symptoms evolve over 2-6 weeks; chronic – symptoms evolve over >4 weeks.

† Diagnosis: **Expectorated sputum** for bacterial culture should have cytologic screening to show predominance of PMN, Gram stain (GS) and Quellung (if GS suggests *S. pneumoniae*). **Induced sputum** often is reserved for patients with non-productive cough and suspected PCP or *M. tuberculosis.* Culture for conventional bacteria gives results similar to expectorated sputum (JCM 1994;32:131). **Fiberoptic bronchoscopy** (FOB) assumes bronchoalveolar lavage specimen (BAL) ± touch preps, bronchial washings, bronchial brush, or transbronchial biopsy; the usual specimen for PCP is BAL. Detection of **fungi** requires stains (KOH and/or Gomori methenamine silver stain) and culture (Sabouraud's media); *Candida* sp. grow on conventional bacterial media. Detection of **viruses** requires cytopathology for inclusions (herpes viruses – CMV, HSV VZV); FA for HSV and influenza; cultures are for herpes viruses and with special request – influenza virus.

‡ Detection of these organisms in respiratory secretions is essentially diagnostic of disease; other organisms may be contaminants colonizing mucosal surfaces or commensals.

Table 7-3: Differential Diagnosis of Pulmonary Complications Based on X-Ray Findings

**DIFFUSE
RETICULONODULAR
INFILTRATES**

Pneumocystis carinii
Miliary tuberculosis
Histoplasmosis
Coccidioidomycosis
Kaposi's sarcoma
Lymphocytic
   interstitial pneumonia
Leishmania donovani
Toxoplasma gondii
Cytomegalovirus

NODULES

M. tuberculosis
Cryptococcosis
Kaposi's sarcoma
Nocardia

**HILAR
ADENOPATHY**

M. tuberculosis
Cryptococcosis
M. avium complex
Histoplasmosis
Coccidioidomycosis
Kaposi's sarcoma
Lymphoma

NORMAL

P. carinii
M. tuberculosis
Cryptococcus
M. avium complex

CONSOLIDATION Common	Rare
Pyogenic bacteria Cryptococcosis Kaposi's sarcoma	*Nocardia* *M. tuberculosis* *M. kansasii* *Bordatella* *bronchiseptica*

*See: NEJM 1995;333:845

PLEURAL EFFUSION* Common	Rare
Pyogenic bacteria (especially *S. aureus* followed by *S. pneumoniae* and *Ps. aeruginosa*) Kaposi's sarcoma *M. tuberculosis* Cryptococcosis *P. carinii* Hypoalbuminemia Septic emboli (IDU) Heart failure Aspergillosis	*Rhodococcus equi* Histoplasmosis Coccidioidomycosis *Leishmania donovani* Lymphoma *M. avium* complex *Nocardia* *Toxoplasma gondii*

*See Ann Intern Med 1993;118:856

CAVITARY DISEASE Common	Rare
P. aeruginosa *S. pneumoniae* *Klebsiella sp* *M. tuberculosis* *M. kansasii* Cryptococcosis Histoplasmosis Coccidioidomycosis Aspergillosis *Rhodococcus equi* Anaerobic bacteria *S. aureus (IDU)* *Nocardia*	Legionella *P. carinii* Lymphoma *M. avium* complex

*Severe: Urticaria, angioedema, Stevens-Johnson reaction, or fever.

Figure 7-2: Cough, Fever, Dyspnea

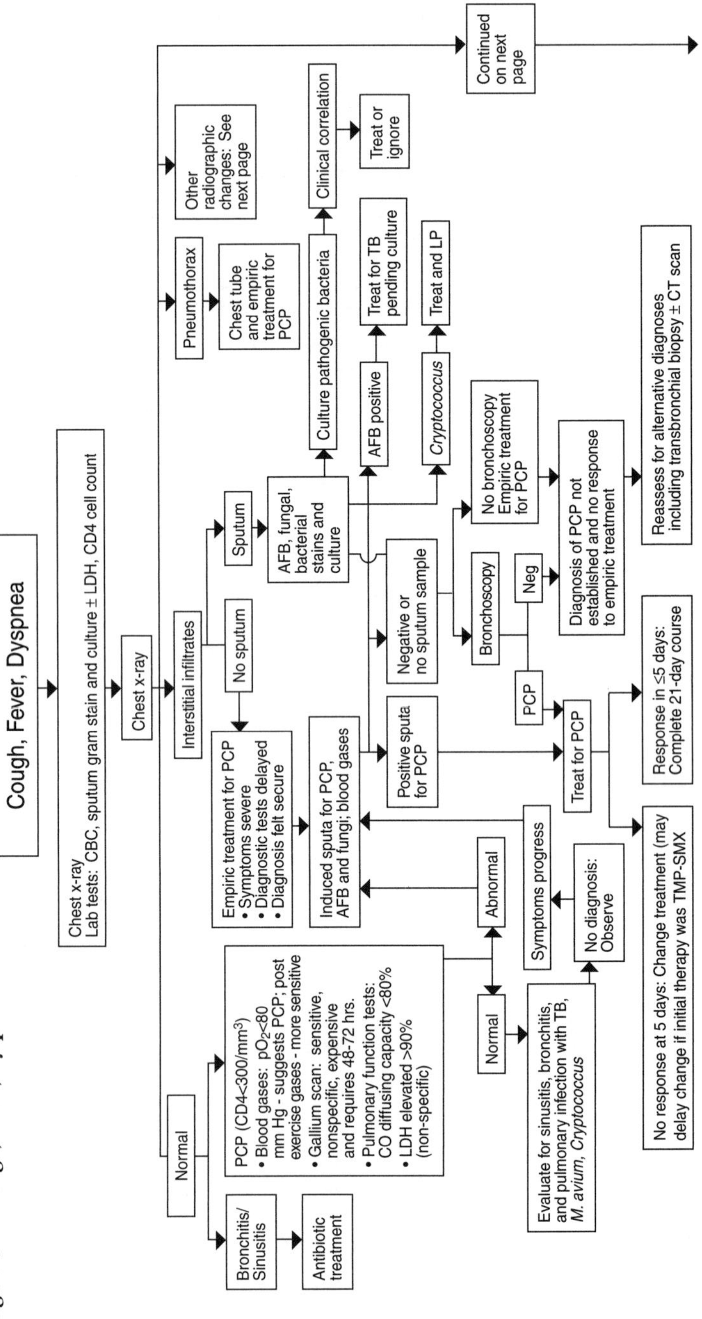

Figure 7-2: Cough, Fever, Dyspnea (Continued from previous page)

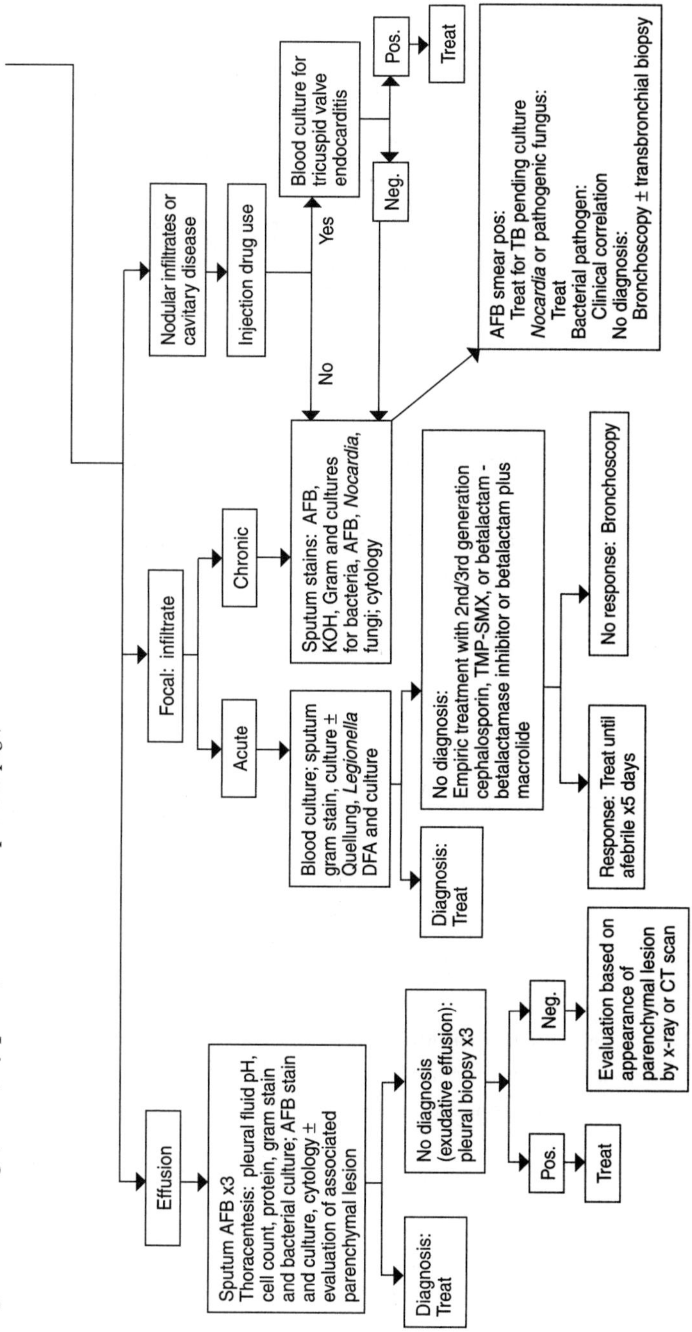

Figure 7-3: PCP Prophylaxis

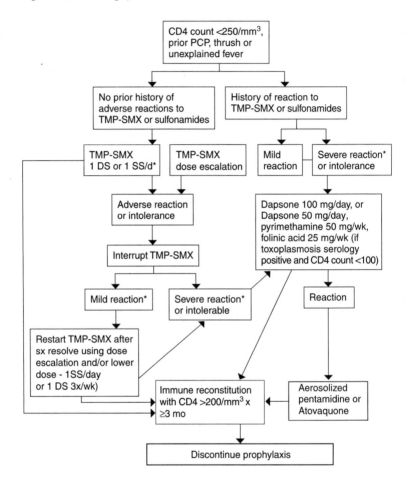

* **Severe:** Urticaria, angioedema, Stevens-Johnson reaction, or fever.

Intolerance: GI symptoms, rash/pruritis.

Mild: Tolerable with aggressive supportive care and/or dose reduction.

Table 7-4: Central Nervous System Conditions in Patients with HIV Infection

Agent/ Condition	Frequency (All AIDS Patients)	Clinical Features	CT SCAN/MRI	CSF*	Other Diagnostic Tests
Toxoplasmosis	2-4%	Fever, reduced alertness, headache, focal neurological deficits (80%), seizures (30%) Evolution: <2 weeks CD4 <100	Location: basal ganglia, gray~ white junction Sites: usually multiple Enhancement: prominent – usually ring lesions Edema/mass effect: usually	Normal: 20-30% Protein: 10-150/mL WBC: 0-40 (monos) Experimental: Toxo Ag (ELISA or PCR)	Toxoplasmosis serology (IgG) false neg. in 5-10% Response to empiric therapy: >85% respond by day 7 (NEJM 1993;329:995) MRI: Repeat at 2 wks Definitive dx: brain bx
Primary CNS Lymphoma	2%	Afebrile, headache, focal neuro findings; mental status change (60%) personality or behavioral; seizures (15%) Evolution: 2-8 weeks CD4 <100	Location: periventricular, any-where, 2-6 cm Sites: one or many Enhancement: prominent – usually solid, irregular Edema/mass effect: prominent	Normal: 30-50% Protein: 10-150/mL WBC: 0-100 (monos) Experimental: EBV PCR or *in situ* hybridization Cytology + in <5%	Suspect with neg. toxo. IgG or failure to respond to empiric toxo. treatment (MRI and clinical evaluation at 2 wks) Additional diagnostics: EBV DNA in CSF (Lancet 1992;342:398) + Thallium SPECT scan
Cryptococcal meningitis	8-10%	Fever, headache, alert (75%); nausea & vomiting; malaise; less common are visual changes, stiff neck, cranial nerve deficits, seizures (10%); no focal neurologic deficits Evolution: <2 weeks CD4 <100	Usually normal or shows increased intracranial pressure Enhancement: negative or meningeal enhancement Edema mass effect: ventricular enlargement/obstructive hydrocephalus	Normal: 20% Protein: 30-150/dL WBC: 0-100 (monos) glucose decreased: 50-70 mg/dL Culture pos: 95-100% India ink pos: 60-80% Crypt Ag nearly 100% sensitive and specific	Cryptococcal antigen CSF: nearly 100% Serum: 95% Definitive dx: CSF antigen and/or positive culture

Table 7-4: Central Nervous System Conditions in Patients with HIV Infection (Continued)

Agent/ Condition	Frequency (All AIDS Patients)	Clinical Features	CT SCAN/MRI	CSF*	Other Diagnostic Tests
CMV (cytomegalovirus)	<0.5%	Fever ± delirium, lethargy, disorientation; malaise and headache most common; stiff neck, photophobia, cranial nerve deficits less common; no focal neurologic deficits Evolution: >2 weeks CD4 <100	Location: periventricular, brainstem Site: confluent Enhancement: variable, prominent – none	CSF may be normal Protein: 100-1000/mL WBC: 10-1000 (monos)/mL Glucose usually decreased CMV PCR positive CSF cultures usually negative for CMV	Definitive dx: brain biopsy with histopath and/or positive culture Hyponatremia (reflects CMV adrenalitis) Retinal exam for CMV retinitis
PML (Progressive multifocal leukoencephalopathy)	1-2%	Afebrile, alert; no headache; progressively impaired speech, vision, motor function; cranial nerve deficit, and cortical blindness. Cognition affected relatively late. Evolution: weeks-months CD4 <100	Location: white matter, subcortical, multifocal Sites: variable Enhancement: negative No mass effect	Normal or changes associated with HIV infection Experimental: JC virus PCR + in about 60%	Definitive dx: stereotactic biopsy – antibody stain to SV40. Characteristic inclusions in oligodendrocytes; bizarre astroctyes
HIV-associated dementia	10-15%	Afebrile, triad of cognitive, motor, and behavioral dysfunction. Early – concentration and memory deficits, inattention, motor-incoordination, ataxia. Late – global dementia, paraplegia, mutism Evolution: weeks-months CD4 <200	Location: diffuse, deep white matter hyperintensities. Site: diffuse, ill-defined Enhancement: negative Atrophy; prominent No mass effect	Normal: 30-50% Protein: increased in 60% WBC: increased in 5-10% (monos) Beta-2 microglobulin elevated (>3 mg/L)	Neuropsychological tests show subcortical dementia Minimental exam is insensitive – use timed tests, eg, HIV Dementia Scale (JAIDS 1995;8:273)
Neurosyphilis	0.5%	Asymptomatic Meningeal – headache, fever,	Aseptic meningitis: may show meningeal enhancement	Protein: 45-200/mL WBC: 5-100 (monos)	Serum VDRL and FTA-ABS are clue in >90%; false neg

		photophobia, meningismus ± seizures, focal findings, cranial nerve palsies **Tabes dorsalis** – sharp pains, parasthesias, decreased DTRs, loss of pupil response **General paresis** – memory loss, dementia, personality changes, loss of pupil response **Meningovascular syphilis** – strokes, myelitis **Ocular syphilis** – iritis, uveitis, optic neuritis Any CD4 count	General paresis: cortical atrophy, sometimes with infarcts Meningovascular syphilis – deep strokes	VDRL positive: sensitivity – 65%, specificity – 100% positive Experimental: PCR for *T. pallidum*	serum VDRL in 5-10% with tabes dorsalis or general paresis Definitive diagnosis: positive CSF VDRL (found in 60-70%) **Note:** Most common forms in HIV-infected persons are ocular, meningeal, and meningovascular.
Tuberculosis	0.5-1%	Fever, reduced alertness, headache, meningismus, focal deficits (20%) CD4 <350	Intracerebral lesions in 50-70% (NEJM 1992;326:668; Am J Med 1992;93:524).	Normal: 5-10% Protein: Normal (40%) – 500/mL WBC: 5-2000 (average is 60-70% monos) Glucose: 4-40/mL AFB smear pos.: 20%	Chest x-ray – active TB in 50% PPD positive: 20-30% Definitive dx: positive culture CSF

*CSF: Cerebrospinal fluid

1. Normal values: Protein: 15-45 mg/dL; traumatic tap: 1 mg/1000 RBCs; Glucose: 40-80 mg % or CSF/blood glucose ratio >0.6
   Leukocyte counts: <5 mononuclear cells/mL; 5-10 is suspect; 1 PMN is suspect

   Bloody tap – 1 WBC/700 RBC
   Opening pressure: 80-200 mm H_2O

2. CSF analysis in asymptomatic HIV-infected persons shows 40-50% have elevated protein and/or pleocytosis (>5 mononuclear cell/mL); the frequency of pleocytosis decreases with progressive disease).

Figure 7-4: Headache in Patients with AIDS

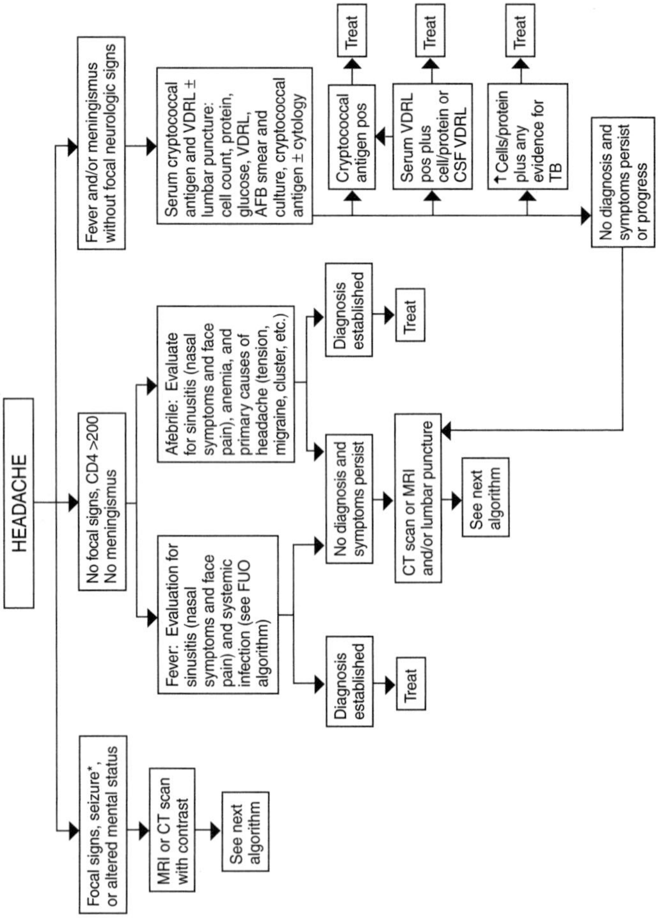

Table 7-6: Oral Lesions in Patients with AIDS

Condition	Clinical Features	Diagnosis	Management	Cost/Wk*	Comment
Candidiasis	**Psuedomembranous lesions** – white, creamy plaques on inflamed base on palate, buccal mucosa, or tongue	Clinical appearance Oral swab, scraping, or rinse specimen for 1) KOH wet mount or Gram stain to show yeast and pseudomycelia, 2) Culture, 3) Biopsy, (usually for leukoplakia lesions to detect OHL)	Clotrimazole troche 10 mg for sucking to dissolution 5x/d	$28	Pseudomembranous lesions are most common; erythematous lesions are most commonly under-diagnosed.
	Erythematous (atrophic) spotty – or confluent red patches (under-diagnosed)		Nystatin oral pastilles (200,000 units) or oral suspension (500,000 units/5cc 5x/day)	$10	Colonization rates for *C. albicans* are 10-40%.
	Hyperplastic – "candidal leukoplakia"; white lesions that do not wipe off but respond to antifungal treatment		Ketoconazole 200-400 mg po/day x 10-14d	$21-42	Most common cause of candidiasis is *C. albicans*, but *T. paraglabrata, C. krusei, C. psilosis* and *C. tropicalis* also implicated; some are resistant to azoles and may require amphotericin B. *In vitro* sensitivity tests: a utility not established.
	Angular chelitis – erythema and fissures at corner of mouth		Fluconazole 50-100 mg po/day x 10-14 d	$30-48	
	All forms are commonly associated with esophagitis		Itraconazole 200 mg po/day x 10-14d	$100	
			Amphotericin B 0.3-0.5 mg/kg IV/d x 3-7d, then oral agent (refractory cases)	$90-200	
			Amphotericin B oral suspension 1 mL swish and swallow qid	$25.20	
Oral hairy - leukoplakia	White plaques with vertical folds in patches or confluent; on tongue, usually lateral surface ± dorsum; may involve pharynx	Clinical appearance Biopsy: epithelia hyperplasia with "hairs" and little inflammation; EBVcan be shown with EM, immunofluorescence, or Southern blot	Usually asymptomatic and not treated Sx – pain, altered voice, difficult mastication, or reduced or altered taste Acyclovir 800 mg po 5x/day x 14 days	$140	Treated patients often relapse when treatment is stopped; maintenance high dose acyclovir is sometimes required. Ganciclovir, valacyclovir and famciclovir are probably effective

Table 7-6: Oral Lesions in Patients with AIDS (Continued)

Condition	Clinical Features	Diagnosis	Management	Cost/Wk*	Comment
Herpes simplex	Crops of small painful vesicles on an erythemous base, most common on palate and gingiva	Clinical appearance Smear – multinucleate giant cells with HSV by FA stain and/or culture	Acyclovir 400-800 mg po 3x/day or 5-10	$42-84 (po) $730-1,460 wk (IV)	May need supportive care to permit oral feedings: 2% viscous lidocaine, Dyclone, Benadryl, or 5% cocaine (severe cases)
			Valacyclovir 0.5-1 gm po bid	$42-84	
			Famciclovir 125-250 mg po bid	$44	
			Patients with advanced HIV and extensive acyclovir exposure may require Foscarnet 40 mg IV q 8 h	$700/wk	
Herpes zoster	Orofacial zoster with vesicles in distribution of trigeminal nerve on one side	Clinical appearance Smear – multinucleate giant cells	Acyclovir 800 mg po 5x/d	$140/wk	Major concerns are pain and ocular involvement Rare cases of oral lesions
			Valacyclovir 1 gm po tid	$126/wk	
			Famciclovir 500 mg tid	$133/wk	
			Acyclovir 5-10 mg/kg IV q 8 h	$730-1,460 wk (IV)	
Cytomegalovirus (CMV)	Oral ulcer usually with disseminated disease	Biopsy and cytopath If dysphagia, endoscopic biopsy of esophageal ulcers	Indications to treat are unclear		Infrequent cause of mouth ulcers.
			Ganciclovir 5 mg/kg IV bid x 2-3 weeks	$340/wk	
Kaposi's sarcoma	Red or purple macules or nodules usually on palate or gingival margin; most have cutaneous lesions	Clinical appearance Biopsy	Treat for cosmetic reasons or symptoms (problems with mastication, bleeding, speech changes, pain): Intralesional vinblastine: 0.1 mg/cm² lesion Intralesional 3% Na tetradecyl sulfate		Radiation treatment often complicated by severe mucositis. Recent report favors intralesional sclerosing agent: sodium tetradecyl sulfate (NEJM 1993;328:210).

Condition	Clinical Features	Diagnosis	Management	Cost/Wk*	Comment
Necrotizing ulcerative periodontitis	Periodontal disease with marginal gingivitis (red band at gum margin); periodontitis – rapid loss of gingival tissue, periodontal attachment, and bone. Patient notes bone pain, bleeding gums, and gum destruction.	Clinical appearance	Debridement and curettage, topical antiseptics (Betadine), mouthwash with chlorhexidine (Peridex 0.12%) rinse x 30 sec bid ± antibiotics	Peridex – $20/480cc	Debridement and curettage by dentist is considered by some to be essential.
			Antibiotic treatment: Metronidazole 500 mg po bid	$2	
			Clindamycin 150-300 mg po qid or	$21-42	
			Amoxicillin clavulanate 875 mg po bid	$56	
Aphthous ulcers	Crops of ulcers (1-10 mm diameter) on oral mucosa	Clinical appearance R/O HSV Biopsy: nonspecific inflammation	Topical fluocinonide (Lidex) 0.05% ointment mixed 1:1 with orabase and applied 6x/d	Lidex – $17/15 gm Orabase – $6/5 gm	Antibiotics x 4-5 days for secondary bacterial infections Oral prednisone, starting at 40 mg/day with taper over one month for severe disease resistant to topical agents.
			Dexamethasone elixir (0.5 mg/5 mL) rinse and expectorate	$2/30 mL	
			Miles Soln (1 mg hydrocortisone, 84,000 units, nystatin 84 mg tetracycline/5 mL viscous lidocaine) swish and swallow 4x/day	$15/140 cc	
			Intralesional injection with triamcinolone 0.1 mL/cm^2		

Table 7-6: Oral Lesions in Patients with AIDS (Continued)

Condition	Clinical Features	Diagnosis	Management	Cost/Wk*	Comment
			Mouth rinse with Dyclone and Benadryl or 2% viscous lidocaine	Dyclone $25/30 mL	
			Severe disease: Oral steroids		
			Thalidomide 200 mg/day po	$30.00/day	Thalidomide: see NEJM 1997;336:1489

* Cost is average wholesale price for a seven-day supply unless otherwise stated (Medi Span Hospital Formulary Pricing Guide, January 1997).

Table 7-7: Esophageal Disease in Patients with AIDS

	Candida	Cytomegalovirus (CMV)	Herpes Simplex Virus (HSV)	Aphthous Ulcers
Frequency as cause of symptoms	50-70%	10-20%	2-5%	10-20%
CLINICAL FEATURES				
Dysphagia	+++	+	+	+
Odynophagia	++	+++	+++	+++
Thrush	50-70%	<25%	<25%	<25%
Oral ulcers	Rare	Uncommon	Often	Uncommon
Pain	Diffuse	Focal	Focal	Focal
Fever	Infrequent	Often	Infrequent	Infrequent
DIAGNOSIS (see footnotes 2-4)				
Endoscopy	Usually treated empirically Pseudomembranous plaques; may involve entire esophagus	Bx required for treatment Erythema and erosions/ulcers single or multiple discrete lesions, often distal	Dx required for treatment Erythema and erosions/ulcers usually small, coalescing, shallow	Similar in appearance and location to CMV ulcers
Microbiology	Brush – yeast and pseudo-mycelia on KOH prep or PAS See footnote #4 Culture with sensitivities may be useful with suspected resistance	Bx – intracellular inclusions and/or positive culture Highest yield with histopath of biopsy and culture. Culture is often not recommended due to false positives	Brush/bx – intracytoplasmic inclusions + multinucleate giant cells, FA stain, and/or positive culture	Negative studies for Candida, HSV, CMV, and other diagnoses

Table 7-7: Esophageal Disease in Patients with AIDS (Continued)

	Candida	Cytomegalovirus (CMV)	Herpes Simplex Virus (HSV)	Aphthous Ulcers
TREATMENT				
Acute	Fluconazole 100 mg po qd; up to 400 mg/d Ketoconazole 200–400 po qd Ampho B 0.3–0.5 mg/kg IV Efficacy of fluconazole is 85% (Ann Int Med 1993; 118:825) (See footnote #5)	Ganciclovir 5 mg/kg IV bid x 2-3 wks Foscarnet 40-60 mg/kg q 8 h x 2-3 wks Efficacy of antiviral treatment is 75%	Acyclovir 200-800 mg po 5x/day or 5 mg/kg IV q8h x 2-3 wks	Prednisone 40 mg po/d x 7-14 days, then taper 10 mg/wk or slower Thalidomide 200 mg po/d (BJM 1989;298:432); JID 1999;180:61). Corticosteroids by intralesion injection
Maintenance	Fluconazole 100 mg po qd (indicated with frequent or severe recurrences) Lower dose or less frequent dosing may reduce resistance development	Maintenance treatment arbitrary May await relapse – then ganciclovir, 5 mg/kg IV/d Possible role for oral ganciclovir	Maintenance treatment arbitrary: Acyclovir 200-400 mg po 3-5 x daily	None

Note:

1. One-third of AIDS patients develop esophageal symptoms (Gut 1989;30:1033). Esophageal ulcers are usually due to CMV (45%) or they are idiopathic/aphthous ulcers (40%); HSV accounts for only 5% (Ann Intern Med 1995;122:143).

2. Diagnostic studies may include barium swallow, but diagnostic yield is low (20-30%) compared to esophagoscopy; with endoscopy a diagnosis is established in about 70-95% (Arch Intern Med 1991;151:1567). Response to empiric treatment often precludes need for endoscopic diagnosis of fungal esophagitis.

3. Other diagnostic considerations – drug-induced dysphagia (Am J Med 1988;88:512) including AZT (Ann Intern Med 1990;162:65) and ddC; infection – *M. avium*, TB, cryptosporidia, *P. carinii*, primary HIV infection (acute retroviral syndrome), histoplasmosis, and tumor – Kaposi's sarcoma or lymphoma (BMJ 1988;296:92; GI Endosc 1986;32:96).

4. Esophageal brushing: Non-endoscopic method to establish the diagnosis of candida esophagitis. Procedure is: Pharyngeal anesthesia → 16 French N-G tube inserted to distal esophagus → sheathed sterile brush extended through tube → brushing is done during withdrawal → brushings for cytopath and fungal stain (Arch Intern Med 1991;151:1567; Gastrointest Endosc 1989;35:102). This procedure is inadequate to establish other diagnoses.

5. Fluconazole is preferred treatment for *Candida* because of better efficacy and better absorption than ketoconazole in patients with hypochlorhydria.

ODYNOPHAGIA IN PATIENTS WITH AIDS

EVALUATION

1. Medication or food related

2. Gastroesophageal reflux disease:
   (heartburn ± regurgitation and dysphagia)

3. Opportunistic infection or tumor

   Common: *Candida* sp.

   Less common: HSV, CMV, idiopathic (aphthous)

   Rare: TB, *M. avium*, histoplasmosis, PCP, cryptosporidia, Kaposi's sarcoma, lymphoma

Figure 7-7:

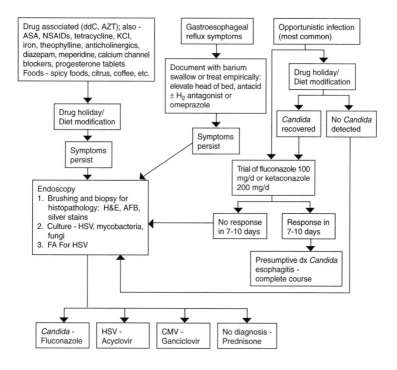

Table 7-8: Acute Infectious Diarrhea in Patients with AIDS

Agent	Frequency*	Clinical Features	Diagnosis	Treatment
Salmonella	5-15%	Watery diarrhea; fever; fecal WBCs variable; any CD4 count	Stool culture Blood culture	Ciprofloxacin 500-750 mg po bid x 14 days TMP-SMX 1-2 DS po bid x 14 days Ampicillin 2 gm po/d or 6 gm/d IV x 14 days Third generation cephalosporin or chloramphenicol Treatment may need to be extended to ≥4 wks
Shigella	1-3%	Watery diarrhea or bloody flux; fever; fecal WBCs common; any CD4 count	Stool culture	Ciprofloxacin 500 mg po bid x 3 days TMP-SMX 1 DS po bid x 3 days Antiperistaltic agents (Lomotil or loperamide) are contraindicated
Campylobacter jejuni	4-8%	Watery diarrhea or bloody flux; fever; fecal leukocytes variable; any CD4 count	Stool culture; most labs cannot detect *C. cinaedi, C. fennelli*, etc.	Ciprofloxacin 500 mg po bid x 3-5 days Erythromycin 500 mg po qid x 5 days
Clostridium difficile	10-15%	Watery diarrhea; fecal WBCs variable; fever and leukocytosis common; antibacterial agent nearly always — especially clindamycin, ampicillin, and cephalosporins; any CD4 count	Endoscopy: PMC, colitis, or normal Stool toxin assay: Tissue culture or EIA preferred CT scan: Colitis with thickened mucosa	Metronidazole 250-500 mg po qid x 10-14 days Vancomycin 125 mg po qid x 10-14 days Antiperistaltic agents (Lomotil or loperamide) are contraindicated
Enteric viruses	15-30%	Watery diarrhea; acute, but one third become chronic; any CD4 count	Major agents; adenovirus, astrovirus, picobirnavirus, calicivirus (NEJM 1993; 329:14), clinical labs cannot detect these viruses	Supportive treatment: Lomotil or loperamide

Agent	Frequency*	Clinical Features	Diagnosis	Treatment
Idiopathic	25-40%	Variable Non-infectious causes – R/O medications, dietary, irritable bowel syndrome; any CD4 count	Negative studies including culture, O&P exam, and C. *difficile* toxin assay	Severe acute diarrhea: Ciprofloxacin 500 mg po bid or ofloxacin 200-300 mg po bid x 5 days ± metronidazole (Arch Intern Med 1990;150: 541; Ann Intern Med 1992;117:202)

* Frequency among patients with acute diarrhea defined as ≥3 loose or watery stools for 3-10 days.

Figure 7-8: Acute Diarrhea in Patients with AIDS

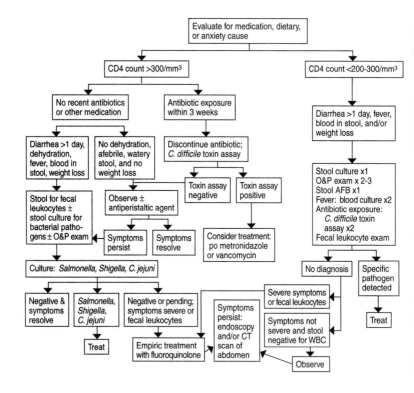

Table 7-9: Chronic Infectious Diarrhea in Patients with AIDS

Agent	Frequency*	Clinical Features	Diagnosis	Treatment
Microsporidia *Enterocytozoon bienensi* or *Septata intestinalis*	15-30%	Enteritis; watery diarrhea; no fecal WBCs; fever uncommon; remitting disease over months; malabsorption; wasting; CD4 <100	Special trichrome stain described (NEJM 1992;326:161) Biopsy – EM or Giemsa stain	Albendazole 400-800 mg po bid x >3 wks; efficacy is established for *Septata intestinalis, E. bienensi*: Best results are with highly active antiretroviral therapy
Cryptosporidia	10-30%	Enteritis; watery diarrhea; no fecal WBCs; fever variable; malabsorption; wasting; large stool volume with abdominal pain; remitting symptoms for months; CD4 <200; CD4 <150 is associated with recurrent or chronic	AFB smear of stool to show oocyst of 4-6 μm	Paromomycin 1000 mg bid or 500 mg po qid x ≥4 wks; efficacy is marginal Best results are with highly active antiretroviral treatment (HAART) Nitazoxanide 1,000 mg/d (not FDA-approved) Octreotide 50-500 μg SC or IV tid (nonspecific) Azithromycin 1,200 mg po bid x 1 day, then 1,200 mg/d x 27 days, then 600 mg/d Nutritional support plus Lomotil; may require parenteral hyperalimentation
Cytomegalo-virus	15-40%	Colitis and/or enteritis; fecal WBC and/or blood; cramps; fever; watery diarrhea ± blood; may cause perforation; hemorrhage, toxic megacolon, ulceration; CD4 <50	Biopsy to show intranuclear inclusion bodies, preferably with inflammation, vasculitis CT scan: segmental or pancolitis ± enteritis	Ganciclovir 5 mg/kg IV bid Foscarnet 40-60 mg/kg IV q8h Results of treatment variable (Ann Intern Med 1990;112:505; JID 1993;167:278); foscarnet and ganciclovir are equally effective (JID 1995;172:622)
Mycobacterium-avium	10-20%	Enteritis; watery diarrhea; no fecal WBCs; fever and wasting common; diffuse abdominal pain in late-stage; CD4 <50	Positive blood cultures for *M. avium*; bx may show changes like Whipple's disease, but with AFB; CT scan may be supportive: hepatosplenomegaly; adenopathy, and thickened small bowel	Clarithromycin 500 mg po bid + ethambutol 15 mg/kg/day +/– rifabutin 300 mg/day.

Table 7-9: Chronic Infectious Diarrhea in Patients with AIDS (Continued)

Agent	Frequency*	Clinical Features	Diagnosis	Treatment
Isospora	1-3%	Enteritis; watery diarrhea; no fecal WBCs; no fever; wasting; malabsorption; CD4 <100	AFB smear of stool; oocytes – 20-30 μm	TMP-SMX 3-4 DS/d; Pyrimethamine 50-75 mg po/d
Entameba histolytica	1-3%	Colitis; bloody stools; cramps; no fecal WBCs (bloody stools); most are asymptomatic carriers; any CD4 count	Stool O&P exam	Metronidazole 500-750 mg po or IV tid x 5-10 days, then iodoquinol 650 mg po tid x 21 days or paromomycin 500 mg po qid x 7 days
Giardia	1-3%	Enteritis; watery diarrhea ± malabsorption, bloating, flatulence; any CD4 count	Stool O&P exam	Metronidazole 250 mg po tid x 10 days
Cyclospora cayetanensis	<1%	Enteritis; watery diarrhea; CD4 count <100	Stool AFB smear – resembles cryptosporidia	TMP-SMX – 1 DS bid x 3 days
Small bowel overgrowth	(Not known)	Watery diarrhea; malabsorption; wasting, often associated with hypochlorhydria	Hydrogen breath test; quantitative culture of small bowel aspirate	Amoxicillin-clavulanate 250-500 mg po tid Doxycycline 100 mg po bid
Idiopathic (Pathogen-negative)	20-30%	Usually low volume diarrhea that resolves spontaneously or is controlled with antimotility agents (Gut 1995;36:283). Typically not associated with significant weight loss and often resolves spontaneously.	Bx shows villus atrophy, crypt hyperplasia + no identifiable cause despite endoscopy with biopsy and EM for microsporidia (CID 1992;15:726). These histologic changes are unlikely to explain diarrhea since they are seen in symptom-free persons with HIV (Lancet 1996;348:379). With pathogen negative persistent large volume diarrhea, must rule out Kaposi sarcoma and lymphoma.	Supportive care: Lomotil or loperamide Nutritional support

* Frequency among patients with advanced HIV infection and chronic diarrhea defined as >2-3 loose or watery stools/day for ≥30 days.

Figure 7-9: Chronic Diarrhea (CD4 count <300/mm³)

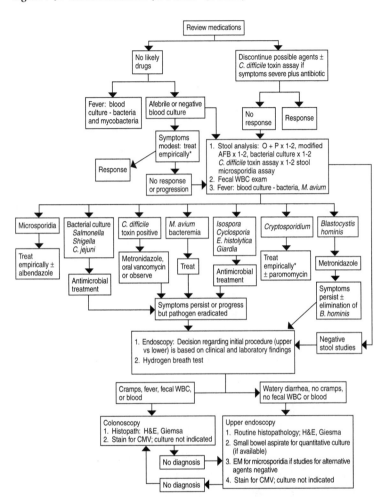

* Frequent small feedings, bland foods, avoid caffeine; low lactose, low fat, high fiber diet. Supplement with polymeric formulas and antiperistaltic agents (loperamide or Lomotil progressing to tincture of opium ± octreotide) as necessary.

Table 7-10: Dermatologic Complications in Patients with AIDS

Skin Condition	Presentation	Diagnosis	Treatment
Bacillary angiomatosis (*Bartonella henselae, Bartonella quintana*) (CID 1995;21:594; Br J Dermatol 1997;136:60)	Erythematous, lobulated with wet-appearing surface occurring anyplace on skin; may resemble pyogenic granulome or Kaposi's sarcoma; visceral disease common involving liver (peliosis hepatis), osteolytic bone lesions, lymphadenopathy, and bacteremia	Biopsy – vascular proliferation in the dermis with varying edema, mucinosis and fibrosis. PMN infiltrate is always present. Warthin Starry stain shows organism	Erythromycin 500 mg po qid Doxycycline 100 mg po bid Duration: ≥8 weeks Repeat courses may be needed. Local destruction or excision of lesions may be useful adjunctive therapy.
Cryptococcosis (*C. neoformans*) (Med Clin N. Amer 1997;81:381)	Nodular, papular, follicular or ulcerative skin lesions, may resemble molluscum; common locations – face, neck and scalp; usual complication of disseminated *C. neoformans* and rarely a primary disease	Serum cryptococcal antigen assay usually positive Biopsy – Gomori methanamine silver stain – shows budding yeast + positive culture. Do LP to exclude meningitis	Amphotericin B 0.7 mg/kg qd ± flucytosine, 100 mg/kg po/day or fluconazole (negative LP) 400 mg po/day x 8 weeks, then 200 mg/d Surgical removal of persistent cutaneous nodules with cryotherapy or electrocauterization may be helpful.
Drug reaction (JAMA 1997;278;1895)	Morbilliform exantham ± pruritis are most common; most frequent onset is 7-10 days after initiating treatment. Less common – urticaria, erythema multiforme, TEN, pityriasis rosea-like eruption	Hx of new drug exposure, clinical features and past history of drug eruptions. Response to drug holiday – rash usually responds at 3-5 days after drug discontinued. Rates with sulfonamides 10-40%, dapsone 10-20%, clindamycin 20-30%, amoxicillin 20%, TB drugs – 10% (JAIDS 1992;5:1237)	Varies according to symptoms extent, patient tolerance and need for implicated drug. Antihistamines ± topical steroids D/C implicated drug or reduce dose Watch for signs of TEN or erythema multiforme major such as blister formation, tenderness of lesions or mucosal lesions. Severe symptoms – discontinue all drugs. Systemic steroids are not useful.

Skin Condition	Presentation	Diagnosis	Treatment
Folliculitis (S. aureus, Pityrosporum ovale, Demodex folliculorum, eosinophilic inflammation)	Pruritic follicular papules and pustules on face, trunk, and extremities; spontaneous exacerbations and remissions; usually seen with CD4 <250 mm³ and >50/mm³	Clinical presentation Biopsy – perifollicular. Inflammation ± follicular destruction and abscess formation. Special stains (PASD, B+B may show agent Eosinophilis in eosinophilic folliculitis.	Varies by etiology S. aureus – topical erythromycin or clindamycin or systemic antistaph agent P. ovale – topical or systemic anti-fungal agents D. folliculorum – permethin cream Eosinophilic – topical steroids, phototherapy with UVB and/or PUVA (NEJM 1988;318:1183)
Herpes simplex (HSV-1, HSV-2) (CID 1995;215:5114; ID Clin N. Amer 1998;12:47)	Cluster of vesicles on erythematous base; common at all stages of HIV infection – more severe, prolonged, and refractory to treatment in late-stage HIV infection. Forms – oral, genital, perianal, periungual (whitlow) and disseminated (late stage HIV)	Tzanck prep (Giemsa stain of vesicle contents) shows multinucleate giant cells and intranuclear inclusions specific for HSV or VZV, but sensitivity is low. Viral culture is gold standard.	Acyclovir 200 mg po 5x/d or 400 mg 3x/d; up to 800 mg po 5x/day or IV acyclovir 5-10 mg/kg q8h x 5-7 days Famciclovir 125 mg po bid Valacyclovir 0.5-1 gm po bid Acyclovir resistance; Foscarnet 40 mg IV q8h or 60 mg q12h or topical trifluridine 5% optic solution q8h
Herpes zoster (Varicella-zoster virus) (Med Clin N. Amer 1997;81:411)	Vesicles on erythematous base in unilateral dermatomal distribution; common at all stages of HIV infection. Most common complication is persistent pain; other complications include trigeminal nerve involvement with possible blindness, disseminated disease, VZV pneumonia.	Tzanck prep shows multinucleate giant cells and intranuclear inclusions; but is insensitive and agent cannot be distinguished from HSV except by viral isolation (3-5 days) or FA stain (1-2 hrs) Viral culture and FA stain	Acyclovir 800 mg po 5x/day or 5-10 mg/kg IV q8h x 7-10 days Valacyclovir 1 gm po tid Famciclovir 500 mg po tid x 7 days Steroids are usually not advocated. Acyclovir resistance: Foscarnet 40 mg IV q8h or 60 mg IV q12h

Table 7-10: Dermatologic Complications in Patients with AIDS (Continued)

Skin Condition	Presentation	Diagnosis	Treatment
Kaposi's sarcoma (Arch Derm 1996;132:327; ID Clin N. Amer 1998;12:63)	Firm, purple to brown-black macules, papules, plaques and nodules; any cutaneous site, especially face, chest, genitals ± oral mucosa; visceral involvement, and lymphatic obstruction are common. Most common in gay men.	Biopsy – shows vascular slits lined by atypical endothelial cells with hemosiderin deposition R/O – bacillary angiomatosis, B cell lymphoma, hemangioma, or hematoma.	Determined by symptoms, cosmetic concerns, and staging based on tumor bulk, CD4 count, and "B symptoms" (J Clin Oncol 1989;7:1201) Local: Radiotherapy; intralesional vinblastine, surgical excision, cryotherapy, or laser oblation (cosmetic purposes only) Systemic: Cytotoxic chemotherapy with various combinations of vincristine, vinblastine, doxorubicin, anthracyclines, etoposide, bleomycin, pachtaxel and liposomal anthracyclines. Experimental: Angiogenesis inhibitors, growth factors, cytokine inhibitors, retinoic acids, anti HHV-8 agents.
Molluscum contagiosum (Poxvirus-Molluscipoxvirus) (Int J. Derm 1994;33:453)	Pearly white or flesh-colored papules with central umbilication; most common on face (beard area), neck and genital region, usually 2-5 mm diameter; > 1 cm – "giant molluscum"	KOH prep, Tzanck smear or biopsy to show intraepidermal molluscum bodies.	Cryotherapy, electrosurgery, curettage, or chemical cauterization (cantharidin, podophyllin, 5 fluorouracil, tretinoin, silver nitrate, phenol) Rarely eradicate lesions Topical cidofovir; imiquimod HAART – lesions may disappear
Psoriasis (Rheum Dis Clin N. Amer 1991;17:59)	Erythematous scaly, sharply demarcated plaques on elbows, knees, scalp, lumbosacral area ± nail changes and arthritis	Clinical features – Histopathologic features distinguish chronic eczematous process or drug reaction	Topical treatment: emollients, topical steroids, coal tar, vitamin A, vitamin D derivatives, anthralin, salicylic acid Phototherapy: PUVA (psoralen followed by UVA) or UVB. Cyclosporin may be useful. Acitretin: 25–50 mg po ± phototherapy

Skin Condition	Presentation	Diagnosis	Treatment
Candidiasis	Skin lesions – moist, beefy red with satellite papules. Thrush is present in >70%. CD4 count is usually <200-300/mm³. Variations: intertrigo, balanitis, glossitis, thrush, angular cheilitis, paronychia, nail dystrophies	KOH prep or fresh mount show pseudohyphae	Topical: ketoconazole, miconazole, clotrimazole or nystatin creams. Systemic: ketoconazole or fluconazole
Photosensitivity	Hyperpigmentation, eczematization and/or blister formation on sun exposed areas Causes – photosensitizing drugs, liver disease, HIV, idiopathic	Clinical features Phototest with UVA, UVB and light may be useful	Patient education – avoid sun and use of sun protection including sunscreens. Topical and systemic steroids Hydroxychloroquine may be useful
Prurigo nodularis	Hyperpigmented, hyperkeratotic often excoriated papules and nodules Usually associated with other signs of chronic pruritis/excoriation – lichen simplex chronicus, patches of hyperpigmentation, linear erosions/ulcerations and scars	Clinical features Lesion biopsy may be necessary	Must interrupt viscious cycle of pruritis → trauma → lichenification → increased pruritis: Use high potency topical steroids under occlusion or intralesionally May need to remove hypertrophic lesions with cryosurgery, laser or surgery. Oral antihistamines, phototherapy (UVB, PUVA)
Warts (Am J Med 1997;102:1)	Common warts – verrucous (hyperkeratotic, yellowish, inelastic irregular surfaced) papules and plaques. Variants – flat, plantar, mosaic, and periungual Genital and perianal – small, soft, pedunculated papules in clusters. HPV types 16 and 18 are associated with cervical and anal cancer	Clinical features Biopsy lesions that grow rapidly to rule out cancer	Indication is cosmetic Cytotoxic agents: Trichloroacetic acid, podophyllin, nitric acid, 5 FU, bleomycin Physical ablation: cryotherapy, electrodessication, CO₂ laser, surgery Immunologic: Imiquimod cream, cantharidin solution, DNCB sensitization

Table 7-10: Dermatologic Complications in Patients with AIDS (Continued)

Skin Condition	Presentation	Diagnosis	Treatment
Asteototic eczema (Med Clin N Amer 1996;80:1415)	Patches and plaques with varying degrees of erythema, scaling, crusting and lichenification (acute, subacute or chronic eczema, usually on extremities) Diffuse xerosis (dry skin) is always present. Very pruritic	Clinical features	Moisturizers, topical steroids, antihistamines Antibiotics for secondary infections

Table 7-11: Treatment of Wasting Syndrome (See NEJM 1999;340:1740)

Agent	Regimen	Cost (/wk)*	Comments
Megestrol (Megace)	400-800 mg/d oral suspension	$90.72-$181.44	Appetite stimulant; most weight gain is fat. Side effects: impotence, reduced testosterone levels, alopecia, hyperglycemia, abrupt withdrawal may cause adrenal insufficiency (Anticanc Res 1997;17:657; Ann Intern Med 1994;121:400). Recommended only if weight loss and reduced intake.
Dronabinol** (Marinol)	2.5-5.0 mg po bid to qid	$42-$168 ($3.02/2.5 mg)	Appetite stimulant and anti-emetic. Studies fail to show significant wt. gain; any wt. gain is fat (J Pain Sym Man 1997;14:7; AIDS 1997;13:305). Recommended only if weight loss and reduced intake.
Testosterone Cypionate* or Testosterone Enathate**	Males: 200-400 mg IM q 2 wks or 100-200 mg q week by self-administration. Replacement dose: 200 mg q 2 wks	$2.65 (200 mg)	High androgenic and anabolic effect. Significant increase in lean body mass (CID 1999;28:634). About 50% of men with AIDS have hypogonadism; benefit is largely restricted to this group (NEJM 1999;340:1740). Optimal results are achieved when testosterone is combined with a resistance exercise program (JAMA 2000;283:763). Trials show improved mood, libido, appetite and energy. Side effects: balding, acne, gynecomastia, virilizing to women, testicular atrophy; may cause worsening of fat loss.
Testosterone patch** (Testoderm) (Androderm)	Males: 5 mg Testoderm TTS or 5 mg Androderm patch q 24 h. Females: Experimental	$17.58 ($2.51/4 or 6 mg patch)	High androgenic and anabolic effect: males only. May have skin reactions with Androderm patch (J Clin Endocrin Metab 1998;83:3155). Trials show improved quality of life, increased body mass and few side effects; best results with hypogonadism.

Table 7-11: Treatment of Wasting Syndrome (See NEJM 1999;340:1740) (Continued)

Agent	Regimen	Cost (/wk)*	Comments
Oxandrolone** (Oxandrin)	Males: 10 mg bid or 20 mg qd or bid po; usually 15 mg/d Females: 5-20 mg/d po	$3.75/10 mg	Most require 20-40 mg/day Low androgenic effect Main concern is hepatic toxicity; peliosis hepatis, cholestatic hepatitis and hepatic tumors; may cause worsening of fat loss Most wt. is lean body mass (AIDS 1996;10:1657) Testosterone is preferred for hypogonadism.
Oxymetholone (Anadrol-50)	Males: 50 mg po bid		High androgenic potential – do not use in women Follow hepatic enzymes; peliosis hepatis and hepatic carcinomas reported (Brit J Nutr 1996;75:129) May cause worsening of fat loss
Nandrolone** (Deca Durabolin) Generic	Males: 100-200 mg q 1-2 wks IM Females: 25 mg/wk or 50 mg/2 wks	$13.78 (100 mg)	High anabolic effect Low androgenic effect – reduced potential for virilization in women Main concern is hepatotoxicity. Testosterone is preferred for hypogonadism.
Resistance training	20 min bicycle or treadmill, then 1 hr resistance training 3x/week	None	Most weight gain is lean body mass Appears to be as effective as growth hormone or anabolic steroids for fat accumulation ascribed to protease inhibitors (Nutrition 1997;13:271; Semin Oncol 1998;25:S112; AIDS 1999;13:1373)

Agent	Regimen	Cost (/wk)*	Comments
Megestrol (Megace) plus Testosterone	Above doses	$92-$184	Rationale is to combine effects of megestrol (appetite stimulant, increased body fat, estrogen effect) and testosterone (increased lean body mass and androgen effect)
Testosterone plus Nandrolone	Testosterone (Above doses) Nandrolone (Above doses)	$16 (for 200 mg/100 mg q 2 weeks)	Popular regimen that has not been studied
Growth hormone (Serostim)	6 mg SC/d (0.1 mg /kg/d)	$1,764	Most wt. gain is lean body mass (Ann Intern Med 1996;125:873) May reverse fat accumulation ascribed to protease inhibitors (AIDS 1999;13:2099) – but may accelerate fat loss Side effects: Edema, arthralgias, and myalgias; less common are diabetes, acute pancreatitis and carpal tunnel syndrome Cost is about $260/day Reserve for patients with severe weight loss who failed alternative treatment
Thalidomide (Synovir)	50 mg bid po or 100 mg hs up to 400 mg/d; usually 100 mg po qid	$30-$120/day	Effect is attributed to decrease in TNF or other cytokines Side effects: Dose related sedation and neuropathy and high rate of pruritic red rash – may be dose-related (AIDS 1996;10:1501) The drug is not FDA approved for this indication.

*Cost is AWP (Hospital Formulary Pricing Guide, Medi Span, August, 1998)

**Controlled substance: Category C-III; pregnant women or women planning pregnancy should not use any anabolic agents

Table 12: Treatment of CMV Retinitis

Treatment	Cost/month	Time to Relapse (median)	Comment
IV ganciclovir: 5 mg/kg IV bid x 14-21 days, then 5 mg/kg IV/d	$1,020/mo*	50-90 d	Side effect: neutropenia, thrombocytopenia, Risk of line sepsis, CMV resistance is more common compared to foscarnet
IV foscarnet: 60 mg/kg IV q8h or 90 mg/kg IV q12h x 14-21 days, then 90-120 mg qd	$2,190/mo*	50-90 d	Side effects: renal failure, electrolyte imbalance, Risk of line sepsis, possible anti-HIV activity, CMV-resistance is uncommon
Oral ganciclovir: 1 gm po q8h	$1,400/mo	30-60 d	Limited absorption Side effect: neutropenia Avoid with vision threatening CMV retinitis: lesions near optic nerve or fovea
Ganciclovir implant: Replace q 6 mo ± oral ganciclovir: 1 gm q 8 h	$1,200/mo ±$1,400/mo	220 d	Lack of protection against systemic CMV disease and protection of other eye** without oral ganciclovir Cost assumes 1.5 implants q 6 mo
Fomivirsen (Vitraven): 330 mcg intravitreal injection day 1 and 15, then monthly ± oral ganciclovir: 1 gm q 8 h	$880/m ±$1,400/mo	90-110 d	Lack of protection against systemic CMV disease and protection of other eye* unless combined with oral ganciclovir etc.
Cidofovir: 5 mg/kg IV q wk x 2 then q2 wks; probenecid, 4 gm with each dose	$1,412*/mo	60-120 d	Side effects: renal failure, probenecid reactions
Intravitreal injections Foscarnet: 2400 μg 2-3 x/wk x 2-3 wks, then q wk		50-100 d	Lack of protection against systemic CMV disease and protection of other eye ** Requires repeated injections
Ganciclovir: 2 mg 2-3 x/wk x 2-3 wks, then q wk		50-100 d	

* Does not include infusion therapy costs

** Frequency of CMV in contralateral eye is 50% at 6 mo; frequency of CMV disease in other organs is 30% at 6 mo (Arch Ophth 1994;112:1531)

Figure 7-10: Fever of Unknown Origin in Patients with AIDS

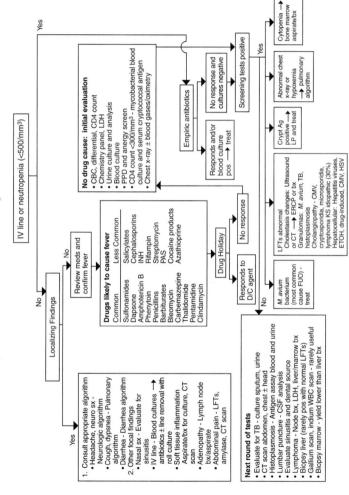

INDEX